I0039094

My Father's
Daughter

(2019 Revised Edition)

My Father's Daughter:
A Story of Survival, Life,
and Lynch Syndrome Hereditary Cancers
Copyright © 2019 TX 8-769-521

by Lindy Bruzzone

Library of Congress Number: 2017939963

ISBN Codes:
PDF   978-1-62274-185-4
Epub   978-1-62274-238-1
Hardcover: 978-0-578-50657-9
Softcover: 978-0-578-50658-6

All rights reserved. No part of this publication may be reproduced, distributed, or transmitted in any form or by any means, including photocopying, recording, or other electronic or mechanical methods, without the prior written permission of the publisher or author, except in the case of brief quotations. No part of this publication may be embodied in critical reviews and specific other noncommercial uses permitted by copyright law.

Although every precaution has been taken to verify the accuracy of the information held herein, the author and publisher assume no responsibility for any errors or omissions. No liability is assumed for damages that may result from the use of the information contained within.

With gratitude to Valdas Miskinis for the cover design.
Attribution: https:www.istockphoto.com/gm492042550-76102187

Printed in the United States of America
Backfire Publications, LLC

Disclaimer

This book tells the story of a family that lives with a defective mismatch repair gene that creates a high-risk disposition of contracting the hereditary cancers of Lynch syndrome.

Written by a layperson and a non-medical professional, consideration of any practices or information given in this book, including specific medical technologies, diagnostic methods, and treatment protocols, should not occur unless accepted and prescribed by a medical professional.

The information provided in this book is not an alternative to medical advice from your physician or other professional health care provider. If you have questions about anything you read in this book, consult your physician or health care provider. If you think Lynch syndrome may affect you, seek consultation with your physician or a genetic counselor to determine if genetic testing is right for you. Do not cease any medical treatment without discussion with your physician.

In this book, there is no intent to represent *current* scientific evidence. Before relying upon it, check to see if recent studies have been completed as research results occur daily in the rapidly evolving field of genetics. The author is a patient advocate diagnosed with Lynch syndrome. The sole purpose of this work is to share the experiences of a family affected by Lynch syndrome and those living with hereditary cancers. This book is a sociological work, not one recommending any specific, professional, medical procedures.

To protect personal privacy, we have changed some of the names. This 2019 edition of My Father's Daughter, A Story of Survival, Life, and Lynch Syndrome Hereditary cancer is a recent version of the original works with the same title published in April 2016 and in August 2017. Differences in versions include changes in technology and updated research findings.

Acknowledgments

To our children: Judith Ruggiero Ferrara and Christopher Hoen, and our grandchildren: Sonny Ruggiero, Scott Ruggiero, Jaycie Ruggiero, and Amaya Hoen. While many are still learning how to navigate through life, I am proud of the manner you are managing the challenges and your supportive way of caring for each other and others during this genetic journey. You are my inspiration.

To Steve Reed, who has been a wonderful father to my grandchildren; thank you for giving them direction; enhancing their lives and teaching them the valuable lessons of survival, and to my son-in-law, Sheriff Tom Ferrara, for providing the support and care for my family that only a father can. Thank you for guiding them into adulthood.

To my brothers, Jim, Bill and David, and my sisters, Stephanie and Donna—this is our story of lives well lived, because of childhood convictions and beliefs that have withstood the rigors of time. Your stories are yet to be told.

With love and gratitude to our aunt, Carole Nelson, and cousins Steve Nelson, Torie Nelson, Julie Lowe, and nieces and nephews who stand together during times of need, Greg, Jill, Alison, Alisa, and Brian.

Thank you to the dear friends of my youth, Sandee and Tom Scovronski, Patrice Niles, Judy Johnson, Bernadine Sam, Helaine Jesse, and Claire Jesse for a memorable childhood and creating fond memories of growing up. I have not forgotten the wonderful childhood memories created. You are always in my heart.

To Maizie Jesse, my Godmother, for your kind, compassionate nature, and the gift of faith. It made life so much better, And for Amy Morton, my dear friend, for the years of friendship through thick and thin.

With gratitude to those at Kaiser Permanente, North Bay, Vallejo, and Sacramento, to Dr. Aradhana Ghosh, my oncologist, who provided me with the strength to continue battling, and to my Kaiser Permanente physicians—Dr. Ralston Martin, my gastroenterologist, who cared us with such passion and skill; Dr. Suzanne Generao, my urologist, for her tremendous skill, in seeking the cancers of my father; Dr. Christopher Walker, our family practitioner, who has been our incredibly positive rock during ten years of this journey, in overseeing my care and making sure every consideration is offered in the way of screenings to make sure we receive what we need to live; George Berndt, M.D., a great surgeon. Thank you for saving my life; to Eugene Chang, M.D., always a kind and patient soul, even when my body does not cooperate; Carlos Perez, M.D. who listened, understood, and removed the fear and uncertainty of breast cancer from our lives; Eileen Crowley, M.D. for enormous hugs; Tim Grennan, M.D., who eliminated the risk of contracting breast cancer from our lives, and Mark Price, M.D. who brought normalcy full circle after eight years of adapting to uncertainty.

To my medical team at Banner Health/MD Anderson Cancer Facility, in Phoenix, Arizona; Boris Naraev, MD; Prathab Devaraj, MD; Iram Ahmad, MD; Amanda Grant, Chinedu Mmeje, MD; Regiana Maria Davis, and to all in the laboratory and imaging departments, thank you. Your smiles and positive attitudes, coupled with your knowledge, and competence gets us through until next year's series of cancer screenings.

We write this with appreciation to Christopher Hamerski, MD, of California Pacific Medical Center's Paul May and the Frank Stein Interventional Endoscopy Center and his staff for outstanding care, and careful explanation of updates of the innovative technologies available to physicians and patients.

It is for those I worked with at the California Department of Corrections (CDC) at San Quentin and the California State Department of Corrections Parole Division. To: Robert Roenicke, Steve Lawrence, Thomas Webb, Ed Veit, Doug Filangeri, Lea Ann Branch, Ron Chun, Betty McCormick, Mike Trott, Steve Schroeder, Jim Haagenson, Art Calderon, Bea Chavez, Jill Brown, and Jeanne Woodford, I am grateful for the opportunity to have worked with you and for the memories we share;

It is in memory of Sam Brown, Jay Dowdy, Jim Hall, and all the others who left us far too soon and who are memorable in my life. Thank you for mentoring me and being the best at what you do. It is also for those who lost their lives while advocating for the best for our families: To the memories of Wolfram Nolte, Kate Murphy, Rachel George, Ashley Lauren Bezdek, Becca Garner, Cody Mading, Averi Mading, Isabella Mading, Stephen Sutton, Marcella Jacob, and Henry T. Lynch, M.D. We miss you all. We will always remember the positive attitudes, and the strength and courage you proved even during the final hours. Thank you for your passion, your commitment, your courage, and courage, and all the good you left in this world that has helped others to live.

I owe a debt of gratitude to those who demonstrated their strength and courage in caring for Lynch syndrome families and experts that we worked with through good times, difficult times and times of devastation as we wove our way through loss: Barbara and Ed Fabiani; Jamie Kennedy; Erin Mading; Beth and David Fairbank; Kristal Mading; Erma Rutter; Micki George; Jennifer Martin; Jill and Ken Chang, Susan Olsen; Brian and Mandy Matthews; Debra Harris; John and Elanne Nelson; Bill Harb, M.D.; Cristi Radford, GCG; Carrie Snyder, CGC; Richard Boland, M.D.;

Douglas Riegert Johnson M.D.; Deb Duquette, GCG, James Church, M.D.; Uri Ladabaum, M.D.; Noralene Lindor, M.D.; Dung Le, M.D.; Steve Gruber, M.D.; Sapna Syngal, M.D.; Sir John Burn. M.D.; Hans Vasen M.D.; Amy Blanco, GCG, Albert de la Chapelle M.D.; Kevin Monahan, M.D.; Sanford Weiss, M.D.; Linda Farkas, M.D.; and Matthew F. Kalady, M.D.

I hold much appreciation to have had the opportunity to work with the thousands with Lynch syndrome, many of whom are still battling through advocacy efforts so others may live: To Reagan Barnett, Sue Caspers Waddell, Cathy Cordero, Cathy Uvanni, Kathleen Perrault, Debbie Sansbury, Shari Borrowman, Oneita Covert, Kathy Douglas, Leanna Daringer, Melissa Mitchell, Robin Braverman, Heidi Lutter, Holly Gillingham, Sarah, and Pete Gilbert, Sarah Ann Moore, Nancy Lehner, Gerri Wetzel Schoutko, Susan Porter Zamanski, Carolyn Watson, Dr. Ivy Razmus, MD; Sharon Bacigalupi-Fuhs, Mark Cooper, Pauline Skarrott, Diane Hardesty, Debbie Harris, Montse Ricart, Tracy Smith, Helen Bufton, Susan Morris, Heidi Lu, and Carolyn Dumond. Thank you for your ever-constant support and being there with passion and commitment to protecting lives.

And, finally, it is dedicated to all who work hard with advocacy organizations, worldwide, Lynch Syndrome UK, Lynch Syndrome Australia, Lynch Syndrome Spain, Lynch Syndrome Netherlands, Lynch Syndrome France, Lynch Syndrome Belgium, Lynch Syndrome Germany, Lynch Syndrome Finland, Lynch Syndrome Scotland, Lynch Syndrome Ireland, and Lynch Syndrome Italy, Lynch Syndrome Canada, and Lynch Syndrome Norway. You are doing amazing things with little, and your passion is overwhelming. You inspire me with your passion, dedication, and commitment toward others less fortunate. What a difference you are making in this world! But that is what living is all about, isn't it?

Preface

Reflection must be reserved for solitary hours;
whenever she was alone, she gave way
to it as the greatest relief...
— Jane Austen

Even as children, my brother, sister, and I knew how we might one day die. It would be like everyone else in our family who died from cancer—my father, his father, most of his siblings, his mother, her father, and others. The concept of "someday" played a significant part in our lives, as it does in millions of others who live with uncertainty as they spend a lifetime playing Russian roulette with cancer.

In our family, hereditary cancer is not something that "just happens," nor can we explain it as a matter of chance; it is a matter of circumstance. We expect it to occur "someday." In our family, it is what it is, and it was what it was, the way those in our family lived, and how they died.

For hundreds of years, familial and inherited cancers were a topic of controversy amongst medical professionals and clinical researchers. However, little research efforts occurred until the early 1900s. Not knowing why loved ones died of cancer, hope was elusive for our parents and grandparents.

When we asked our parents when someone would discover a cure for cancer, they always answered, "Someday, by the time you grow up."

We believed them because they trusted in the clinical researchers and the scientists who made public assurances, printed in newspapers with bold headlines. There was always some cure existing around the corner.

Our parents spent their lifetimes waiting for it to happen. As years passed with little or no advances in technology, both lost hope. For them, someday" happened the day they contracted cancer.

For us, "someday" was light-years away. We were not willing to put our lives on hold, waiting for what may or may not occur then. We wanted to live now. There was much we wanted to do that conflicted with sitting and waiting for cancer to strike.

We were the children of the 1950s and the 1960s, the free-range kids who sought adventure and roamed the hills freely. Growing up in a time of prosperity and not during the Great Depression, when our parents grew up fearing eugenic sterilization laws.

We saw rapid technological changes daily, televisions, stereos, computers, microwave ovens, pre-prepared foods, cassette and eight-track players, electric typewriters, movies, and dishwashers had become commonplace in homes. We rode up and down the first escalator in Reno, Nevada, and watched in awe while road crews installed stoplights in our small town.

We were the first on our street to sit on the patio and listen to music sounding from a portable radio. Air travel expanded. Traveling into space became a reality. Medical research was booming. Watson and Crick discovered the molecular structure of DNA. Researchers founded vaccinations for polio and childhood diseases, and everyone was excitedly anticipating a cure for cancer.

Then, our parents were learning to trust our physicians and not to fear them. While we lived in an evolving world, hope appeared everywhere. We did not have time to worry about the future. We were busy filling our days with adventure.

My siblings and I were risk-takers. In our youth, there was nothing more exhilarating than the feel of adrenaline surging through us as we raced one another through the foothills, where we played. The sense of empowerment and the confidence we grew up with kept us energized.

Those were the moments when we felt most alive when we realized we could do anything anyone else could do and more. From an early age and throughout our childhood, our parents encouraged us to explore, to take risks, and conquer what we could, but to avoid those situations where we could not. Their wish for us was to grow up confident and independent, to know we could do anything we wanted. The only thing needed was our best effort.

It was not the result of their concern due to the cancers that struck their family members, but it was so we could become successful in our own right when we reached adulthood. They lived with a sense of uncertainty of life. Our parents did not know if we could count on them to be around.

We ran a footrace against time as we tried to fill our lives with as many experiences as we could. Jim swam across the Potomac River and back on a bet. He paddled into the ocean alone, hunting sharks while I lived around the country and faced dangerous challenges with my career in the criminal justice system. Our sister pounded the streets as a private investigator.

The confidence we gained from our risk-taking endeavors empowered us. Believing there are as many ways to live as there are to die, we reminded ourselves living with uncertainty is often a matter of perspective. While our parents were readying themselves to die, we were preparing ourselves to live.

Much of what we learned about survival came from our grandmother, who shared with us the history of our ancestors' risk-taking struggles. A woman born during the Victorian era, her stories were first and second-hand accounts of the ordeals and the triumphs of our ancestors.

Grandma brought to life the character of ordinary people, doing extraordinary things. Telling the stories of the challenges they faced that were far more difficult than those we would ever experience during our lifetimes, she would later drive us around Southern California and show us where several had once lived and where they had died.

"Most of your grandfather's family died young," she revealed. "When we married, he and a few of his nieces and nephews were the last alive. Don't be afraid. Someday, knowing this will help you."

Revealing this to us was a risk. In the 1950s and early 1960s, eugenics laws allowing the mandatory sterilization of "defective persons" were still in existence. Physicians were often careful to document less than eight percent of deaths by cancer on death certificates, to protect the family members of the deceased from sterilization and public harassment. People living with Cancer feared treatment due to the extreme paternalistic practices of the eugenics movement. Many with cancer chose to die than to take the chance of risk to their loved ones.

This book focuses on the survival of the generations of our family, the risk-takers, and who settled a new country and those of us who contracted the same cancers, generation after generation. It tells the story of ordinary people, under extraordinary circumstances, fighting to survive. It details what we have done and are doing today to remain cancer-free. It tells of what we did to protect our family members and to live in a hereditary cancer family.

Within ten-years, Dad, Aunt Marcella, Jim, and I contracted nine cancers between the four of us. Collectively, we shared our hereditary cancer history with fourteen physicians. Despite the patents for genetic tests for Lynch syndrome filed in 1993, the first diagnosis of Lynch syndrome did not occur in our family until 2008, following my diagnosis of cancer, fifteen years later. By then, my father had died.

With that first diagnosis, we discovered the reason behind the family cancer. In our bodies, a microscopic gene in our DNA is defective. The mismatch repair gene no longer corrects errors in cell replication. Simplistically put, "Errors stack upon errors," "rogue cells" develop, and they eventually become aggressive cancerous tumors."

My Father's Daughter reveals the gritty details of the generations of a family caught within a crisis in living with an unknown hereditary cancer syndrome. It tells my story of learning to survive while engaged in a risk-taking profession of protecting public safety on the streets, in the correctional institutions of California, and later as a high-profile investigator. Applying the lessons learned in street survival to that of surviving cancer saved my life. Finally, it is the story of our family as we waited for "someday" to come when the "unnamed cancer thing" would strike.

Many of us, affected with Lynch syndrome or another hereditary disease, are risk-takers. It is not surprising to find a large number working in public safety, our military, and in the medical profession. Often, we attempt to compensate by living outside ourselves and hoping to provide a difference in the quality of life of others.

Life is messy in families facing crises. Seldom is any of it as clear and organized as the desktops and laboratory benches in the scientific institutions of those who try to define us. Once diagnosed, everything changes. We are different. Our way of living is different. Everyday life is different. When changes occur, it takes time to adapt, and ordinarily, it happens at one time with everyone adapting together. Not so, with Lynch syndrome. Then, everything occurs step-by-step. A continuous requirement to adapt exists not only for those affected but also for those who care for them.

Following diagnosis, my husband, Steve, and I dedicated five years of our lives toward full-time advocacy issues to address the needs of those with Lynch syndrome, after founding the international organization, Lynch Syndrome International, to protect families from hereditary cancer.

Volunteering full-time services to develop and stabilize the organization, we worked with thousands to improve the situations of our families. A dramatic increase in diagnoses and novel treatment approaches occurred once more were identified with Lynch syndrome. This streamlined access to more affordable genetic testing options and better access to genetic counseling and testing for Lynch syndrome. At last, we, with Lynch syndrome, had a voice. After realizing a dramatic improvement in circumstances, my husband, Steve, and I resigned after five years, with hopes the organization would develop further in the hands of others.

Evenings are now far different than those we knew while growing up in a family with an undiagnosed hereditary cancer syndrome. Then, chaos filled our days. Racing in different directions seeking distractions from the fear and uncertainty had only put a band-aid upon our level of anxiety. We lived with a constant underlying sense of uncertainty.

Today, between my two siblings, a nephew and me, who contracted cancer, we, along with the nine others diagnosed with Lynch Syndrome of the seventeen in our family, are still alive. We intend to outlive our parents and meet the age of our aunt, who lived with Lynch syndrome until age eighty-five. We are thankful for genetic testing, annual screenings, the ability to practice preventative measures, receiving cancer detection at a younger age, and consulting knowledgeable medical teams.

Today, living is far more comfortable. Our children have grown up and are gone. Their children are finding their way into the world with one less worry. On nights like tonight, a peaceful silence accompanies the occasional creaking of walls and the ticking of a grandfather clock that no longer serves as an ever-constant reminder that time is lapsing. That sense of urgency we once felt is no longer intense. It is simply something that keeps me moving.

Upon completion of this book, and after pressing the power button on my computer, the screen at once darkened. Bathed in the golden glow of the fire, the glistening cinders captured my attention as they sparkled upon the last smoldering log. My eyes intently watched as it battled for life, discharging a few courageous flames.

Suddenly, the log broke into small pieces, falling to the bed of the firebox, and a brilliant display of fiery rubies erupted, sparkling brightly as the cinders swirled behind the glass. Dancing joyfully, for a few moments, one by one, they tired and drifted upon a bed of deadened black and gray ashes. Though extinguished, I could still feel the warmth they had once radiated.

It reminded me of what occurs with the natural progression of life when the bright glow of our days tarnish, and our spirits fade. We quietly disappear, leaving little but the bitter chill of loss for those we love, then later, we return as the warmth of loving memories for them to keep as they continue onward. It is then we realize life *is* uncertain.

But, even toward its end, like the fire, life still sparkles. When those sparkles diminish, a vibrancy radiates, and with it, comes faith. Not only does faith live on, but today, so do we, just as our ancestors still very much exist within our hearts, through the legacies of the stories, the inspiration, the memories, and the DNA we inherited from them.

By all odds, I should not be alive. I hold an immense amount of gratitude for those who once cared for me, and for those who still do. The encouragement they offer has proven lifesaving as I continue traveling through this ever-twisting journey toward a cancer-free life.

Written with the hope that <u>My Father's Daughter</u> will offer inspiration to anyone who is facing a challenge in their lives, this book intends to serve as a roadmap for all living with hereditary cancer syndromes.

Geared toward those facing challenges with cancer and for the genetics and medical professionals so they may better understand us and realize who and what we are, living with Lynch syndrome and its cancers. Still, it is also for the governmental leaders responsible for health legislation so it can assist in providing essential services to the people.

Authoring this book was far from easy. I have done many things that were challenging during my lifetime, but this topped them all. Having to be brutally honest about the past and to write out the intricate details of our family's story was one of the most painful experiences I have ever faced.

There were times I would type fast, just wanting to get past a section because reliving it was far too emotional and difficult to handle. Time does not take care of all ailments. All I wanted was to get through each revision. What helped is viewing each one through a distinctly objective perspective, which I had to do when writing this.

Especially emotional for me was discussing family relationships of a mother and her children, and those of a father and his, and to do so from the viewpoint of being their oldest daughter. It was something I had always avoided. At times it broke my heart to realize what they endured and how the helplessness they experienced affected them throughout their lifetimes. What I learned from them was how fortunate I am in that we, of the next generation, have more opportunities at life and in living than either of our parents ever did.

It helped me realize who and what I am and what I can change and what I cannot. It is my hope our story helps others in understanding who they are and what they can do to find a way to adapt and to live with their circumstances.

For me, it is now a remembrance of being my father's daughter. I am a part of everything my father and his family once were. I have his skin, his hair, his eyes, and his DNA, even the part of him that is defective. He and the others who came before us are also a part of us, just as we will always be a significant part of all those who have followed us into this lifetime. No one can ever attempt to take that away from us. Their courage and inspiration live within us. It is our legacy. This is our story.

Contents

Contents

Dedication

For my husband Steve, who is the best of
everything imaginable and who
makes life an adventure.
You are my rock;

For all who have given my family and me
excellent care at
Kaiser Permanente, North Bay,
over the past thirty-five years;

For all at Banner Health Care
MD Anderson Cancer Center
for taking us in and offering us comfort
with world-class care;

We are so incredibly grateful for all you do
and for what you have done;
Without you, we would be nothing.

MY
FATHER'S
DAUGHTER

A Story of Survival, Life and Lynch
Syndrome Hereditary Cancers

Lindy Bruzzone

Chapter One

A MATTER OF FINALITY

*There are things that we don't want to happen but have to accept, things we don't want to know but have to learn and people we can't live without but have to let go. —*Criminal Minds

Whirling through the Carson Valley, the icy March winds were spinning dust funnels and sending tumbleweeds sailing across the desert. Standing outside, my family and I quietly watched mourners poured through the double doors, stepping past us with their hushed whispers and respectful nods. Some I recognized. Most I did not. I had not been home much over the past twenty years.

Awakening early that morning, it was a relief to find the sun had not broken through the blanket of ominous clouds that had rolled in from the northwest. Hurled across the endless Nevada sky, their shadows swept across the sand and sagebrush that covered the high desert. Shivering beneath a pewter sky, the grayness of the day blended with the overwhelming grief I felt. Our father was no more.

Earlier, upon rising, I gazed out the window upon the snow-covered peaks of the Sierra Nevada. I wished for the same comfort their beauty had once brought to a troubled soul. Then, Dad used to say, "Look toward the mountains, Lindy. That is where you will find strength."

But the comfort once received as a child was evasive. Even the splendor of its blue and white sculptured pinnacles, reaching for the skies, could not quell the agonizing feeling of loss that was churning inside. The one last bit of hope that continued to exist within us that had kept us hopeful through all those years was finally gone, leaving behind nothing but the emptiness of loss.

Carson City, where my father lived, sets in the middle of where the mountains and the desert collide. The two opposites merge into a peaceful coexistence with the surrounding land. Sprinkled with towering cottonwoods rooted into the banks of a winding river, its rolling hills, and the ever-changing tapestry, woven of sand, rocks, and pines, which have endured the elements of time.

It seemed only right that they were burying him in the small town where he had remained after our mother had fled. He died, having lived with as many extremes and contradictions, like that existing in the land surrounding him. He, too, was always in the middle, juggling the demands of two families while living a lifetime riddled with uncertainty. Creating difficulty was the ever-constant conflict always brewing in the wings, created by the constant needs of others that created a barrier between a father and his children.

Uncertain of his future, our father not only lived with the lifelong fear of contracting cancer; but with the uncertainty of whether he would ever be able to afford to retire. Storing away the dreams of a working man, for the day when he would be debt-free, cancer-free, and financially free to live his dreams, he continued trying to meet those goals while enduring cancer treatments. Finally, facing the uncertainty of survival, those simple dreams that he clung to diminished and fell by the wayside. Realizing the end of his life was near, he replaced them with a nagging need to seek redemption and to clean up loose ends with my siblings and me.

It was Easter morning when we received the call of finality. I was in the kitchen of our North Bay, California home, preparing our annual holiday brunch for my husband and his family. Turning off the water in the sink and quickly drying my hands, my heart sank as I glanced upon the Caller ID. Pausing, I prepared myself for the worse, knowing who was calling and why.

"Your father passed away early this morning," our stepmother reported matter-of-factly. A few seconds of uncomfortable silence followed. I don't think either of us knew what to say.

"I'll let everyone know," I quietly assured her.

I had just seen Dad thirty-six hours earlier. Then, I prayed for his death to come quickly. Emaciated and in pain, he was struggling to hang on to life, facing difficulty letting go. Before leaving their home, I visited with his wife for over an hour, encouraging her to permit him to die.

Our father had battled cancer for seven years after living a life filled with the uncertainty of whether it would take him down, as it had taken the lives of his father, all of his aunts and uncles, his grandfather, his great-grandmother, and all those in-between who had lived and died with the mysterious "family cancer thing." No one could figure out what caused everyone to contract cancer and die. Following his diagnosis, he set about living on his terms, in a studio apartment above his shop, while navigating through cancer treatments and passionately embroiled in a legal battle with his estranged wife over community property.

My siblings and I were his only natural children from his first marriage. We once knew a father who was young, bold, and full of confidence. Later, from a distance, we watched as he developed from an aging workaholic into a kindly, weathered man whose only wish was to retire and embrace life. Despite his circumstances, he didn't wear the tarnish of the disappointments that come with age that most sixty-seven-year-old men wore. Dad worked hard at remaining hopeful.

Earlier that morning, and vivid in my mind, were the memories that flashed. Images of Dad were etched, building fences, mowing the lawn, playing his ukulele, sitting on the banks of a mountain lake, fishing, laughing with friends in the coffee shop, and pouring over building plans. Dad loved the simple life.

Warming my heart was the image of our father at his best, wearing worn leather boots and a silver dollar belt buckle. His olive-toned face lit with joy, we would sing to the radio while bouncing down dirt roads. Sliding back and forth across the enormous vinyl bench seat, my brother and I hung onto one another for dear life, as Dad, his son, and his daughter spent the day driving the backroads of Nevada, in Dad's old, flatbed truck.

Deeply rooted in grief, I kept seeing him as he was during those final hours of life, laying hollow-eyed and wasted, in a bed filled with pillows, battling to maintain his grasp on whatever remnants of life were left, while I desperately wished the day to be over so I could curl up in the car and go home where I would feel free to grieve as only a daughter does following the loss of a father.

Glancing upon the rooftops of Carson City below, my heart winced as the memories of living here played over and over in my mind. It was here that our father taught us how to navigate our way through life and to pick our battles. A quiet man, Dad seldom spoke unless he had something of importance to say. When young, we learned life lessons through the parables, fairy tales, and folktales he told. Clinging to every word, we instantly understood the underlying moral behind each of his stories. Working hard at preparing us to grow up, and to be independent someday, he was worried we may, one day, contract cancer.

Then, our father was a giant, solid and immortal... that is until reality reared its ugly head. Brutal with life's truths, at his end, Dad was merely an ordinary man who, like everyone else, held little control over his fate.

This morning, I felt his spirit everywhere during my drive through the sleepy town. He had lived here for half a century. It had changed since we were children. Developing into a mid-sized city, I did not recognize many parts of it, except for the timelessness of Main Street, the Capitol Building, the beautiful old trees, and the Victorian homes in central downtown.

I felt Dad's spirit alive at the baseball field, where he spent a few years coaching Little League and Babe Ruth baseball teams. And I could feel it at Mills Park, where he dreamed of one day making it a reality for the townspeople, while involved in its planning. But where I felt it most was at the modest home that he and my mother built together in the 1950s, when we were young. It's color, and the facade had changed, but the fence we once climbed upon was there, as was the lawn where we spent our childhood.

It was while stopping in front of the 1800s built Victorian bungalow, where we last lived, I felt a sense of despair. It had been our father's dream and our mother's demise. Intended as the last step to a forever home, sprawled upon acreage in Genoa, it was where our family ended, and a new one began for him.

Here, we discovered how Dad managed heartbreak, uncertainty, and fear, where he learned to walk away from the pain of divorce and everything and everyone related to it. It was from here that Mom ran as fast and as far as she could, leaving the memories of everything behind.

During his illness, Dad often called several times a week. As his oldest daughter and chief confidante, we spoke on the phone for hours, making up for the years of silence. There were the conversations when he was despondent and depressed and the ones when he was feeling triumphant, eager to share his test results after completing session after session of exhaustive cancer treatments.

"Baby Doll! They zapped it away!" he exclaimed, excited over his cancer tests. "It's all gone!"

Cheering him on, my brother and I realized his challenges were immense. During Dad's journey with cancer, we made it a point to see one another as often as possible. Initially, Dad and I crossed the Sierra Nevada and met halfway once or twice a month to share a cup of coffee and visit. And he visited my brother and me at our California homes when he felt strong enough. We saw him often during those final six years of his life.

The last time we had visited was four months earlier, during autumn. Steve, my husband, and I spent a short while with him while he was working in his shop. Dad had tried to conceal the ragged weariness he wore as he sank into an office chair. So as not to exhaust him, we kept our visit short. He was tired. Unfortunately, our conversation was guarded as the opportunity to speak alone, without his wife present, was not possible. As usual, she sat possessively perched next to him, intently taking in every word spoken.

Walking us to our car, Dad opened the passenger door for me. Turning to him and extending my arms for the usual farewell hug, he embraced me tightly, not letting go as quickly as he had before. Lasting longer than usual, it conveyed a sense of finality.

Steve flipped the ignition key. After sliding inside and closing the door, Dad bent his head through the open window. Eyes tearing, he said, "I love you, Baby Doll. Don't ever forget that."

"As I do you, Dad… always," I whispered.

"My father is dying," I murmured to Steve, as I caught a glimpse of him below, still standing alone in the clearing, watching as our car passed along the highway above him and his business.

Weakened by surgeries and treatments, after six years of battling his cancers, he reconciled with his estranged spouse and returned to the home he built with his own hands, twenty years before, to die. The calls stopped.

Eventually, the positive energy that earlier radiated from him dissipated, and his voice transformed from one of hopeful enthusiasm to that of quiet resignation. Soon, his weariness became accompanied by a diagnosis of esophageal cancer, and shortly after, bone metastasis. It erased all hope. His wife issued instructions that all contact with him, from then forward, would be through her.

I checked in with his wife often, sending my loving thoughts to him. Finally, at the end of February, his wife allowed us to visit with Dad. With death imminent, Dad summoned our family to gather for a final farewell. A bittersweet day, again, little opportunity existed to be with him alone, until his spouse finally stepped away for a few brief moments to speak with her two daughters in the kitchen. Turning his back to where everyone had gathered in the family room, his eyes searched mine as he quietly said, "Listen closely. I do not regret anything, Lindy. Nothing. Don't ever forget that. You have to keep in touch with your stepmother."

"Okay, Dad, I will," I promised. "As long as she wants me around."

I didn't want it to be our last conversation. On Thursday night, three days before Easter Sunday, I couldn't sleep. Thoughts of Dad wove in and out of my mind while a nagging little voice kept rewinding, "You have to see him." Despite our stepmother's discouragement from visiting, I called and asked for permission to see Dad.

Early the next morning, I drove over the pine-studded Sierras, singing most of the way there. When I am alone and troubled, that is what I do. I sing every song I can think of to stay on top of difficult and challenging times. The calming effect of music has always kept me balanced and comforted in times of need. By late morning, from the summit, the beautiful Carson Valley could be seen below.

"Dad," I whispered, standing over the large bed. My heart broke as I saw the frail wisp of what remained of my father buried beneath a mountain of blankets. He was hardly recognizable. Flickering open, his eyelids revealed glazed and faded eyes, set deep into a sunken face. Though his body had wasted away to little more than a skeleton, his mind was still crystal clear.

"Hey darling," he said, with earnest effort, his voice weak and breathy. "You're here!"

Kissing his forehead, I said, "Yes, how are you doing there, guy?"

He groaned as he struggled to reposition himself within the mountain of pillows surrounding him.

"Do you hurt?" I asked.

"Yeah," he whispered.

"May I get you something?"

"Just time."

My heart wrenched. "I wish I could give you that, Dad."

"Lindy," he uttered, patting the side of his bed, signaling for me to come close. Sliding my chair next to him and grasping his icy hands in mine, I could feel his hot labored breath upon my face as I bent forward to listen.

"Yes?"

"They think it is hereditary," he whispered.

"What?"

"The cancers."

"They?" I asked, whispering back. I glanced toward the door. It was closed, yet he was still whispering. It was clear he intended the conversation to be between us.

"The doctors."

My heart stopped. At last, someone in the medical profession knew what was occurring in families like ours. Dad's revelation was huge. It added more pieces to the puzzle of the cancer mystery that Mom had always mentioned that existed within our family.

"Do you know what kind of cancer your father had?"

"Stomach," he answered.

"Okay," I mused. "But I remember Grandma saying that it was tuberculosis, and he died of a heart attack."

"Some got both. Grandma and your aunt didn't want to admit it."

"Why?"

"Long story. Eugenics stuff."

"Ah, okay," I said, understanding. Mom had revealed to us the fear they felt during that awful time of eugenic practices in our country. The tens of thousands of offenses against innocent people that occurred created immense fear that they too would be removed from their homes to be institutionalized and sterilized so as not to reproduce and bring children like them into this world.

Black, brown, red, white, and yellow, color didn't matter. Entire families turned out in their churches to condemn and shame members of their congregations for being born "physically different" from them.

"Be careful," Mom cautioned us, always carefully in a low tone of voice. "Don't discuss your personals with anyone."

"Who all contracted it?" I asked, holding my breath.

"Everyone."

"Everyone in your family got cancer?" I uttered. I had not realized how prevalent it was, fearing more the breast cancers that plagued the women in Mom's family.

"Except a few cousins," Dad said.

"Do you know what they call this hereditary cancer thing?"

"No," he replied, sounding exhausted. "Get yourself checked, okay?"

Checked for what?

"Okay. I'll figure it out, Dad."

"Good. Knew you would."

Our father had opened the door to a closet we had always kept locked, discussing something taboo. Now, instead of feeling fear, an immense sense of hope was spilling out. Someone, somewhere, had discovered what was wrong with us and why so many in our family had died of cancer. All we had to do was to chase that clue down and figure out who it was. As an investigator, my mind was spinning, wondering where to start.

"Tell your brother and sister to get checked, too, okay?" Dad instructed.

"You can count on it."

"Good," he uttered, laying back in relief and closing his eyes. It had taken immense effort for him to share what he knew. Taking a few seconds to wipe away the straggling tears that escaped a failed attempt to brush them from my eyes, I didn't want my father to see me cry, not now. Holding his hand, I tried to embed his image in my mind.

Don't forget. You cannot forget.

While sitting in silence, my mind filled with childhood memories. We used to dance to the radio, Dad, and me. Whirling across the floor, with my feet on top of his, laughing and singing loudly, to the rhythm of lively fifties music, he would bounce me about like a rag doll.

Tossing me on the sofa, he would pull Mom out of her chair. My siblings and I clapped as they spun and twirled. Now, with children and grandchildren of my own, and with Dad at the end of his life, I glanced toward him, noting a faraway gaze in his dull, hazel colored eyes as he silently laid in his bed, staring upon the wall. I wondered if he, too, was reliving yesterday. Did he remember it as vividly as me?

Without fail, another memory hit. Catapulted back to 1960, I saw a much younger Dad was running alongside the Nevada Bell Telephone Nevada Day float. Having turned eight years old, just two weeks earlier, I was wearing my pink party dress, with a taffeta apron that tied with a satin sash. Mom had sat at her sewing machine for two weeks, sewing it for my birthday, and making another identical one for my sister.

Now, I was sitting on top of the world, in a swing that was hanging in the middle of an enormous bell that employees at the phone had built for that day.

"Lindy," he called out to me. "Smile and wave. Remember, like a princess."

Nodding and giving him a big smile, my little hands, covered with white gloves, waved to the crowds gathered on the sidewalks, precisely in the manner he had earlier instructed.

"That's my girl!" he called to me, laughing.

The efforts of Dad and those he worked with won an award that year. He was proud of it. For years, he kept a photo of it and us, upon his desk, next to his telephone. Whenever I visited him at his office and looked for it, it was always there.

I had not thought about that day in over thirty years, and suddenly, the memory was vivid in my mind, even down to the crackling of the float's crisp paper flowers waving in the breeze. Memories are funny things, as they hide deep in the endless caverns of our minds for decades, and, then, out of nowhere, appear just when we need them most. I sure needed them that day, as I sat next to my father as he was dying.

"Lindy," Dad mumbled. I startled and turned toward him, seeing his eyes darting back and forth between me and one of his dresser drawers.

Our eyes again met. "What, Dad?"

"I have no regrets. Please, always remember that."

"I will, Dad."

It was the same cryptic message from weeks earlier that he had also said to my brother. Neither of us had a thought to ask what he meant then. Now, it was too late.

"Don't forget it," he whispered, his watery, reddened eyes softening.

"I won't." Again, I watched as they traveled toward his dresser, and his head again nodded toward the same drawer as earlier.

Does he want me to open it?

Before I could ask, Dad sank back into the pillows while regrets, all those lingering feelings of sadness I felt as a child, flew through *my* mind, as I thought of all we had missed during the tumultuous post-divorce phase of life as others set court-ordered rules for how we would live. Written in cold, calloused, legal terminology that families were to follow, they redefined dates, hours, and the manner of contact that ended family traditions forever.

With a simple piece of paper filed in a courthouse, not only did the untangling of marriage occur but the end of our family. Within a year after its finality, Dad had erased us from his present and left us to travel down our own paths. Disappearing from our lives, he reinvented a new one, without us.

It was not until his diagnosis with late-stage cancer that changes occurred. Leaving his home, he moved into the small studio apartment he developed with funds he received from our grandmother's estate. Then, he was seeking redemption.

Grandma had left Jim a small inheritance, with the rest to Dad and some for Aunt Marcella. To make certain Dad and his sister each received an equal amount, Jim gave his part back to the estate. It allowed for the development of Dad's storage business and workshop. As a result, Dad referred to Jim as his business partner, often saying he had invested Jim's part into the "family business."

We welcomed Dad back into our lives, as he made an earnest effort to reconnect with us. Now free to do so, we called one another often. Dad was seeking forgiveness for years of neglect. It wasn't necessary. Like most children, we continued to hold a belief in our parents, that circumstances would one day change. Most kids are flexible in offering second, third, and fourth chances at making relationships with their parents work, despite their whatever experiences they may have faced. Children never want to give up on their parents. A relationship between a child and his or her parent is lifelong. Sometimes, as with us, it is spent suspended in time, from the first devastating letdown to the next.

While speaking on the phone, I envisioned him lying upon the hard mattress of his futon, which set against the far wall of his studio apartment. His image fixed in my mind, I could envision him with his head propped on pillows and cradling the phone to his ear.

Dad faced difficulty sleeping. The long, lonely evenings were stressful for him. It was then he felt vulnerable and frightened. That was when he mostly called, seeking a compassionate voice to hear him out. Now free to open himself up to us, he revealed his fears and frustrations.

Hours were spent, speaking of his days with his lawyer, formalizing an end to his marriage, separating joint assets, and dealing with legal matters. Dad dreamed of the day when it would all be over, the cancer treatments, the marriage, and everything else holding him back from living the way he desired. It was exhaustingly emotional, and our father worried about his financial state. He had never expected another divorce, especially later in life. For a man who spent a lifetime planning every step he took, the two things he wasn't ready to deal with while preparing to retire, was a diagnosis of cancer and living alone.

Gathering a lifetime of regrets, Dad tried hard to fix each. Putting out of mind thoughts of the day when the cancers would take his life, he wanted to make the most of what life remained within him. It was important for him to resolve what he could.

"I didn't do what I promised you I would," he confessed during our late-night talks.

"Don't worry about it, Dad. We all get caught up in things," I said.

"Yeah. But whenever you kids called, she made my life hell."

"It's okay, Dad, it's in the past."

"Still, I should have done more. I ran out of time."

"We have now," I offered.

"But is it enough?"

"I treasure every minute of it." Though he could not see the tears filling my eyes, I was sure he could hear the break in my voice, giving away the sheer agony I felt.

"We both know there should have been more," he finally decided. "All I want is to get past all this and to live again, Lindy. I mean, really live. I am so tired of being tired. I've worked so damned long; there doesn't seem to be an end to it. I can't afford that lifestyle anymore. I don't need or want big houses and expensive vacations. I just want to live."

At the end of life, Dad was simply a man filled with disappointments. I worried about him living alone, trudging up the old wooden stairs to the top of his shop and flopping upon his bed after enduring session after session of difficult cancer treatments. Coupled with the stressful hours he spent at the office of his attorney dealing with the legal matters of his separation from his wife, much of the final years of his life were emotionally stressful.

Reminding him, he had a home with us; Dad insisted his quaint studio apartment was comfortable. He liked living alone in the beautiful, small town where he had spent the final two-thirds of his life. Dad grasped tightly to whatever stability was available was before him.

"Can we hold that offer open? For later, maybe?" he asked.

It was clear he was uncertain who would care for him when it became too much for him to do it for himself. Dad needed to know he had options to be with people who loved him; that we would not abandon him, and he would not be left alone.

Living as he did, was a cause of significant concern. I faced difficulty imagining being alone while battling cancer, with only a telephone as a lifeline to reach out to others. Receiving support and feeling a human touch is vital to survival, as is relief from stress. Though depressed, Dad insisted he was content with his situation. He wanted to live as his parents had when his father was preparing to die from cancer.

The seventh year of his cancer battle was Dad's last. Unable to care for himself any longer, he returned to the home he had built twenty years earlier. Taking a stab at treatments, he underwent a last gasp surgery to remove cancer from his esophagus. It wasn't successful.

Translating Dad's cryptic message of "I have no regrets," as one of love, Dad had said he was not sorry he had married our mother and for the over twenty years that they were together. Nor did he feel any remorse for fathering us, and the forty-five years we, the natural children of his first family shared with him, or the twenty-one years he had lived continuously with his second wife and their family. Caring for all of us equally, Dad tried to embrace life with whatever terms were available, and many of those were dependent upon what others were willing to accept.

During our lives, we do many things, some for good and some for wrong, but when the time comes to leave this world, a common phrase is "I have no regrets." Toward its end, when assessing life experiences in their totality, we accept life as it is, and as it was, realizing it to be the only one we will ever experience.

The silence in the room was deafening. Studying Dad's face, I watched his eyelashes flutter, and his eyes suddenly opened, as his hand tightly gripped mine.

"I'm scared," he whispered to me.

"It's okay, Dad," I whispered. "I am too."

I can't claim to know what it is like to be at the final stage of one's death. I haven't been there. But seeing others die from violence and cancer, the thought of dying a devastating death as had Dad, terrified me. I had spent years investigating matters involving public corruption, civil rights violations, workplace discrimination, violent crime, homicide, and counterterrorism. I knew victimization well. I was familiar with what it was like to confront death, like the time a drug dealer pointed a gun to my head and fired, or when working on the streets of one of the most violent cities in the nation, alone, and with living a lifetime in a family affected by unknown hereditary cancers.

During our father's seven-year battle with it, Dad never mentioned death or dying to us, not until the eve of his demise. He planned to differ from his father, his grandmother, her father, and all those in between. He wanted to live. Now, our final conversation had evolved to discussing his uncertainty of what lay beyond. With old business finished with the disclosure of the hereditary nature of his cancer, Dad could move forward.

"It's natural to fear the unknown," I said.

"Can't imagine *you* scared," he teased.

Laughing, I stated, "Oh, I've had my moments."

The empty sounds of silence screamed to help him with whatever he needed. I just didn't know what it was.

Damn it, Lindy. Just go for honesty.

"You know, Dad, I'm certain there is something more to all of this than life itself. I don't think this is all there is," I said, taking a stab at it. "Then, again, I don't know what's out there, no one does."

"Not sure I quite believe that," he whispered.

Okay, we hit upon one concern.

Emitting an uncomfortable laugh, an avalanche of thoughts tumbled through my mind.

Keep going. It is not the time to worry about approval.

"It is my belief I think you will still be around for a long time. It will just be in a different way."

"But how do you know that?" he asked.

"Remember when I called and asked *you* the same thing?"

Seconds of confusion occurred, then a glint of remembrance flashed in his eyes.

"Yeah, I do," he said, his voice lifting. "Think it's like that?"

"Without a doubt," I answered.

"That would be nice," he said, managing a weak smile.

"Yeah, it would," I agreed.

One morning, while caught in that early morning sleep, all my burdens evaporated. I found myself alone, with nothing existing around me — no sounds, no hot or cold, only a gentle, airy atmosphere. There was no stress, no expectations, no heightened emotions — just an aura of incredible peace and comfort from nothing as I walked. To where, I didn't know.

The fog and filtered light began to fade. Familiar images sharpened into focus, the rough plaster upon the ceiling, and the blue cobalt vase I grabbed while I was down in Mexico, now filled with pink daisies, and sitting on the dresser. Nothing had changed. Wherever my spirit was, it had returned.

I had called Dad. He urged me to go to the emergency room, concerned I was experiencing a problem with my heart. He was right. But it was nothing modern medicine could fix. It stemmed from the stress and the shattering of heartbreak while working the calloused city streets.

"Do you think dying is like that?" I had asked him.

"I don't know, Lindy. But I sure hope so," he had answered.

"But how *do* we know?"

Taking a deep breath, he said, "We don't. That's why you need to get your heart checked."

I promised I would, but I didn't. There was nothing wrong with my heart. I just needed some peace and comfort that morning. Glancing down upon Dad, a realization hit that he needed permission to die.

"Dad, are you worried about what will happen to her and the kids?"

"Very much so," he said. "Mostly, just the kids, though."

There it is.

"I'll be around if they need anything," I offered.

"You will?" he asked, his voice lifting.

"I always have," I said.

"She thinks none of you care."

"I've *always* been here for all of you whenever you all have wanted me around."

"I know, Lindy. She's just insecure. Just make sure you stay close, okay?"

"If she and the kids want me here, I'm only a phone call away as I have always been. It's up to them, Dad."

Lifting my arms over my head, I stretched. There was no sense in discussing it further. Despite everything, I was the most forgiving of her acts, and I worked hard to maintain a relationship with both. I couldn't understand how she could say that. Something wasn't right. My wedding was just around the corner, and I had asked her to be my maid of honor. If that didn't display respect for family, nothing did.

I shook my head. The cruelty of the past, her attacks upon us, and the decades of attempts at alienation to distance us from our father created nothing less than pure devastation for us. Any justification of its occurrence, especially discounting it because of "her insecurity," didn't change anything.

I wanted for Dad and me to keep our last hours together, making it about him and me. We didn't have time to discuss his spouse. Even while dying, his focus was trying to mitigate her cruel actions. The occurrences that created pain, hurt, and years of abandonment, spanning three decades, was never resolved. Discussion only compounded it. The only option we had was to move forward and become anesthetized to her comments. I tried hard to focus on filling my life with substance, keeping a relationship with her and Dad, without exploring the past.

"Tired, Dad?"

"Yeah."

"How about I go downstairs and let you rest a little?"

"Just a little," he murmured as I ran my hands through his hair and kissed his cheek. Dad closed his eyes.

"I love you, Dad."

"Love you, too, baby doll." His voice faded as he drifted to sleep.

Lingering, I memorized Dad's face, the wrinkles on his forehead, the scar above his left eyebrow, and the same soft texture of his fine, dark hair that I had inherited.

His breath heavy, Dad emitted groans of pain. I wished for him to be free. Free of the agony, free of the pain, free of cancer, and free of his fight to remain in this life. I wished his soul unleashed, to soar in the wind, so he would not have to live the cancer legacy of his family. Glancing upon him one last time, I quietly closed the door and went downstairs. Dad was still asleep when I left late that afternoon. The tears weighed heavily upon my heart as well as my face, as I sang while driving home.

Thirty-six hours later, early Easter morning, with the television screen flickering and "Amazing Grace" droning in the background, Dad sat straight up, uttering, "Oh, my God!" as though he had seen something incredible. He then laid back down and breathed his last.

Chapter Two

LETTING GO

The dove on silver pinions, winged her peaceful way.
—James Montgomery

The bitter winds bit through our clothing. Noticing I was shivering, Jim tossed his arm over my shoulders and pulled me close. Though wearing dark glasses and working to keep a stoic expression, my brother recognized my grief. Not expecting the loss of Dad to hit this hard, I dearly wanted the day to be over. I longed to curl up in the car and release the anguish boiling inside; the minutes spent standing outside the mortuary seemed like hours.

"You don't have to be tough all the time, you know?" Jim consoled.

Wishing he had not acknowledged my attempts, the human kindness of a touch, a caring word, or sympathy-filled eyes kept opening the floodgates of emotion. While my siblings were internalizing their feelings, those I tried to conceal, tumbled out.

Gazing upon my family and watching them standing around and converse quietly with one another, I noted a bit of Dad reflected in each of our children and grandchildren. Jim had received Dad's levelheaded practicality, his love for building, his humble demeanor, and his dark complexion. Chris, my son, looked the most like him. Inheriting Dad's eyes, his build, his facial features, he shared Dad's love of working with his hands. Scott, our grandson, possessed Dad's guarded heart, his brown eyes, and his thoughtful manner, while our granddaughter, Sonny, inherited his practical resourcefulness and shared his love for country music and art. Jason, our nephew, possessed his dry sense of humor and Dad's love of simplicity; our youngest granddaughter, Jaycie, an infant, never knew him but was bequeathed with his same diligent work ethic and Dad's sound, common sense.

Of all the grandchildren, my daughter, Judi, was the only one to receive the strong memories of his loving attention. His DNA that flowed through those of us, in his first family, made certain a part of Dad would exist and carry forward through the generations.

Throughout the morning, during his memorial service and after, Dad's emaciated image continued to appear. When I closed my eyes, all I could see was the ghostly remnants of the man I loved. It haunted me as I looked upon my loved ones. We shared Dad's genes, the good and the bad.

I wondered which of my children and grandchildren would contract the family cancer. Which would die as my father had, and his father had, and his father and his mother and how everyone who died because of the family cancer before them? The thought saddened me. It was far too much to consider, especially now.

We will deal with all this when it is finally over.

My gaze again focused toward the mountains, praying for the return of a distraction. It still offered none. Edging close to my husband, I needed to tuck into the warmth of his body. Saddened, I sighed in resignation.

With us, it is never over.

The intrusive thoughts kept whirling. I was no longer an investigator, a composed wife, a mom, or a grandmother. I was my father's daughter, grieving the loss of him. Memory after memory, thought after thought, continued to present themselves, offering uncontrollable flashes of insight into our father's life.

Dad had worked hard to make sure our childhood was better than his. The first twenty-one years of his life, he spent sleeping upon a rickety bed at one end of the screened porch of the tiny cottage in Altadena, California, where his family lived. His parents slept at the other end, while his sister was afforded the privacy offered to girls and slept in the only bedroom of their home. Dad never knew a room of his own until his separation from our mother. He had never lived alone anywhere, and when he finally did, it was for less than a year, following his divorce with our mother.

Dad loved being part of a family. He had spent most of his life living with others—first, twenty-one years with his parents, and then twenty years with my mother and us. After a year of their divorce, a girlfriend moved in with him, and a few years after our mother remarried, he married her.

Facing retirement at the end of their twenty-one years together, after being diagnosed with cancer, Dad was confronting the uncertainty of whether his battle would be successful. They separated. His wishes were simple. All he wanted was to live longer than sixty-eight years old and to experience a comfortable retirement. None of his desires appeared to be much of a possibility.

Returning to the humble lifestyle, he knew growing up; he did not want or need more. His goal was to clean up loose ends, and his priorities were to make sure the youngest of his second family was able to get through college.

He regretted not being able to fulfill those same promises to us when we were young. At the end of life, he set out to make it right.

Dad began thinking of himself for once. Fishing with us in the mountains, visiting cousins in Washington, traveling a bit, spending time with *all* his children, and getting acquainted and reacquainted with his grandchildren was important to him.

"I have worked so damned hard all my life; I don't want to die like this, not doing what *I* want to do," he confided. "When I get better…"

But by then, it was too late. There was no "getting better." The clock had stopped ticking. Diagnosed with late-stage cancer, Dad began preparing for the end of his life. The son who spent a lifetime longing to live in the humble manner of his father, as an everyday man, was still working as hard as he did when we were young children. While preparing to leave this world in the same manner his father had, he was dying of cancer and fading into obscurity, without fulfilling his dreams.

As a young father, Dad worked two to three jobs to support our family and save for the future: one fulltime with the telephone company, and the others part-time, hand-painting signs for businesses and building fences. Jim was his partner on nights and weekends, from third grade through junior high. Sitting right alongside Dad in his old, 1950s flatbed truck, he wanted to be just like his father. Then, success mattered. It stopped mattering when Dad realized the value of life after the loss of a child, having a heart attack, and later contracting cancer. He realized there were more important things than big houses and hefty bank accounts.

Now, at his memorial service, and glancing past the crowd, I contemplated how very right it was to be here memorializing our father; and how very wrong it was, coming out of the closet once again trying to appear as a family unified by his death. His second wife and their adopted children had never accepted us as a part of their family.

Here we were, standing beside them, again providing our staunch support. It was the same we had done through the years whenever Dad's second family had summoned us to be a part of their family crises, despite the fact, none had been there when we needed them.

Dad's wife beckoned. Leaning close, I heard her voice quietly state, "The doctors think the cancer was inherited. Poor kid," she said, glancing toward her son. "Now, *he* has to go through lots of testing."

Jim, Steve, and I glanced at one another, sharing our amazement. Her comment was baffling, especially stated at Dad's memorial service, when everyone was deep in grief and were vulnerable.

Why would she say that now?

A long-standing pattern, since meeting Dad, she had again erased us as Dad's only natural children and minimized the hereditary cancer condition existing in *our* family. For some reason, she felt compelled to make her family a part of *our* circumstances.

"All he said was his doctors thought it was hereditary, and to get checked," I had shared with Jim earlier that morning.

"But for what?" Jim asked, frustrated.

"That's the million-dollar question," I answered.

Emitting a deep sigh, he returned to reviewing the eulogy he was writing for Dad, while I toyed with my food. Setting the fork down, I had lost my appetite.

"I'll get on it as soon as I get home," I said, rising. "We have to find out, and nobody here wants to discuss it."

"We can do it together, Lindy, if you want," Jim offered, as though he had the time, with everything else that he was facing.

A single parent of five children, our brother struggled to get ahead. Returning from Vietnam, he worked hard putting himself through college and then did the same through law school. Taking a position as a professor, teaching contract law for the United States Department of Defense Contract College, Jim settled into a situation he loved.

He was always moving, finding challenges, and mastering them, one after another, clearing his land, building a home for himself and his children, working sunrise to sunset planting avocado trees, and developing watering systems on his ranch. When it all became too much, Jim would put his kayak into the back of his truck and headed for the beach. Putting his kayak into the water alone, he fished for sharks.

Once, he sealed a bet with a friend that he could swim across the Potomac River. Jim hopped into its icy springtime flow and swam a few miles to the other side. He then turned around and swam back.

I learned to become a risk-taker from Jim while exploring in the mountains with him. Not allowing myself to give up or to cry, I openly competed against him in basketball, races, and in baseball. From him, I learned perseverance.

In Vietnam, Jim often worked alone, occasionally remaining behind to capture messages and report enemy movements while others retreated from battle. He did the years later, when his neighbors evacuated their homes during the Southern California wildfires, making sure their property and animals were safe. Jim placed others first, ahead of himself. I worried for him; that he would wear himself out. With Dad's death, the days ahead would be difficult. There was still much left unresolved.

The two of them once did everything together; partnering in work, fishing, camping, and being the best of friends as they played baseball and basketball in the front yard.

As adults, they shared more in common. Father and son were both veterans of war; each had constructed their own homes, and each had fathered a flock of children. Jim adopted Dad's work ethic of dogged determination, and like Dad, was a perpetual workaholic, even perfecting Dad's tendency of using work as a distraction from conflict and problems.

It was a coincidence that he and Dad became estranged from their wives at the same time. The years the father and son spent apart were heart-wrenching. Dad's second wife was the wedge that pulled them apart, and Dad's separation from her was the glue that bonded them back together. During the six years, Dad lived alone, he and Jim reestablished their relationship without her constant negative undercurrent playing into it. Jim and Dad shared and accepted truths and regained trust in one another.

Glancing toward Dad's former spouse, I felt bad when I realized she was awaiting a response. "Dad told me about it on Friday," I whispered to her, apologetically.

"I'm sorry. I didn't know your father had done that," she said. I worked hard to hide the fact her comment had me furious.

If you did not know, when did you plan to tell us?

We had been in town for four days, spending most of it in her home. Every opportunity existed to discuss what the doctor told him about the hereditary cancer syndrome, but she did not mention it. The unanswered question, especially since our lives were at stake, was, "Why?"

Two days before Dad's memorial service, she stepped into the family room, with her purse slung over her shoulder. "I have a hair appointment this morning, and then I'm going to the attorney's office to start taking care of things," she said confidently. Patting her handbag, she continued, "I've got everything all ready, right here."

Her first concern was finally getting Dad out of her life. With the efficiency of a hospice facility, the day after he died, before she picked up her daughter at the Reno airport, she went shopping to buy a new bed and bedding, to replace the one in her guest room, where he died. Delivered that same night, two days later, she was heading to the attorney to finalize the details of his estate, while we were dealing with the details of his service.

Something was amiss. Though it didn't seem right, nothing ever does when our loved ones die, and we are rooted deep in grief. Still, despite the days spent in our stepmother's home, Dad's wife had said nothing to us about Dad's cancer being hereditary, or anything else, for that matter.

Glancing upon the dust that had settled on the tops of my shoes, I wondered how to clean them. Like Dad, I used methods of distraction to avoid dealing with matters until I was ready to confront them. What is, is and what was, was. Time ordinarily resolves much of the everyday problems that face us. And, through the years, like my father, I stuffed the ugly, the sad, the painful, and all the other inconvenient matters into little compartments, deep inside, waiting for time to take care of it so that I could keep everything and everyone around us together.

Uncomfortably edging past us, mourners moved toward the embankment where a lone dove sat in a cage. Scanning their somber faces, I watched as our loved ones prepared for the concluding chapter of Dad's life.

Aunt Marcella, the matriarch of our family, and her husband, Karl, had come from Florida, our sister, Donna, from Oregon, and my children, Judi and her three children, along with my son, Chris, traveled from Northern California. Jim and his son, Jason, drove up from Southern California. Everyone still alive had come, except four of Jim's other children. Dad's sister and we and our children and grandchildren were all that remained of Dad's natural family.

My eyes caught upon close family friends, Pat and Frank Holub, and those who worked with our father, even the servers and Dad's friend, John, from the coffee shop that Dad frequented were present. Maizie Jesse, my Godmother, approached and wrapped her arms around me in a comforting hug. The loving gesture unleashed another flood of tears.

"Let's talk later, okay?" she offered before catching up with others. I nodded, unable to speak.

As a man unlatched the door of a small wire cage, set upon the ground, I watched. A few seconds later, a silver dove cautiously peeked through the opening. Blinking his eyes to adjust to the morning sun, he carefully stepped onto the sparse sprigs of grass that shot up amongst the dirt and weeds.

Releasing a dove was my wish for our father. The ancient ancestors of our mother believed it to be a messenger of the Creator that delivered our souls to the other side. Wishing for our father's spirit to be free and to live in the wind, I longed for Dad to follow his dreams and to go and do whatever it was he wanted, wherever he wanted.

Pacing back and forth, the bird stopped for a moment and longingly gazed toward the Sierra Nevada. Fluttering his wings, the crowd of onlookers startled, suddenly stepping back. Taking a few careful steps to the embankment, he glanced around. Then, suddenly spreading his wings, the dove began running and taking to the air, soaring westward, into the morning sky.

My eyes intently followed, watching as it winged across the billows of clouds and drifted into the distance. Eventually, appearing little more than a tiny dot, the dove slowly melted into the beyond, disappearing with the last of what was once our father.

Chapter Three

ANCESTRAL BEGINNINGS

We're all ghosts. We all carry, inside us,
people who came before us. —Liam Callanan

We are all the products of our parents. Fifty percent of our DNA comes from our father, and fifty percent comes from our mother. Since we can only inherit fifty percent from each parent, my brother and sister were born with variations of our parents' DNA that I do not have. Even if identical twins, DNA may differ from one another. The inherited DNA that passes through the generations, coupled with the passing down of traditions, behaviors, thoughts, memories, value systems, and other influencing factors, affects who and what we are.

Our mother was the child of a third-generation, Swedish and Norwegian American father, and a homespun southwest Arizona rancher's daughter, of Irish, English, Scottish, Black, and Native American ethnicity. Her ancestors had been the first settlers of North Carolina, with one being an early Governor, appointed by the King. Others followed as planters, long-hunters, preachers, individuals fleeing religious persecution, and adventurers seeking an opportunity.

The diverse cultures blended into one another, creating a distinct culture of mountain folk who headed westward from North Carolina into the southwest Appalachian Mountains. Many farmed; some preached the gospel, and the "long hunters" traveled mountain trails with Daniel Boone and others. Stalking game and trading furs from North Carolina to Pennsylvania and Ohio, they hunted in pairs, often embarking upon their hunting trips in October and leaving their families behind to fend for themselves until returning in the spring. The independence of the southern men and women, with their unassuming, resourceful, and humble manner, made it possible to endure their lifestyle.

The survival instincts, characteristics, and the traditions they developed offered a respite from the rugged mountain environment. Living in Southwestern Appalachia was challenging, especially for the women. Not only bearing many children wore upon them, but many did not survive the harsh winters.

Nonetheless, they managed the homesteads during the absence of their men who returned from their wilderness treks just long enough to help with the planting of the crops and to father another child. Gathering the family, they headed for the forts, to avoid the Indians who used the mountain lands as summer hunting grounds.

Mom's kinfolk worked and played hard. Nobody paid much attention to the patched, faded clothes they wore or their simple cabins. Appearances in the mountains of colonial America meant little to those as equally modest as their neighbors. Treasured were personal relationships, faith in God, music, traditions, and life.

The Appalachian way of life was demanding. Women wore the years of arduous labor upon their faces. Weathered and weary, most died young, after giving birth to large numbers of children and keeping up with the ever-constant struggle to survive.

The men lived much longer. Our ancestral grandfather, Charles Cromwell Addington, when celebrating his hundredth birthday, hopped down from his wagon unassisted and stepped inside the Nickelsville, Virginia frame church, where he spent a few minutes preaching. After, he walked a quarter of a mile to where the members of his family gathered.

Sitting at the head of a table extending two hundred feet, Grandfather Addington joined those descendants who hadn't yet fled from the mountains. Sixteen children, and six-hundred and seven of their spouses, grandchildren, great-grandchildren, and great-great-grandchildren, were present to celebrate that day. The old preacher lived another four years past that hallmark celebration when his family eventually buried him in the Addington Cemetery, next to his three wives.

The Virginia settlers expressed their passion for living through their music. At night, playing their guitars, fiddles, and banjos and singing the folk songs of their ancestral England, Ireland, and Scotland, bluegrass mountain music evolved in the newly founded land. With it, came a lively jig called "flat-footing," its steps again combined with the original folk dances of the Irish, the Scottish, the Africans, and the Native Americans. The long-lasting traditions passed down through generations, included some insisted upon by our mother. The homes she owned always had a front door that faced the east. She was adamant about it.

"All good things come from there, Lindy," Mom would say. The Native American traditions passing down from generation to generation dictated that the east is from where the sun comes, and from it, we receive life, energy, knowledge, and warmth. It is there, our spirit originates.

In our home, a cast-iron frying pan set upon the stove, along with a large matching kettle that sat in the cupboard. It was another longstanding tradition. They were the heart of our kitchen. Mom's blackened skillet was smooth to the touch from the thousands of meals cooked in it and passed down from daughter to daughter. The recipes passed from a mother to her daughter often began with "Go fetch the old black frying pan and..."

In the Southwest Virginia Mountains, living was difficult, and dying was a part of life. When the time arrived for Mom's kinfolk to leave this world, it was without fanfare. Doctors seldom wandered through those parts of the country, and hospitals were mountains away. Death certificates were rarely issued. Until the 1950s, documentation of death was not reported unless the decedent was a veteran, or it was a requirement for social security benefits.

The place to find the cause of death was in newspapers or family bibles. They usually read, "Heart stopped," "Old age," "Died," "Passed," or, "Wore out." It didn't matter how or why they died. All that mattered to them was being able to pass into the next world after leaving this one.

Though many of our distant cousins still live in Appalachia, our branch of the Addington's moved from the Virginia mountains following the Civil War. Refusing to take up arms against their government, the Addingtons remained neutral. At its end, our ancestral grandparents John Doty Addington and his wife, Sarah Ellen Jesse, left where they had always lived and pioneered westward.

First, they settled in Kansas and later owned and worked a cattle ranch in Bonita, Arizona. Still, working hard, playing music, and brewing moonshine, they raised twelve children in the Arizona Territory. In the 1880s, they moved further west, following the sunshine to Santa Ana, California, where they farmed and lived their final days basking in its warmth.

It was there that Velda, our grandmother, married our grandfather. Grandmother was an independent, no-nonsense Arizona ranch girl working as a sassy waitress in a coffee shop. The daughter of a preacher and his Canadian born Scottish wife, she significantly differed from Grandpa, who was the son of parents of Swedish and Norwegian ancestry. Their lives collided when they met while he was arranging and delivering flowers in downtown Los Angeles.

Quiet and strong-willed, Grandmother was looking for a responsible, lifelong husband. Grandpa was not one, but it was 1931, during the Great Depression, and pregnant with his child, Grandmother settled for him anyway. Her wedding was not a joyful event; it was one that resulted in a lifetime of regrets while parenting a daughter and a son, alone.

Grandpa was adventurous and flighty, a wild partner who loved whiskey and beer. He brought out the hidden, fun-loving, impulsive nature in Grandmother. To him, she was the one with the contacts that supplied him the alcohol he desired, during prohibition.

Mom was born four months after they married. Her brother, Henry, came a year later. Few people were partying. It was hard enough for most to get enough work to keep food on the table. Life in Los Angeles was difficult for the young couple. While she worked, he did not.

Grandmother harbored high hopes that he would "grow up" and be a good husband and father. Opposites attract but seldom remain together, having to compensate for one another's idiosyncrasies. Their marriage was a recipe for disaster. After the repeal of Prohibition, they divorced.

Alone, Grandmother faced the responsibility of two hungry mouths to feed. Working long, hard hours to support Mom and Henry, Grandmother rented out one of the two-bedrooms of their apartment, to get through the tough times. Often, there was little to eat and no money to buy food, except for those rare occasions when Grandpa blew into town, flashing cash and blowing it on extravagances for the children.

Mom and Henry grew up playing on the gravel driveways of the small court apartments, typical to Southern California. His visits never lasted long. He soon vanished until the next time. He broke their hearts, but, as children do, they forgave him and never gave up on their father.

Mom distracted herself from life's challenges by singing. It provided her with comfort during tough times. Blessed with a beautiful voice, she left high school during her junior year. With her father's help, Mom enrolled in professional voice training. Like her Virginia cousins, Maybelle Carter, a founder of country music, her daughter, June Carter, and her husband, Johnny Cash, Mom wanted to "make it big." She took a job as a server at a lunch counter and performed gigs and recorded demo records at night. She was determined. Nothing would stop her, that is until she met Dad. She did not count on falling in love with him.

* * *

Our father was the product of a culture far different from that of Mom. Descending from a lengthy line of risk-takers of English, Scottish, and Irish ancestry, they were some of the first to settle in our country. Added to his pedigree was a rich, diverse heritage from his ancestral grandparents. Family members believed his great grandmother, Hutoka, to be of Native American descent. His fifth and sixth great-grandfathers had been free mulatto soldiers who served in the French and Indian and Revolutionary Wars. Dad's family was a rainbow.

The Snellings of Ipswich, Suffolk, England, descended from Robert Snelling, a linen merchant who set out an enormous fleet of merchant ships that held royal charters to trade in Spain, Turkey, and the Baltic countries. After he and his descendants became involved in the Separatist movement during the seventeenth century, many fell from favor with the King and fled England to avoid persecution.

The more religious family members moved to Holland, where they followed family member and Separatist leader William Ames, a nephew under the guardianship of Robert Snelling. Ames worked with Francis Brewster, another leader of the Separatist movement. In the early 1600s, the Separatists arrived in the new country on a small fleet of three ships, with many followings, shortly after that.

The elders kept the stories of our early American ancestors alive, passing them down from one generation to the next. As children, we sat upon the hardwood living room floor of Grandmother's beautiful, little arts and crafts bungalow, carefully listening as she told of the challenges our ancestors faced.

It was there that Grandma introduced us to our notable ancestral grandparents, the three early governors of Massachusetts, Thomas Dudley, Simon Bradstreet, and John Endicott. She read us the poems of our ancestral grandmother, Ann Bradstreet, America's first woman poet, and told us the stories of adventure and courage of others.

Grandma's stories captivated us, who lived in a tiny Nevada town, at the base of an enormous mountain range. Living far from where our ancestors once resided in their castles and English manors, Grandma rooted us in the history of our country. Providing us with a sterile version of the lives and deaths of notable white ancestors who died of tuberculosis and heart attacks, we didn't hear about the "everyday people" who immigrated from England and Ireland or of the trials of those who were of color or who contracted cancer. It was the 1950s, and the practices of eugenics were in full swing in the first half of the twentieth century. Secrecy was imperative. It kept the family insulated from being a target for mandatory sterilization actions that were actively promoted by California's growing eugenicists.

Claiming ancestral descent from the John Porter family of Salem, Massachusetts, was of utmost importance to her. Born into nobility, Porter held the respect in the colonies as one of their local leaders and their largest landowners. Porter's reputation was legendary for being fair and standing firm as a defender of the women accused during the Salem Witch trials.

Following the Revolutionary War, John Porter's descendant, Israel Porter, pioneered from Massachusetts, westward. First settling and co-founding Gouverneur, New York, he and his family headed west to Ohio for a brief period, then led an expedition to Wisconsin, becoming a founding father of Milwaukee (Pewaukee), Wisconsin, and the first pioneer settler to die there. Remaining, his son, Israel, settled there with his wife and children, including our second great ancestral grandfather, William Berkeley Porter, named in honor of *his* ancestor, Robert the Rebellious.

Robert owned Berkeley Castle, where the Forty Barons of the West, known as the Rebellious Barons, met before continuing to Runnymede to present the Magna Carta to the King in 1215. Robert had stood firm in insisting King John of England sign the document that limited the King's authority and power over the people.

After many generations and being as common as everyone else in America, the Wisconsin farm boy grew up as a risk-taker. Accompanied by his brother, Volney, in 1849, he ventured with a hundred other Wisconsin men to the California gold fields as investors in the "Genoa Company." Traveling in a wagon train, trailed by the small battalion of men headed west to California, they mined for gold for over a year. Mildly successful, but unable to receive their part of the company's profits until arriving home, Berkeley and Volney found themselves in need of raising money to pay their fares back home.

Noting an opportunity in horse-trading with the men in the mining camps, rather than engaging in the back-breaking drudgery of breaking ground with pickaxes and shovels, they became entrepreneurs. Over the next two years, after they made a small fortune, far more than they would have earned digging for gold, the two returned home with cash in their pockets. After retrieving what was waiting for him there, Berkeley secured a small pharmacy in Black River Falls, Wisconsin, and after a few years, he became a civic leader. At thirty years old, he married seventeen-year-old Harriet Lucy Thorpe, who was known as "Hutoka."

At eighteen, Hutoka became a mother, eventually having four children. As a young child trained by her mother to learn the methods of medical treatments, she offered medical care for those on the frontier. Hutoka, and others, known as "Indian doctors," botanist physicians, and midwives, provided medical attention for most of those residing in the pioneer towns.

Experienced physicians were rare and difficult to find in the remote regions of the country. The only difference between midwives and physicians (known as regulars in the 1850s) was the eight months of formal education physicians underwent.

Hutoka was compassionate. She dedicated her efforts toward those who didn't have the means to pay for services of a local doctor, primary, the members of the Winnebago tribe, and the less fortunate in the community. Berkeley was more focused on profit. His advertisements for the Porter Pharmacy covered the pages of the local newspapers with the same extravagant claims of treatments and cures of those snake oil salesmen hawked in the east coast papers.

Nonetheless, the Winnebagos trusted them. For years, Berkeley and Hutoka worked together, protesting the removal of the Ho-Chunk, and attempting to find homesteads for the tribal members to claim that would prevent them from having to leave their homeland.

Before the government removed the rest of the Winnebago onto out-of-state reservations, tribal members approached Berkeley and Hutoka, asking if they would keep their weapons safe for them until they returned. Advising he did not think the government would allow them to come back to Wisconsin, they told him not to worry; they would be back, and they would see one another again.

During the winter of 1873 and 1874, when the government finally acted, Grandfather stood at the train station, with tears rolling down his face as he bade his Winnebago friends goodbye. After, he sent his wife and children to live in Vineland, New Jersey, where his parents and other family members had moved. Suffering from prostate cancer, his father needed Hutoka's help.

After situating them in an operational farm, Berkeley headed back to Wisconsin to settle financial matters. He did not return, as promised. Falling in love with a local woman, he filed for divorce from Hutoka, leaving her and their children in New Jersey. With his former wife and children out of mind, Berkeley began a new life without them.

It wasn't long before Hutoka and Berkeley remarried following the death of his second wife. Their marriage was tenuous, at best. Six years later, Hutoka found Berkeley unconscious in his bed. He had taken a self-prescribed overdose of morphine because he "was feeling melancholy." His breathing labored, Berkeley never gained consciousness and died of the drug overdose after a few days.

Hutoka arranged for a marching band to escort Berkeley's body to the cemetery. She had him buried next to his second wife, and a young son he and Hutoka had lost. After installing an enormous monument in his honor, she settled his estate. Moving from Black River Falls to Ann Arbor,

Michigan, she attended the University of Michigan, Homeopathic Medical School. After graduation, she completed her residency at the Philadelphia Women's College, then opened a practice in Chicago, Illinois, as one of a few of Illinois' first women physicians.

In old age, Hutoka moved to Altadena, California, where her daughter, Lottie, and her husband, Adam Long, ran a boarding house with our then twenty-year-old Grandma. There, she died of natural causes at eighty-nine years old, on January 28, 1924.

* * *

Settling in Massachusetts in the 1600s, Dad's paternal ancestors first settled in Boxford, Massachusetts. They moved into Maine, then pioneered across the country, west, to Columbus, Ohio, south to Iowa, north to Chippewa Falls, Wisconsin, southeast to Urbana, Illinois, then to Kansas, across the frontier to Las Vegas, New Mexico, westward to Phoenix and, finally, settling in Los Angeles.

Our first known American ancestor of Snelling descent was Mark Snelling, the illegitimate mulatto son, or the brother of a widow known as Mary Snelling, or Mary Dowen. A tragic character, in 1730, she lived a difficult life supporting three children alone while living in a fruit cellar built into the incline of a hill, in Boxford, Massachusetts.

Mark worked as a laborer on a nearby farm to earn food and money to care for them, while she grew crops and stole sheep that she slaughtered, hiding the remains in the nearby Mare Pond.

In the 1730s, Mark married a woman, only known to us as Jane, who died in 1739 when their son, Asa, was a year old. Mark raised his child alone. Finally, in 1744, when persons of color were allowed admission into the Congregational Church, Mark offered the First Congregational Church of Boxford his Confession of Sins. A prelude to baptism, it was his rite of entry into the faith of those who lived in the community. His written and signed declaration indicated he had been educated and was able to read and to write well.

Regardless of his education, Mark spent most of his life working as a laborer before serving with the Essex County militia at the Scarborough Blockhouse in Maine during the French and Indian Wars. In 1747, the new country was facing a crisis, and times were difficult for the settlers and the soldiers. Food shortages occurred for the troops. Captain Joseph Frye of Andover, Massachusetts, fed his small battalion until the community was able to help. Mark died later that year, at the approximate age of thirty-six years old. Buried in the ancient Newbury cemetery, nine-year-old Asa, was now an orphan, spending the rest of his childhood bonded out to work on the farms of others and learning to tailor clothing.

Often, Asa dreamed of joining the British military and becoming a soldier as his father had been. Upon coming of age, Asa received an English pound for enlisting and spent the next few decades of his life serving with the British in Quebec.

In 1776, word came to him and his cousins from the Colonies, calling them home to fight for freedom. Responding, the three deserted, trekking through the snow and the wilderness, pursued by the British. Fearing the penalty of hanging for desertion, if apprehended, they hid until the British soldiers gave up their search.

After ensuring they were safe, the three began the long walk toward home, traveling through forests and swamps from Canada to Boston. It was a difficult journey. Indians captured one cousin, and finally tattered and starving, Asa and his other cousin finally reached Cambridge, Massachusetts, only to find military regulations precluded Blacks from enlistment.

Along with Salem Poor and other notable black American patriots from Essex County, the black soldiers volunteered their services until February of 1777 when they could muster into the Continental Army. Thousands enlisted. Asa served in the war for six years, longer than most patriots, discharging in 1783 at the war's end.

Through the generations, parents and grandparents passed down the family stories of Asa's exploits. Some revealed Asa was a "bodyguard" to Israel Putnam, who had grown up with his father in Boxford.

With Asa's tall stature, dark skin, tailoring skills, and prior military experience, the truth is more likely that he was a "body servant" to the General. The Continental Army issued Uniforms to military soldiers in pieces. Asa possessed all the skills Putnam desired in a body servant, including being able to tailor his uniforms, as well as provide service and protection to the General. Most of all, Putnam chose Asa to work beside him because of a long-termed personal relationship of trust.

At an age when most colonial men were preparing for retirement, Asa found himself unmarried and battling the British throughout New England. Walking to and from West Point, New York to Essex County, Massachusetts each winter and returning each spring was grueling. Nonetheless, he continued to enlist term after term, serving his country, often without pay, food, warm clothing, and conveniences.

The thought of freedom and equality meant more to Asa and the other soldiers of color than it did to most. For the free and enslaved black patriots, it was worth spending six to seven years of their lives fighting for freedom, especially for Asa. The term, "all men are created equal" is mighty powerful for those who never experienced equality.

After the war, Asa married Elizabeth Hope, an Irish servant. They started a family. Asa became one of the many heads of families whose children labored in the fields alongside their fathers. Labor was scarce in New England when compared to the South, which depended upon slaves to work in their fields. When their children became adults with families of their own, the small tracts of land held by colonial parents, like Asa, could not support their numbers. The sons moved on, seeking opportunities.

Asa lived to old age, receiving a pension of $23 a month from the government for his service in the Revolutionary War, after giving his testimony to Justice Samuel Putnam, the grandson of the now-deceased General Israel Putnam. In his final years, General Putnam's granddaughter cared for Asa. The recorded age of his death, reflected upon his military and town records, occurred at eighty-six years of age, on July 15, 1823.

Only as successful as everyone else who fled to the colonies, Massachusetts colonists faced the same challenges in survival as others. Parents died, leaving children penniless and orphaned. With several generations of pioneers settling upon the new lands, fathers had little to offer their sons in inheritances, after fighting in the wars of a young country. The transition from English merchants to farmers was difficult, during colonial times, due to the scarcity of farm labor that existed.

With a small amount of seed money from their fathers, and a family Bible to pass down through the generations, young men left their homes and families in large numbers, often with others with whom they had grown-up. Heading west, they carried with them, the legacies of long-standing family traditions and their family names.

In 1810, Asa's son, Aaron Snelling, lived in Livermore Falls, Maine. There, he developed his acreage into a prosperous farm founded on the Androscoggin River. A successful farmer and cattleman, he was an early investor of the Durham stock, introducing it to the agricultural community in New England. He was also a stockholder in the local railroad.

Aaron married Mary Perry, the daughter of David Perry, of Wayne, Maine, a veteran of the Revolutionary War and a descendant of Elder William Brewster of the Mayflower.

Their son, Moses Perry Snelling, left his home in Livermore Falls, Maine, at eighteen, to attend vocational training in Leominster, Massachusetts, to become a carpenter. Upon completion, he migrated west to Columbus, Ohio, then a booming town.

There, he married Sarah Truman, an eighteen-year-old orphan from England. Moses and his bride moved to Southern Iowa and birthed a son. Moses named him David Perry Snelling, after Moses' older brother and his maternal grandfather, David Perry. The use of the name Perry, as a middle name, passed through generations.

Tragically, she died at the age of twenty, as did most of her brothers and sisters. Sarah Truman and her family are the probable roots of what we know today, to be Lynch syndrome.

As what occurred with Mark with Asa, Moses found himself raising an infant alone, fathers caring for young children following the deaths of their mothers was not unusual. A lieutenant in the Wisconsin militia, Moses leased David out to one farmer or another while he was on active duty or when building homes in another town.

After an unsuccessful remarriage, Moses eventually moved to Illinois, near his brother, David Perry Snelling, who, by then, was a judge. Moses married and settled in Urbana, Illinois, where he became a deacon in the Congregational Church, where he dedicated himself to the causes of abolition and prohibition. He and his wife held services in his home until he built a new structure for the congregation. Dedicated to his beliefs, Moses assisted runaway slaves to escape to Canada and offered support for his friend, Abraham Lincoln, who often spoke at the Goose Pond Church, while campaigning for President.

David remained in Wisconsin, working in the lumber camps until 1861 when Lincoln called for troops. He enlisted as a federal soldier, promoting to First Sergeant, in charge of Company G in the 13th United States Infantry, under the personal command of General William Tecumseh Sherman. Occasionally, he served on his staff.

The stories David grew up with about his great-grandfather, Asa Snelling, inspired him while engaged in the Battles of the Tennessee. They motivated him to continue trudging through the Mississippi Valley swamps, hunting down Confederate soldiers, while suffering from tuberculosis and malarial fever. Wounded on three occasions while fighting in Black River and Champion Hill, David honorably discharged in October 1864 upon completion of his term of service. Then, working as a police captain in Nashville, Tennessee, he saved enough to buy a small plot of railroad land in Illinois.

Suffering from war disabilities made his attempts at farming impossible—David, his wife, Harriet Ford, and their son, Austin, headed to Kansas. There, David and his father, Moses, farmed, developed a telephone service, and brought coal and building materials into Olathe.

In Kansas, David's tuberculosis worsened. Moses cared for his son's family while David traveled to a tuberculosis rehabilitation center in Las Vegas, New Mexico, for a prolonged period of treatment. He returned home, feeling able to run his business, allowing his parents to pioneer to the west.

Now old enough to be involved in David's business, his daughters ran the telephone switchboard while the boys set the poles, strung the wires, ran as messengers, and worked on the farm. During summers, David continued the tradition of leasing his children to farmers as had occurred with him. A letter from one of his sons told a story of young men dreaming of running away and joining the circus.

It wasn't long before David's illness returned. Finally leaving Olathe and his four oldest behind, he, his wife, and the two youngest again headed back to New Mexico, for further treatment. After a while, feeling better, they continued west to Phoenix for a brief period, and then traveled to Los Angeles, California, they settled there until his death, a few years later in 1901, at sixty-two years old.

Our grandfather, Harrie, David's youngest son, grieved heavily when his father died. After his mother went to live with her daughter, he traveled to Sonora, Mexico, to work for his older brother Dumont who now managed a local telephone exchange for Colonel Tom Mix.

Grandfather loved living with Monty, as he was known. Riding his Indian motorcycle up and down the desert, installing and repairing phone lines granted him a sense of freedom that he embraced. Grandfather was fond of the simplistic Mexican lifestyle, its spicy food, colorful southwest furniture, and the soft roll of the Spanish tongue.

Their project complete; he returned to Los Angeles, where a brother-in-law hired him at Home Telephone Company. Later merged into Pacific Bell Telephone Company, with the advent of World War I, Grandfather volunteered with other Pacific Bell Telephone employees to serve in the 411th Telegraph Unit of the Signal Corps.

Mustered into military service at the Presidio of Monterrey, Grandfather quickly adapted to military life. Shortly after deploying to Vancouver, Washington, with his unit, they returned to Monterrey, readied to ship out to the European front. There, he managed German-speaking agents who crossed enemy lines to capture and decode communications, he and his unit engaged in the battle at Aisne-Marne, France, where Germans released mustard gas into the trenches.

Resulting in the tragic casualties of over 4,500 troops, Grandfather never once spoke of the horror he experienced as he adapted to a return to civilian life. Armed with a positive nature and a desire to look forward, he returned to his work at Pacific Telephone Company, camped in the Arroyo, and danced at clubs with friends.

His ability to adapt proved to be an invaluable characteristic after 1918, when tragedy began to hit his family. From then until 1932, every one of his five siblings, except for one, died of cancer between the ages of fifty-four and fifty-six years old, leaving eight, young nieces and nephews behind. Grandfather could do little more than watch as cancer wiped out his entire family.

Living in Southern California was challenging in 1928 when my father, Harrie, was born. With a population of two million, only twelve percent were minorities. Intolerance existed against any person with dark skin, the Native Americans, Blacks, Mexicans, Asians, and those of mixed race.

The Klu Klux Klan was active, with John Porter, a used automobile parts dealer, served as its president. Becoming the Mayor of Los Angeles in 1928, he fostered an anti-minority climate. No one in our family spoke about the deaths from cancer, outside of themselves. It was too dangerous with the roots of racial discrimination and eugenic practices in operation.

In 1943, Grandfather Snelling contracted stomach cancer. After applying for a social security disability, he was devastated when he received a notice threatening deportation to Mexico unless he proved United States citizenship.

Despite being a California resident for over fifty years, a fourteenth generation American, a World War I veteran, and the son of a Civil War veteran, rather than provide him with the benefits he earned, the government relayed an intent to deport him. They believed him to be Mexican because he had dark skin and spoke Spanish fluently.

Anger overtook Grandma as she engaged in a letter-writing campaign to the city officials of Olathe, Kansas, and others, requesting help. In 1887, Olathe, Kansas, was the gateway to the Santa Fe Trail. When Grandfather was born, birth certificates were not issued. Friends and relatives sent dozens of signed declarations of personal knowledge of Grandfather's birth. Those documents, accompanied by the Civil War records of his father, listing the names of his dependent children, supplied the needed evidence of citizenship.

The roots of eugenics dated back to the 1882 Act to Regulate Immigration. It was two-fold. First, it disallowed the immigrants' entry into the country. Second, it opened the doors to a movement that gave immigration officials the power to deny persons they believed unfit to come into the country. Those who did not have the means to care for themselves returned to their native countries.

The eugenics movement was running in full swing in California, following its start in the early 1900s at Cold Springs, New York. Its mission focused on removing negative physical traits in human beings by practicing actions of mandatory sterilization upon persons the geneticists considered as being "undesirable. Their efforts created an ugly division amongst Americans.

Led by medical professionals, politicians, the socially elite, and others, many were involved in advocating for the mass sterilization of the ill, the poor, the uneducated, the addicted, the criminals, the alcoholic, the disabled, and the deformed. Directly in their sight were immigrants, minorities, and those with hereditary conditions, including blindness, alcoholism, diabetes, epilepsy, deformities, and family traits of contracting cancer. Funded by the Carnegie Institute and the Rockefeller Foundation, American researchers, and the social elite worked to develop ways to improve a "better breed of people."

Pasadena, California, was the epicenter of the California based movement developed by Paul Popenoe in 1908. A marriage counselor who edited the Journal of Heredity, he later headed up the local eugenics' organization, The Human Betterment Foundation. Its members included top educators of the University of California system, political leaders, and even ministers of churches. Pastor Robert R. Freeman, of the Pasadena Presbyterian Church, was a member of the Board of Trustees. It was the church my father and his family attended.

Their publication stated, "Strong, intelligent, useful families are becoming smaller and smaller. Irresponsible, diseased, defective parents do not limit their families. There can be but one result. That result is race degeneration; there is one outstanding, practical, humane measure which, administered, will go far to change this trend toward human deterioration. This measure is the sterilization, by a harmless surgical operation, of men and women who are so seriously defective that, for the protection of themselves and their families, of society and posterity, they should not bear and rear children."

Promoted to a leadership role with the American Eugenics Society, Popenoe's movement inspired the radicalization of a society that supported the mandatory sterilization of over 20,000 Californians. That same radicalized philosophy formed a base of support for the Nazi government, praising Hitler, and republishing the German Sterilization Law of 1934 in the Journal of Heredity. That same year, Popenoe arranged for the display of Nazi exhibits at the annual meeting of the American Public Health Association at the Los Angeles County Museum.

A simple everyday man, Grandfather was the last living survivor of his immediate family, he did not focus on politics or anything else outside his work or his loved ones. Grandfather lived as others did during the Depression. He was hard working and was never a burden upon society. Nonetheless, the Pasadena eugenics movement considered Grandfather and his children imperfect because they came from a "cancer family." The pressure on Grandfather, and Dad, to undergo voluntary sterilization so as not to produce offspring like them was strong.

Following the experiences he had with the horrors of World War I and facing the wrath of the local eugenics movement, Grandfather's priority was protecting his family. He worked hard to ensure their survival while he lived with the uncertainty of his fate.

Living frugally in one bedroom, as the family grew, added on a sleeping porch. Owning a car, a milk cow, a few rabbits, a couple of sheep, and some goats, Grandfather farmed his small plot of land on evenings and weekends, developing a good-sized orchard of fruit trees and a rotation of ground crops.

Working long days at the telephone company was difficult. Having fallen from a pole, he had previously suffered a permanent injury to a leg. But motivating him to continue working as a repairman was the ability to increase the amount of savings in his bank account, to protect his family if he died in the manner of his brothers and sisters. Purchasing life insurance policies naming his family members as beneficiaries, Grandfather's priority was making sure his wife and children could support themselves, and his son and daughter could attend college if he were to die from cancer.

More critical, Grandfather focused his energies upon teaching Dad how to become independent and to protect himself. He spent considerable time with his daughter, encouraging her to get a good education, and a respectable job, so she would be able to live autonomously.

As feared, "someday" struck in 1944 when Grandfather became the last of his direct family to contract the same cancers as them. Fifteen-year-old Dad and Marcella grieved his loss. Refusing to believe he died from cancer, Dad's sister convinced herself that her father had a heart attack, as stated by his physician. Dying from cancer would have cast a shadow upon her and her entire family.

Following his death, Dad begged Grandma to allow him to transfer to Cathedral High School in Los Angeles with his friends, where he could start anew. Many of the boys attending the school were Hispanic Catholics who were commuting from Pasadena and Altadena to Los Angeles. They, too, were vulnerable to the eugenicists' campaigns.

Founded by the Christian Brothers, whose mission was to educate the working class and the poor with an intensive, high-quality education that would prepare the young men for college, Cathedral High School was a welcome change for Dad. With his olive skin and being a member of a "cancer family," he had much in common with other students.

Grandmother did not want him attending school outside Altadena. Finally, she gave in to his pleas. The Christian Brothers offered Dad the attention he needed and missed from his father. Completing the tenth grade, Dad transferred from Cathedral High School to Pasadena Junior College to finish high school.

Grandma realized the good that came with change. Being away from Pasadena and Altadena, filled Dad with an immense sense of relief and confidence. A natural tendency for young men to seek protection and comfort is to gravitate toward that which is familiar.

For those living with a folk history of cancer, Pasadena was a frightening place to live. This fear was lifelong. In our family, a steadfast rule was not to discuss private matters with others. It was not just for privacy; it was to ensure survival.

Chapter Four

GROWING UP IN THE FOOTHILLS

What was silent in the father speaks in the son
and often is found in the son is the unveiled
secret of the father. — Friedrich Nietzsche

Graduating from his last two years of high school at Pasadena Junior College in 1945, Dad enlisted in the Army. At seventeen years old, they assigned him to a construction detail at Camp Beale, in Northern California, and later promoted him to sergeant. Assuming the responsibility of processing the discharges of World War II soldiers, Dad supervised the unit in 1948. It was after he discharged, that Dad spent his lunch hours perched upon a stool at the lunch counter of a drugstore where sixteen-year-old Mom worked.

Enamored with her feisty demeanor, a strong work ethic, and intense beauty, Dad returned daily to capture her attention. One day, as Mom presented him with his check, he placed a cigar band on her ring finger.

"Will you marry me?" he teasingly asked. Mom laughed, but she continued to look forward to Dad coming by for lunch. After a year of dating, he again asked her the question in earnest.

"Dad. I want to settle down and have a family," Mom confided to her father. "I don't want to sing anymore.

Though disappointed that his daughter wanted to give up her dreams to marry Dad, Grandpa offered his blessings. Dad surprised Mom with a diamond ring, and after she converted to Catholicism, they asked for permission from the Catholic Church to wed.

Two and one-half years after meeting, on July 15, 1950, the seventeen-year-old soft-spoken woman with a beautiful voice, gave her hand to Dad. With the promise of one day having a piano so she could keep singing, they began their Catholic life and their dream of raising six children.

Sharing much in common, the two decided to move to Auburn, California, located on the western edge of the Sierra Nevada Mountain Range, where Dad frequented while in the Army. Captivated by the romanticism of the "old west" small towns, he dreamed of one day settling in that area.

Living a modest lifestyle as that Dad experienced as a child, they played Scrabble and card games; and sang and danced to the radio. Fishing, hiking, picnicking, and saving for their first home, the young couple were busy planning their future.

While Dad still grieved his father's death from stomach cancer, Mom understood. Her father had survived the same. Shortly after, her mother contracted breast cancer, not long after her mother had died from a breast cancer-related stroke. Mom and Dad supported one another through their grief and shared fears of cancer.

Upon receiving a transfer to Auburn, California, with Pacific Telephone Company, Dad bought an old camping trailer and made a move north while Mom was pregnant with Jim. It was there; my brother was born ten months after they married, and while they were living in that little trailer. I came into this world eighteen months later.

"What's her name?" Dr. Joy, the physician who delivered me, asked.

"Mary Lou," Dad told the doctor as he rocked me in his arms.

"Why don't we just call her Lindy, Hap?" Mom asked. "She doesn't look like a Mary Lou."

Dad conceded. Girls named Mary Lou had light-brown hair, sparkling blue eyes, freckles sprinkled across fair skin, and wore pigtails. Like Dad, I had olive skin. The small bit of soft fuzz on my head was dark. Chubby and mostly bald, with a café au lait mark, the size of a silver dollar embossed upon the back of my right calf. Dad called me his American beauty with the short, stubby, beauty.

By then, they had moved out of the trailer and into a small, dilapidated, two-bedroom, rural bungalow with chipped linoleum floors. Located in the western foothills of the Sierra Nevada, outside Auburn, California, the rent was inexpensive, and the young couple was saving to build a home of their own.

After, my sister, Donna, arrived fifteen months later. Mom and Dad gave up the dream of having six children following Mom enduring a series of miscarriages. They decided to settle for us three. The costs of delivering babies and caring for more children were mounting.

Each morning, Dad hopped into his old, green 1940s pickup truck, tossing his metal lunch bucket onto the bench seat and praying it would start. Dearly loving that old truck, he spent a lifetime telling us stories of the nightmares he would have, fearing it wouldn't get him to work.

His truck sputtered as he pulled into the driveway at dusk, and as usual, squeaked to a stop. Upon hearing the screen door slam shut when he entered the house, it burst with activity. Mom always described those early days of their marriage as their best, while Dad focused upon the family unity as one of the beloved memories of his life.

Every day, without fail, when Dad returned home from work, the first thing after entering the door was to kiss Mom. It was a tradition that continued through their marriage. After showering, he would wearily flop on the sofa while Jim raced in circles around the living room. I would crawl up on his lap and insist upon his sole attention as he read the morning paper to me. I was a Daddy's girl.

* * *

In early 1954, Dad received a transfer with Nevada Bell Telephone Company to Carson City, a quaint town of 4,500 people. The little village offered more than rustic charm and beauty. It supplied protection to families like ours.

Following passage in 1911, Nevada's eugenics laws had become unenforceable following a federal circuit judgment in a 1918 case. A judge had sentenced a young epileptic male to prison, and to undergo mandatory sterilization. The federal court decided the judge's order to be out of compliance with the State of Nevada Constitution and its ban against the use of cruel and unusual punishment. As a result, Nevada became a safe place for us to live.

We settled into temporary veterans' housing. Covered with dry, weathered wood, when we played upon the porch, we ended up with splinters in our fingers and feet.

In the mornings, Mom would stand at the front door and watch as a four-year-old Jim raced to where other young children stood in line, waiting to pump kerosene into a small pitcher. Placing it beneath a spout, Jim slid a nickel into the slot, and the cooking fuel poured into it. Done, Jim ran back to the porch to give it to Mom.

Playing barefoot in the dirt parking lot that separated the rows of housing, the afternoon winds would kick up, the dust would fly, and tumbleweeds danced across the parking lot. Knocking us to the ground and stabbing through our skin with their dry spines, we always ran home, crying.

At 5:00 p.m., each evening, dozens of vehicles, filled with weary fathers, wheeled into the parking area. When the first arrived, we ran for dear life, to reach the safety of the porch and into the tiny apartment. It was Mom's signal to prepare dinner.

Despite living a humble lifestyle, Dad was grateful. We had a roof over our heads. Living in veterans housing, residents faced two choices. They either moved onward after a while, or they moved upward. Most did the latter, finding jobs and permanent housing in the small town.

Then, life was simple. Folks did the best they could with what they had, which after World War II, and the end of a long depression, was little. Families worked hard, played hard, lived quietly, and listened to their radios. In the evenings, the same song played in stereo from all the radios in the housing project, from the only radio station in town.

It wasn't long before our parents found a two-bedroom Cape Cod home in the foothills upon the southwest side of Carson City to rent. Our living situation dramatically improved. It was small, but it was home, a temporary stop while Mom and Dad were planning to build their own home up the hill.

Inside that little house, we spent our mornings listening to Mom as she sang to the radio. Like other families, we did not watch television for another two years until 1957. Clustered around the sofa at night, we would close our eyes and allow our imaginations to run rampant, creating the scenes, while intently listening to the radio announcer.

During the weekends, Dad took us to the drive-in theater, where everyone in Carson City frequented. In awe, we would watch the news clips of President Eisenhower riding in a Jeep while visiting our troops in Korea, and seeing the USS Nautilus, the first nuclear-powered submarine, patrol ocean waters. We seldom saw the actual movie. By the time it started, we were usually asleep, bundled tight in the back seat.

No longer bald, little pigtails sprouted from each side of the top of my head. Strong-willed, I refused to wear shoes, wanting to look just like my Mom, who also preferred being barefoot.

Our world now existed far beyond that of a wooden porch loaded with splinters. Surrounded by a white picket fence, velvety grass sprouted from beneath a large willow tree. Beneath it was where I kept my favorite toys beneath it—a wooden telephone; my book, The Three Little Pigs; and a little red wagon.

For hours, with Daisy, our cocker spaniel, I would stand in the front yard, gripping the fence tightly and rocking back and forth, peeking through the pickets upon the neighborhood kids playing baseball in the street. I fell in love with the little red-headed kid who lived up the road who would stop and speak with me. Whenever he rode by on his bicycle, I raced outside. Telling Mom that we would marry when I grew up, she laughed, never knowing two decades later, we would again meet and consider it.

Mom and Dad socialized with friends and family members and became involved in the community. They loved the simplicity of small-town life and the little two-bedroom home where we three kids and the dog slept in one room, while our parents slept in the other.

At five, Jim attended kindergarten at Gleason School and was learning to read. Eager to keep up with him, I insisted on doing the same. Captivated by the story of <u>The Three Little Pigs</u>, I asked Dad to read it to me every night.

It told the story of three little pigs and the Big Bad Wolf who terrorized them. Each decided to build their own home. The first was lazy. He constructed his home of straw while the second built his home of sticks. Finished before the third, who was busily building his house of bricks, the two laughed and played all day. But it was the little pig who built a home of bricks who survived the huffing and puffing attacks by the Big Bad Wolf. His home kept him safe.

Identifying with those little pigs, our parents were also building a house. At three years old, I clearly understood the underlying moral of the story. Prevention is the key to survival. Deciding we needed a home constructed of bricks as our neighbors owned, and like the one built by the little pig. I hounded Dad unmercifully.

"Are you building our house with bricks?" I nagged whenever he studied and restudied plans for the home that he and Mom were building.

"I'm gonna use wood, Lindy," he always answered.

Concerned, I continued to badger him, hoping he would change his mind. It never happened. Dad's patience with me wore out first.

"Dang it, Lindy. Quit bugging me about it!"

"But it is bugging me too, Dad," I grumbled. His decision to build our home of wood instead of bricks disturbed me for months.

Following one exceedingly grueling day for a three-year-old, I decided enough was enough. Not being able to keep straight pins held between my lips as my mother did when she was sewing, I kept swallowing them by the dozens. It frightened Mom.

"You will not get shots," she promised, carrying my sister while dragging Jim and me across the street and up the brick steps to the back door of the doctor's house.

We didn't enjoy going there. Whenever we went to the Doctor's house, we always left vaccinated. After poking his finger into my tummy, the doctor felt I would be okay. He then turned to Mom and suggested, "Why they're here, why don't we just give them their vaccinations?"

Jim melted into a wall, praying for invisibility, while I begged for a reprieve. Despite Mom's promise that we would not get shots, the doctor inoculated Jim and me. Walking back home, Mom didn't talk to me. She was mad because I caused them another bill that they couldn't pay, and Jim held me accountable for getting shots.

"Wait until your father gets home," Mom threatened.

"You're in big trouble," five-year-old Jim added.

Shadows were forming overhead. I didn't want to be there when Dad got home. Knowing it would not be long before it would become dark, and Dad would be pulling into the driveway, I decided to run away and build a house of my own, one made from bricks.

Placing some clean panties, and few treasured items, including my book, I grabbed a few bricks from the garage and put them all into my little wagon. Daisy and I were ready to roll.

"I'm running away," I announced, standing at the gate.

"Goodbye. We'll miss you," Mom called from the front porch as she waved farewell. It only fueled the tantrum. Jim followed as I sat on the curb, a few houses down from ours and across from where workers were building a brick house. Everyone seemed to have one, but us. He begged me to return, but I did not listen. Intent upon watching the workmen as they constructed a home with mortar and bricks, I was learning how to do it. I was dead set on building my own house.

As children, we learn much from watching others. It is how we gain most of our longstanding behaviors. It was not long after following the processes of how they constructed a brick wall; a realization hit as I glanced upon the contents of my wagon. I did not have enough bricks to build a house. Unknowingly getting myself into something I couldn't get out of, I cried, not knowing where I would live.

Our neighbor, the doctor approached. Sitting beside me, we talked. He walked me back home, but I refused to go inside. Staying in the yard, as promised, I arranged and rearranged bricks, under the willow tree, until the sun set over the mountains, and twilight fell. Though becoming dark, I continued humming and singing, underneath the dripping branches of the tree. Dad pulled into the driveway and parked. Stepping through the gate, he stopped and smiled down on me.

"Hey, there. Like your new place?"

I stopped singing and shook my head no, trying not to cry.

"Come here, kiddo." Dad sat down, patting the ground next to him. "Aren't you scared out here all alone?"

"Uh-uh," I shook my head. "The Big Bad Wolf can't get me here."

"Okay, that's good. We can just sit here for a while, then."

Wrapping his arms around me and pulling me close, Dad and I talked a bit. We tried to catch a few falling stars and capture a glimpse of the man in the moon. We were unsuccessful. All I remember is awakening the following day in my bed. Dad always made challenging times better.

As we age, we recompose our pasts with bits and pieces of the memorable moments of our lives. We carefully tuck them away into the far reaches of our minds, hoping we can reconstruct them later, to share with our children. As a three-year-old, I learned several valuable lessons, though it was not until many years later, I realized their importance.

I made it a point to defer to Dad's advice that we always have a plan. If it did not work, he drilled into us to always keep another one in our pocket to fall back on. The Pollyanna notion that following one's heart never leads one astray is misleading. As the story of the "three little pigs" reinforced, learning lessons, the hard way, has its consequences.

When young, Mom and Dad read to us every night. Upon growing older, we devoured more of those tales written centuries before our birth, reading them ourselves. Their storylines of characters facing peril prepared us to be ready for the circumstances we would face in the world well beyond our childhood and taught us how to deal with the more complicated issues of living.

Fairy tales and parables reinforce a notion that consequences result from actions, setting a clear boundary of good and evil, weakness and strength, and right from wrong. That one little fable, the Three Little Pigs, taught me that prevention was vital to protecting one's self. In retrospect, what I learned as a child was one of the most remarkable lessons that I had ever learned in survival. It was lifesaving.

In January 1956, Mom and Dad were busy building our new home. While Jim and I attended school and Dad was at work, Mom, at five foot, three inches tall, and weighing one hundred and thirty pounds, with a toddler in tow, shuffled through slush and ice, hauling heavy panels of Sheetrock from the back of the truck into the house that she and Dad were building. Wearing a tool belt and good at swinging a hammer, Mom spent her days in a freezing half-built home, tacking insulation into the crevices of walls, aligning Sheetrock, and taping, sanding, and texturing it.

Mom's capabilities impressed me. When young, she had always assured us we could do anything we wanted if only we believed in ourselves. That year, she proved it. She dearly wanted her own home, even if they had to build it themselves.

Mom differed from other mothers who spent their days inside, cooking, cleaning, and watching daytime television. Fresh and wholesome, she wore jeans rolled up at her ankles and Dad's long shirts.

In summer, Mom never wore shoes. Like Dad, she preferred to live simply. It was what attracted Dad to her and what she loved in him. The child of a single mother and an absent father, Mom learned to make do with whatever was available. A hard worker, without a sense of entitlement, she wasn't afraid to get her hands dirty. Mom seldom asked for anything and never complained. She felt blessed for her simple life.

Dad shared Mom's humble manner. Like his father, he focused on saving money, having learned to set dreams aside while preparing for the uncertainty of life. Between what Dad brought in from his wages, and what Mom made offering daycare for two to four more children she cared for during the day, besides us three, they could put cash into a special fund for "someday." They were preparing to build a home in Genoa and construct a summer home on their property at Twin Lakes. Like his father, Dad was also putting savings away for our college educations. Mom and Dad worked well as partners. Mom was proud of paying her way in their relationship.

Every morning, Dad arose, dressed, pulled on his boots, grabbed a cup of coffee and a bowl of cereal, and barked instructions and reminders to Mom, before rushing out the door before seven.

Mom prepared us for school and dropped us off at the little six-room brick building, named Martha Gleason Elementary. Like most kids, our fondest memories were recesses when we played on the monkey bars and slid down the slide. Loving the weekly spelling bees and tolerating the school nurse who vaccinated us, we adored our teachers, Mrs. Watson, and Mrs. Brown.

In the mornings, Mom worked alone in the partially completed house until Dad arrived for lunch. Inhaling a dry sandwich and taking a few swigs of coffee, Dad helped her with what she needed and returned to work while she put three more hours into the home's construction before picking us up from school and taking us home.

Once off work, Dad went to the construction site, continuing the building of our home. We helped as much as we could at our age, on weekends. For a year, our parents spent every spare moment they had, building that little house, and working day and night. They would bundle us up in sleeping bags and put us to sleep in the back seat of the car while they often worked until midnight. We learned a tremendous work ethic by watching what they did and by cleaning up after them and fetching items.

Steadfast determination paid off. By Christmas, our home was ready for occupancy. As Dad put a small eighteen-inch-wide copper box labeled Zenith and adjusted the rabbit ears atop it, we squealed with joy as we watched our first television show.

Growing up as everyday kids during a time of rapid technological and social change, we viewed history as it occurred on television. Elvis Presley and the Beatles performed on The Ed Sullivan Show, and we saw news reports of Rosa Parks refusing to give up her seat on the bus to a white man when returning home from a long day at work. We intently watched the civil rights marches in the south and repeatedly saw the 1963 assignation of John F. Kennedy in Dallas.

Magic brewed in Southern California when Disneyland opened its doors, and Mickey Mouse debuted in *his* television show. Howdy Doody, Captain Kangaroo, and Mr. Green Jeans soon followed. On Saturdays, Shirley Temple, and Tarzan movies dominated weekend programming, along with cartoons featuring Yogi Bear, Huckleberry Hound, Bullwinkle and Rocky, and Tom and Jerry.

Waking early, we sat for hours, sitting on the floor in front of the television, waiting for the Indian Head test pattern and its annoying buzz to disappear. Suddenly, lively music burst through the wires. Watching intently, until Captain Kangaroo was over, we raced to our rooms, tossed our clothes on, brushed our teeth and hair, and ran down the hill to school.

With our house finished, Mom and Dad burst onto the Carson City social scene. Besides Dad managing Nevada Bell Telephone Company's services in Nevada's rural areas and Mom working fulltime, caring for three to four other children in her home daycare service, both were busy. Mom worked at the Winter Olympics in Squaw Valley for a few weeks and became involved with state and local political campaigns.

During our elementary school years, she was our Cub Scout and Brownie pack leaders, our 4-H leader; and she organized school activities as the "room mother" for all our classrooms. Sitting on the fundraising committee for the PTA, she planned events and arranged the end of the year picnics at our schools. She also served on the Board of Directors of the Leisure Hour Club.

During summer, Mom volunteered alongside Dad at the Little League field, selling food in the concession booth, and playing women's softball, while Dad coached. He served on the Carson City Planning Commission, founded the Carson City Jaycees, and both worked hard at becoming a contributing toward the development of Carson City.

On summer mornings, Mom dedicated her efforts toward working with us to keep up with our studies and not grow stagnant during the months we were out of school. Teaching us basic arithmetic and grammar skills in the mornings, she had us reading in the afternoons for an hour each day.

"Be careful. Watch out for the mountain lions and the Bobcats. They can see you, but you cannot see them," Mom always called out to us when done, as we headed for the hills.

We were the only children we knew whose mothers took us fishing, hiking, and taught us how to skip rocks. She took us to the Carson and Walker Rivers, but we never caught fish there. At Spooner Lake, high in the Sierras, we caught a few small ones. But it was at Twin Lakes, outside Bridgeport where we found the fishing to be the best. Often, we caught our limit using salmon eggs and bait we found under rocks. It became our traditional family vacation spot during summers.

The woman who left school at sixteen to seek fame and fortune regretted her decision. Despite not attending further education, she and Dad remained inquisitive, becoming self-educated. Any time there was a question of how to do something, one or the other would race down to the library and find a book instructing them on the steps to take to get it done.

Fascinated after reading everything she could on the Russian and United States 1950s mind experiments, Mom wanted to see if they would work on us. She took turns flashing pictures before each of us and quickly covering it up, she asked us to describe what we saw. Those efforts taught us skills in observation, perception, and memory. Our grades improved, which was a good thing. Mom and Dad held us to coming home with straight A's on our report cards. Devastation struck hard when any of us received a B.

Neither our parents attended college. In Pasadena, high school ended in the tenth grade, though teens could continue to Pasadena Junior College to continue and complete the eleventh and twelfth grades. Mom chose not to do so while Dad completed his high school education at the junior college at seventeen years old, wishing to enter military service, instead.

Mom worked hard to make our summers an adventure. Showing us how to walk on pine needles and how to cross hot rocks while barefoot, without burning our feet, she taught us to master firing slingshots and to flatfoot, a traditional Appalachian dance of her ancestors. Insisting we sing from our diaphragms, we were always singing together, in the house, and while in the car. She even taught us how to stand on our heads. As children, we knew a loving, involved, active mother, who made a legendary chocolate mayonnaise cake.

Teaching us what occurred in the past and the current events happening today, she rooted us into current events. She felt it was important that we were attentive and involved in what was going on around us.

Mom particularly loved art and music. Spending an hour each morning with us, she showed us the works of the great art masters. From books she pulled from the library, Mom shared the stories of the artists. She told us, "someday," we could see them for ourselves in Europe. Then, for us, "someday" meant living dreams and having hope.

In the afternoons, we would lay upon the carpet, closing our eyes, and listen to classical music. In the autumn, she took us up into the mountains to harvest pine nuts and play in the leaves.

Mom was intent on making sure we had a well-rounded socially conscious perspective, and that we were comfortable discussing sensitive and controversial issues most children didn't even consider. As we watched the 1960s television coverage events unfolding in the deep south during the Civil Rights movement with her, she explained to us that everyone is a part of those who came before them.

"You must remember we are all different. Someday, you may have a black child or an Indian child, or you could get cancer like others in our family," she explained after it became public that Dinah Shore, a 1960s entertainer, had given birth to a black child. "Don't let anyone make you feel like a lesser person because of it. In America, we are all equal. Only those who are ignorant refuse to recognize the beauty of it."

When Grandmother was dying, we discussed death. "Death is a part of living," Mom told us. "Our thoughts and our souls are energy. Energy lasts forever. We become forever free and can live anywhere. Even in our hearts. We never really die."

It was reassuring. Being able to understand the "family cancer thing" that existed in both our parents' families was comforting. As children, we never viewed our differences as being shameful. Proud of who and what we were, as children, the only difficulty we faced was not knowing a name for our cancers and when and if they would come.

But we didn't ponder upon it much. Our family was a rainbow. Both our parents came from multi-racial backgrounds, with some grandparents being white and Southern Baptists, others being Presbyterians, and us, Catholics. We even had an Arab Muslim uncle, who we adored. We were far more fortunate than many others who had nobody. Despite having a family history of cancer, we had plenty of food to eat, and we slept in our own bedrooms of a permanent home. Finally, blessed with an ancestry that was rich with risk-taking involvement of those who came before us, we were rooted in our nation's history. Not only did the stories of our ancestors inspire us, but our father consistently reinforced, "You don't have to look far to find someone worse off than you."

Living the same as everyone else, we were not the poor victimized kids, living tragic lives, as children who live in a hereditary cancer family are often viewed to be. Like others, we had parents who loved and prepared us to face future difficulties.

It was when the Johnson family moved into the neighborhood; it became a child's haven. Of the twelve home sites on our street, children only lived in two, with the one other family having younger children who were not old enough to play outdoors. That first year, our street had been a lonely place to live.

One day, after spotting moving trucks pull up at the house on the corner, we raced to investigate, eager to know if kids were moving in. They were. Their family was tailor-made for ours.

Frank Johnson, a newspaper reporter for the Nevada State Journal, later appointed as the State Gaming Commissioner by Governor Paul Laxalt and Dad, became good friends. Their mother, Joyce, and our Mom shared a love of art. Their son, Frankie, was Jim's age; their daughter, Judy, my age; and Susie was the age of my younger sister.

Judy and I could have been twins if we were not like day and night. Slim, Judy had fair skin, long blonde hair, and blue eyes. In second grade, I was chubby, with dark skin, long brown hair, and brown eyes. The two of us were young aspiring cowgirls who wore jeans, sweatshirts, and cowgirl boots. Our love of horses and our disgust for boys was what we shared.

There were no city parks. The only playgrounds in Carson City were at the schools, and they were not as much fun as the empty fields, a few houses up the street from where we lived. Bordering upon the thousands of acres of foothills, filled with adventure, they served as our playgrounds. After completing chores, we ran up the street to the fields where we reenacted battles between cowboys and Indians. The boys were always cowboys. Judi and I were the Indians defending ourselves and our land.

As second graders, preparing for third grade, seven-year-old Judy and I did everything possible to torment our eight and nine-year-old brothers. It prompted Jim and Frankie to recruit a little army of boys to combat us.

One day, Judy and I stood our ground against an entire squad of them. After ending up in a camouflaged ant hole that they had dug up and covered with sagebrush, and Mom was through with cleansing the bites and the wounds, we declared revenge upon them. After recovering from that, we declared an all-out war upon them.

In the mornings, while they slept, Judy and I prepared for guerilla warfare by collecting crab apples, small rocks, dirt clods, and other forms of ammo to hurl at them. Distributing it throughout our little network of forts, we dug in, deep beneath sagebrush while waiting for them to pass on the trail. Leaping up from the middle of it and letting out a battle cry, we let our slingshots loose upon them. Then, screaming, we ran for home as fast as we could, with our brothers on our tails.

On one of those occasions, stepping into the midst of the stampede through the front door, Dad grabbed Jim's arm as he tried to capture us.

"How many times did I tell you, don't harass the girls?" Dad asked, holding him back.

"But Dad, we aren't. They're doing it to us."

"Come on, two little girls?"

"They were hiding in the sagebrush and shooting at us with their slingshots, Dad."

"Two little girls were hiding in sagebrush and shooting at you?" Dad asked in disbelief.

"I swear, Dad. You do not understand. They're not girls," Jim explained. "Girls don't act like that. Something is wrong with them."

"I don't care what they do. I am talking about you. Do not do it. If the girls do it again, you tell me. Do not chase, fight, or grab girls. Got it?"

Jim left, pushing past me as he slid out the door of the garage where Dad had taken him for the one-on-one discussion. It was my turn for judgment. Creeping into Dad's darkened cave, he set me upon his makeshift workbench. Dad was resourceful. It was merely a board that connected two sawhorses into a table.

A moment of painful silence prevailed as he looked upon me with a stern expression upon his face. "Okay, Lindy, what happened?" he finally asked after an agonizing minute or two.

"We were just little kids playing, Dad."

Viewing the nonreactive expression upon Dad's face, I could tell he did not buy it.

"Playing what?"

"Indians."

"Indians doing what?" His voice became firm as he expressed his frustration with my lack of detail. In turn, I was frustrated with his questioning.

"Creeping up on them. They were cowboys, Dad."

"Lindy, did you throw rocks at them?" His face tightened.

"No, Dad. I didn't."

"You didn't?" he asked, sounding relieved.

"No. We just shot them with our slingshots. We didn't throw nothing." In our family, throwing rocks was equivalent to committing a cardinal sin.

Dad sighed with resignation, then looked me square in the eyes, his eyes narrowing as he asked, "Why would you want to shoot your brother with a slingshot, Lindy?"

"'We're little, and they keep trying to scare us."

"So, you try to scare them back?"

"They're scared when we hide in our forts," I admitted. Dad sank his head into his hands; I suspected it was to mask laughter.

"You and Judy have forts?" he asked, lifting his head in disbelief.

"All little kids have forts, Dad."

I guess the thought of his seven-year-old daughter having a fort in the middle of giant sagebrush from where we hid and attacked our older brothers, was too much for our father. Dad looked upon me in silence, his facial expression serious.

"What, Dad?"

"Okay, Lindy, this is what we will do. First, give me your slingshot. Having one does not allow you to shoot at anyone. From now on, it is only for target practice when Mom or I can watch you."

"Huh?"

"Hand it over," he insisted. Reluctantly, I pulled it from my back pocket.

"Here, Dad," I said, tears filling my eyes.

"Thank you. Now, you will take a bath and put on a nightgown, and when you get up tomorrow morning, you will dress like a girl, and you will act like a girl. Understand?"

"What?" I shot at him, not believing what I was hearing. My father was sentencing me to the house and a life of playing with paper dolls. He was drop-dead serious.

"Do you understand?" he reiterated.

"Okay, Dad," I said, my lips trembling.

"Do you understand?" he again asked. "Yes or no?"

Nodding, I uttered, "Yes," while fighting tears. Sliding onto the ground, I ran to the door. Hollering back at Dad, I yelled: "It isn't fair!"

By the next morning, the day before was nothing more than a faded memory. Tossing on old jeans and boots, I raced to Judy's house and found she had received the same lecture as me. Her father authored an article in the Nevada State Journal about it and the talk *she* received.

The lectures of our fathers did not affect us. We did not care. For a while, we missed our slingshots. We were dependent upon them. But, as girls, we were living a lifestyle that prepared us to become the strong, independent women of the 1970s during a time when there was a tremendous amount of change that occurred in the traditional roles of women. Once again, we two little girls headed for the hills, and our Dads gave up on us.

When older, we received recognition of becoming accomplished lizard and snake hunters. The snakes we caught were older garter and gopher snakes, but one day our friends and we found a baby that had been sunning upon a rock alone. We took it home to foster it until it could care for itself. Taking turns, we cared for the snake. At night we tucked him in with us or under our beds in a shoebox. We fed him, petted him, and played with him in the yard.

We named him "Baby Snake." As he matured, both Dad and Judy's father became concerned. They called the state wildlife department to look at it to verify its species.

When the truck pulled up, neighbors gathered to watch. Asked to present the snake, Jim proudly handed the shoebox to the game warden. The warden opened the lid, and his eyes widened as he saw Baby Snake lounging upon a bed of plucked grass.

"My God," he cried out as he snapped the lid back on. "They have been playing with this?"

"Get in the backyard, kids," Mom ordered.

Waiting to know what was happening was agony. The boys spent most of their time peeking over the fence and reporting what they could see. After the game warden pulled away, solemn appearing parents came to the patio, one by one, to retrieve their children. Mom and Dad arrived. Looking grim, Dad set the box holding Baby Snake on the concrete. After a few agonizing seconds, he spoke.

"Baby was a rattler, kids. We had to put him down."

For a moment, a stunned silence prevailed. We were in shock. Grief and immense anger followed.

"Why didn't you protect him? He didn't have rattles," I demanded, crying.

Dad explained Baby would have developed rattles, and though a baby, he was as dangerous as an older snake. We did not believe him. After they left the patio, Jim expressed his insistence in getting justice. He planned to file a police report. He felt they should arrest our parents and the game warden for murder. Donna leaked it. Dad called another family meeting.

"But Baby Snake was a good snake; he was innocent," Jim said.

"He hurt nobody," I added.

Negotiations began. We never filed charges. We worked our way through the grieving process of the first loss we ever experienced.

"Death is a part of living," Mom reiterated, taking us out for ice cream.

Driving us to the movies, Dad said, "Nothing lives forever. But he *was* a good snake. Try to remember the good times with him."

Jim claimed the body and planned his funeral. Children throughout the neighborhood attended, taking part in the funeral parade. We buried Baby in Mom's flower garden. Jim marked his grave with a crude wooden cross reading, "Here lies Baby Snake. Cruelly murdered by Mom and Dad."

Afterward, Mom and Dad enforced new rules. The hills were off-limits until we learned more about the natural predators that wandered through the surrounding area. We rebelled. Though it did not do us much good, our parents did not mind our speaking out. Mom felt it was great; we were learning to protect ourselves and others. They encouraged us to think for ourselves and to make the right decisions.

Judy's father arranged for her to visit a herpetologist who taught her about the different poisonous species of reptiles. After picking up a few books from the library, Mom taught us the basics of Nevada herpetology on the patio of our backyard. In retrospect, I suspect those lessons resulted as diversionary methods, insisted upon by the game warden.

There is nothing like a summer in Carson City for those of us who grew up there. We were the last of the "free-range" children raised in the foothills. Every day was an adventure. It was better than any playground found in any developed park—the freedom we experienced taught us how to take risks and how to embrace life.

The surprise visits from Grandpa during our summers made it even more special. He would spend two or three days with us while passing through town during his gambling trips, arriving with a repertoire of tall tales tucked into one pocket, and a roll of silver dollars stuffed in the other.

We loved hearing the stories of his past, of working with the mob in Cicero, Illinois, and then later with General Claire Lee Chennault of the Flying Tigers in China in the late 1930s. We could never decide if he was a crook or a hero. Not that it mattered, we adored him. His experiences left us wide-eyed and speechless as Grandpa impressed us with his tales of his later mishaps and close calls as a cowboy and a rodeo-rider.

To Mom's chagrin, we staunchly defended Grandpa. We wanted to be just like him. Often, she would come into the room while he was telling one of his wild stories and stand, leaning against the door, shaking her head, saying, "Kids, he is only kidding."

But we did not believe her. We believed *him.* Though sixty years old, anyone could see Grandpa was still a cowboy. He wore boots, a hat, and a silver belt buckle to prove it. It was good enough for us.

Now, with all that in the past, instead of running beer for the mob, Grandpa was drinking it. Still appearing ruggedly good-looking, Grandpa always chewed upon a cigar that dangled from his mouth. And, no longer managing a stable full of horses, he was adept at performing a delicate balancing act of managing his time between the dozens of the young fillies who adored him.

Grandpa's love for women, gambling, drinking beer, chugging Jack Daniels, playing cards, and living a life of inconsistency was the only consistent things about him. He moved from job to job and wife to wife. It complicated his life. Having as many ex-wives as earlier careers, Grandpa could not stand still. He had to keep moving and could not afford to stop. There were several he wished to avoid that I am sure he owed spousal support.

Years earlier, Grandpa had contracted cancer. His surgeon performed a partial gastrectomy, the removal of part of his stomach. Grandpa recovered quickly, facing no problems with eating.

Mom was still worried. The morning hollering and nagging were almost comical. She insisted Grandpa's cancer would come back, and he would die if he kept eating Limburger cheese on toast and drinking beer for breakfast. Grandpa laughed and ignored her rants. Life held little meaning if it did not include spicy sausages, garlic, onions, cigars, or the smelly Limburger cheese. Grandpa lived vicariously.

It never happened; cancer never came back. Our grandfather did not even get a stomachache. He shoveled down his food, took a big swig of beer, and emitting a loud burp, would heartily laugh. Grandpa was a lot of fun when he was eating.

Watching him carefully, he always offered me a bite of his toast, but I wrinkled my nose and shook my head no. I had no intention of eating anything that brought on cancer.

"You need to experience more of life, kid. It won't kill you," he scolded.

Grandpa never let on that he knew he was under surveillance when visiting us if he knew. Constantly tailed, we spied upon him, each of us wanting to be the first to spot his cancer. Thoroughly searching the house and underneath it for Grandpa's cancer, we carefully examined toilets and drains. All we found were spiders, scorpions, snakes, and other creepy-crawly things. We never found Grandpa's cancer.

"It must not be contagious," Jim determined.

"Maybe it went somewhere else," I reasoned. It made sense to me. If we could not find it, then perhaps it could not be as bad as we heard on tv.

Thanksgiving rolled around, my eighth. Donna and I helped Mom cook. She was teaching us to prepare our dinners, "someday," when we were older and had children of our own.

Dad relaxed on the patio, sipping wine while reading. Holidays always released a bittersweet sentiment from him. Two or three days earlier, he had undergone removal of skin tumors from his face, neck, and back. Mom reassured it was nothing serious but said to be careful when we touched him. Dad was sore. Her assurances didn't ease the worry I felt.

Needing fresh air, I took my "princess cocktail" (7-up with cherry juice) and our big white cat, Tammy, outside and sat in a chair across from him. Curious about his father, whom I never met, I asked, "How come your Dad never comes to our house?"

"He died," Dad replied.

"When did that happen?" I asked, surprised.

"A long time ago. When I was young."

"What'd he die of, Dad?"

"Cancer."

"Like Aunt Marcella had?"

"Yeah. How do you know about that?" Dad asked, surprised.

"Grandma told Mom."

"Grandma talks too much," Dad said.

"Mom said you got it too."

"Great. She did, huh?"

"Yes."

Again, an uncomfortable silence prevailed until I got up the nerve to ask the big question.

"Dad, are you going to die?"

"We all are, Lindy," Dad sputtered, choking on his wine.

"No, I mean now."

"I sure don't plan to," he said, continuing to laugh. "Not anytime soon."

"Good," I said, heaving an enormous sigh of relief.

"What did I tell you earlier, Lindy?" Mom asked from the front door.

"But, Mom, I just…"

"Sweetie…"

"I know, Mom. But it worries me."

"There's no need for worry. Get in here and help me and stop bothering your father."

Getting out of my chair, I ran over and kissed Dad. As I hugged him, I whispered, "I'm glad you're not going to die."

Though difficult for Dad to speak about his father, it was not for Aunt Marcella. She loved telling us stories about him. He had brown eyes like Dad. His hair was the same color as ours, and it was also fine. Kind and easy-going, he spoke in a soft voice and walked with a limp, the result of that injured foot from falling from a telephone pole.

Grandfather's biggest dream was to build an adobe mission style home in Santa Barbara one day. His biggest hope was to live long enough to get it done. Now, Dad was living his father's dreams, hoping to make them a reality with the homes he built.

The first snowfall appeared, blanketing Carson City in white and announcing the countdown to Christmas in early December. Our Christmas tree sparkled where it set in the living room. Living with an artist, like Mom, we found she always made certain each was more beautiful than that of the year before. Stockings hung upon the fireplace that Dad had built that fall, and the aroma of fresh pine and cinnamon wafted through the house.

Baking for days, Mom sang as she rolled out cookie dough and frosted homemade cakes. We spent Christmas Eve caroling throughout the neighborhood, then returning home to hot chocolate and cookies. Guests always visited that evening. A family tradition was before heading off to bed; our parents allowed us to open one gift. It was always a warm flannel nightgown to sleep in on Christmas Eve.

On Christmas morning, we awakened early, waiting for what seemed to be "forever" until our parents awakened. The celebration began with homemade coffee cake and orange juice, coffee, and hot chocolate while we opened gifts and checked out what Santa left. It was always ten books, a jacket, and toys. The books were my favorites. The fairy tales, whose characters, when confronted with adversity, always triumphed at the end.

As *her* annual tradition, sixty-six-year-old Grandma drove her old Ford sedan over the snow-covered roads of the Sierra Nevada, alone, to spend the holiday with us. She filled the trunk of her car with used children's library books to us to read throughout the year. We loved them!

Later that year, after finishing them and those I got for Christmas, I begged Dad to allow me to choose from the basic adult paperback books from his bookcase. He was fussy about what I read. Once, catching me picking one of his adult novels, Dad grabbed it from my hands, stating *he* would decide what I would read.

"Okay, Dad. Please don't forget I like books about cowboys," I begged.

Spring arrived, with its chilly Nevada winds sweeping down from the mountains. While howling and kicking up fallen snow outside, we curled up in large chairs, next to a roaring fire, and read books by Zane Grey and others that carried a consistent storyline of gut-level survival.

Dad plucked the strings of his ukulele and sang with Mom as she prepared dinner. Outside, the wind was howling in harmony, but we did not care. Safely tucked inside, we were warm.

That spring, Judy and her family moved to Lake Tahoe. Without her, I was lost. But the loneliness did not last long. The redeeming grace was Helaine and Claire Jesse, who had moved in down the street. Helaine was a grade younger than me, and Claire was Donna's age. Bright, earthy, and humble, they became wonderful friends.

Helaine was thoughtful while I was impulsive. We hiked in the hills, played with Barbie dolls, and shamed my brother while playing twenty-one in basketball and catch on the front lawn. On Christmas Eve, we caroled through the neighborhood. We were both big sisters, charged with the responsibility for watching over the younger children in our families and for those cared for by our mother in her daycare business.

Dad would bring scrap paper home from work. We spent the day sitting on the shady side of the garage, scribbling stories, designing houses, and making clothing for our paper dolls. Writing and directing puppet shows in our garage, Helaine produced a few friendly little shows. I was the stage crew and the ticket seller. Her little brothers were the audience.

When we needed extra cash, we went on scavenger hunts to get empty coke bottles to cash in for candy. And, in the evenings, at dusk, we played "kick the can." Every kid in our neighborhood abided by an unwritten law. We all ran for home when the streetlights came on.

The oldest and the bossiest, I was the leader. Age had its privileges. Helaine was bright, thinking things through before deciding to act, while I was more impulsive, acting first. Her manner was calm while mine raced. She considered her words before she spoke. Reckless, I had no problem expressing what I felt and often spoke before I thought.

The year passed quickly. Dressing in period clothing, we took part in a pageant in Virginia City, directed by Helaine's mother, Maizie. Mostly, we played by the tiny spring in an old apple orchard tucked in the foothills behind our home. The grass surrounding it was like velvet, and we would sit for hours in our special little place.

That year, Jim and I began attending mass on Saturday evenings at the beautiful little St. Theresa church, close to our home. Surrounded by lit candles and colored stained glass, silent whispers would emit from the depths of my heart, without fear. It was where someone always listened, bringing comfort when needed.

The encouragement to practice our faith was the best gift we could have received from our parents. In later years, it offered me strength when I needed it most. The church was often the one stable place I could call home, no matter where I was. Often, after a critical incident, or when I was out of the country, I would drop into a church to seek peace or pray for others in solitude. It was where faith infused me with massive doses of hope and comfort.

Chapter Five

GRANDMOTHER'S DEATH

*It's so much darker when a light goes out than it would have been
if it had never shone.* — John Steinbeck

During the fall of 1961, when nine years old, our lives began to unravel. Autumn had always been my favorite time of the year. The air heavy with the aroma of burning pine, we would spend our time outdoors, our cheeks reddening from the crisp, refreshing breeze that sent a shiver through us as it swept through our hair.

A rich tapestry of copper, burgundy, red, amber, and gold leaves drifted to earth, covering the ground. Hearing the soft whistle of bare trees shuddering in the wind and their dried remnants of the once green leaves of summer crunching beneath my feet, I loved our autumn walks through our quaint, village. It brought as much warmth to the heart as did the hot chocolate we sipped on while covered with warm blankets as we lounged on the patio.

On Saturdays, Dad granted Mom a short reprieve away from herding the half a dozen kids that she cared for during the week, allowing her three or four hours of peace, to paint without distraction. It was her time of freedom, away from the responsibilities of caring for children. And, it was our time with Dad. On "Dad days," he would load us up into the back of his old pickup truck and take us to A&W for "a beer." With bellies full of soda, we hiked and played with him all afternoon.

Halloween lurked around the corner, along with Nevada Day. Excitement built through October. Anxious for the weekend to arrive, everyone was filled with anticipation, that is, everyone except for Mom. She was not into the autumn celebrations.

Pacing the house all night and sleeping during the day, Mom was out of sorts. Grandmother was facing the end of her life after enduring seven and one- half years of battling ductal carcinoma of the right breast. Mom mistakenly felt more than enough time existed for them to resolve the issues creating the barrier that had kept them apart and had put off visiting her mother. Her mother's death looming, Mom regretted not acting sooner.

Having a greater attachment to an absent father who had twice as much money as her mother and hungering for her father's love and approval, Mom had placed the responsibility of his disappearance from their lives upon Grandmother. She was only capable of showing loyalty to one or the other parent. Complicating matters, Mom felt alone. She was not comfortable around her mother's family, who were staunch Southern Baptists who worshipped, speaking in tongues. That, along with their strong religious beliefs and judgmental attitudes, frightened her. The illegitimate child of her mother, the unwanted result of a shotgun marriage, she did not feel welcome in their homes.

And, while her mother's family did not offer much support or acceptance of them, her father's family embraced her as a part of their family. Living close to six uncles and two aunts, Mom loved being in their much larger homes, filled with children.

Her Scandinavian grandparents, aunts, and uncles provided her with the attention that she craved, and they lovingly doted upon her. When her father could not help with her support, or when our mother needed something, they were always there for her and her brother, making certain they felt like a part of the family.

Having a dependent nature, Mom did not share her father's willingness to take risks, nor did she inherit her mother's keen sense of independence. Not having the gritty "can do, will do" spirit of survival of either; her sole desire was to become the same as many women of her time... a typical, small-town, 1950s wife who stayed home to raise a family.

Our mother felt as though she was the unloved, unwanted bastard child. Longing for the attention of a "here today, gone tomorrow" father and the acceptance and approval from an exhausted, overworked single mom, she was unhappy. As an adult living four hundred and fifty miles away was a relief for her. It offered Mom the opportunity to escape from her family and the past.

We visited Grandmother until I was six years old. After she became ill, Mom stopped, making excuses not to see her. As a child, she had watched her great-grandmother die a devastating death from breast cancer. It frightened her. Mom's fear of the disease created a tremendous barrier in the relationship she shared with her mother and the other women in the family. Mom feared she would be next. Holding no doubt, Mom knew it would also be her fate, "someday."

Five years after Grandmother received the first diagnosis of cancer, it metastasized through her body. Receiving a terminal prognosis, she battled it for two and one-half more years, when Grandpa called on that October morning in 1961.

"You better get here now if you want to see her," Grandpa said.

"If you don't do this, you *will* regret it," Dad said as he tossed her suitcase upon the bed. "Go," he insisted. "We're going to be fine here."

Dad understood Mom's fear. Haunted by the constant reminder of the deaths because of cancer in his family, he constantly relived that of his father, while his sister lived in denial that he died of cancer. Parroting her mother's insistence, that their father and that the others died of tuberculosis and heart attacks, she made herself believe it. It was a far more acceptable cause of death. Tuberculosis and heart attacks were acceptable methods of dying by eugenicists.

Overcome with guilt, Mom relented. Accompanied by Jim, she tossed their bags into the car and sped south to the City of Hope Cancer Center in Duarte, California, to be with her dying mother.

No matter how much we may think we have prepared ourselves to see someone suffering from cancer during their last moments, most of us are not ready to view the battle that one goes through during the end of life. Mom certainly wasn't prepared for it.

Entering the cold, sterile room, she saw a woman she did not recognize, who she had always known to be healthy and vital. Hooked up to tubes and attached to breathing apparatuses, Grandmother was in pain. Suffering from brain damage, she faced difficulty speaking. But what affected Mom most was her eyes no longer sparkled. They were dull and red, set into a sunken face.

Mom's heart broke to find her mother confused and unable to recognize her. She sat silently alongside her, later telling us she could feel her mother's soul drifting from her body as she was dying.

Now, too late to say or do anything else, Mom returned home a different person, a woman filled with conflict and regret. Deep in grief, she spent her days sleeping and crying. A week and one-half later, Mom received another telephone call. It was one of finality.

"Thank you," she murmured, dropping the phone back into its cradle. Drifting into her bedroom, she closed the door. Dad followed and remained with her for a while, then came out onto the patio.

In a solemn tone, he instructed, "Kids, please be quiet tonight. Your grandmother is no longer with us. Your mom needs peace."

Jim and I were sad. Donna was confused, wondering why she had not seen our Grandmother, thinking she had visited. She asked if our Grandmother would be coming back. I found myself wishing I were young, like her, so I would not have to understand death, either.

Awakened early the next morning to the sound of singing in the backyard, I peeled through the curtains that covered the patio door. Amid the smooth gray gravel pebbles covering the ground, stood Mom. She was in tears. Mom's display of grief was heartbreaking.

Turning toward Dad, I asked, "What's Mom doing out there?"

"She's expressing gratitude for the day," he casually stated, as he sipped on coffee.

"But why, Dad?"

"It's for your Grandmother," he casually answered.

"But she's dead," I retorted, confused.

Frustrated, Dad stated, "Lindy, it's complicated. It's what your mother needs to do right now."

I did not understand, but the raw emotion displayed by Mom singing quietly so early in the morning was heartrending. Placing the curtain back, I picked up the glasses from the table and put them in the dishwasher and tossed the empty wine bottles into the trash. Some of Mom's friends must have stopped by after we had gone to bed.

Putting our suitcases into the car, I hopped into the front seat next to Mom, who again drove the four hundred and fifty miles down to Southern California for Grandmother's memorial service. Tears streamed down her face as we passed the big pines lining the shoulder of the bumpy two-lane highway hugging the Eastern Sierras. I silently gazed out the window so I would not have to see her cry.

Reaching Grandpa's house, Mom slid out of the car and walked toward the door, while we pulled out our luggage from the trunk. As Grandpa stepped onto the porch to greet her, I looked away as she sank into his arms and began sobbing uncontrollably.

"I should have been there," she cried.

While Grandpa consoled Mom on the patio, Donna and I sat inside the living room, across from Great-Grandpa John. Sitting so straight, he was as stiff as a sculpture. Assessing us through his stern, faded eyes, Grandpa John finally softened, telling us *his* story of having cancer. Pulling up his shirt, he showed us his colostomy bag. Offering a polite excuse, Donna and I quickly escaped the house and sat upon the front lawn. Whispering to Donna, I said, "I sure am glad we live in Nevada because there's a lot of cancer here."

Chapter Six

MOM'S CANCER

How shall a man escape from that which is written; how shall he flee from his destiny? — Ferdowski

Everyone experiences a challenging year in their lives. Toward the end of 1961, while Mom was trying to resolve her grief over the loss of her mother, her physician recommended that she undergo a hysterectomy. He was concerned that she might have contracted cancer.

Amazingly, Mom wasn't worried. She expected it. "Someday" had just arrived for her sooner than she hoped and decided to have a hysterectomy. Mom had held off long enough and no longer shared Dad's desire to have six children. And, she did not want to take a chance of contracting cancer.

The first thing she did was to go shopping for what she needed in the hospital and during recovery. Putting away the nightgowns, the bed pads, and a frilly negligee she hoped would make her look pretty in the hospital, she called me into the kitchen.

"You're old enough to take care of things now, Lindy," she said, handing me her apron. "I don't know how long it will take to get better, but I'll need to depend on you until then."

"Okay, Mom," I said, rolling up my sleeves and tightening the apron strings the same way as I spent years watching her do.

"First, we have to teach you how to cook. So, get out the cast iron frying pan," she instructed.

Before she finished speaking, it was on the stove, along with the small saucepan she used to cook vegetables. That day, I learned how to prepare fried chicken, mashed potatoes, gravy, and vegetables. The next, we made meatloaf, and later, spaghetti.

With the cooking lessons completed, we went to work on learning the proper housekeeping chores that we would need to do while she was away, washing windows, cleaning floors, changing linens, and sanitizing the bathrooms in preparation for Mom's return home.

The day before she left, Mom taught us how to set the table for formal dining. The enormous number of utensils she placed on each side of the plates was overwhelming. Explaining in detail how every fork, knife, and spoon used, we learned dining etiquette. During lunch, she how to use each utensil, where to place them once done, how to properly how to use a napkin, to chew with our mouths closed, drink beverages without gulping, when it was appropriate to speak with adults, and when to stay silent, and how to cut our meat with a steak knife.

We learned to sit like ladies, with our legs crossed at our ankles. Mom taught Jim that the man opens all doors for ladies and always pulls out their chairs for them to sit. Instructed to address adults as "M'am" and "Sir," she taught us when to say "may," "can," and please, to say "yes" instead of "yeah." We learned the difference between "shall" and "should." In three days, we received a crash course in preparation for adulthood.

"If you are going to succeed in life, you must be polished," Mom insisted. "Proper etiquette is something every mother should teach their children. You need to learn this now. I can't guarantee how long I will be around."

The day Mom left for the hospital, I felt prepared to care for the family, that is until I arrived at school. Then, all I could think about was what I needed to do once I came home. Overwhelmed, I spoke with Dad. Understanding my dilemma, he changed the menu and planned to take us out to dinner one night. Maizie saved the day with a casserole that covered us for two meals.

We had no problem with my cooking. I did well with making hot dogs and spaghetti, but the frying of chicken was a challenge. Mom was far better at it. Red on the inside and blackened on the outside, I needed a lot more practice. As usual, Dad came to the rescue, bringing home hamburgers and milkshakes. We liked them better.

Two days after they admitted Mom into the hospital, my sister and I raced home from school on our bikes. Getting our chores done quickly, we raced off on a mission, quickly zipping across town, past the Governor's Mansion, and to the small hospital where Mom was recovering.

Donna was unable to sleep. She was worried and unable to stop thinking about Mom. Dad's consolations were not working. Tired of listening to her cry, I decided to show her that Mom was fine. We parked our bikes and tiptoed to the side of the building. On tiptoes, we peeked through the various windows of the rooms of patients, searching for her. At last, I felt immense relief as I saw our mother sleeping in a tall metal bed.

"Is she dead?" Donna asked, peering at her, her brown eyes enormous with fear.

"I don't think so, Donnie," I answered, as I softly called out to her.

"Mom, are you awake? Mom?" Finally, when she stirred, a weight lifted from my shoulders as she opened her eyes.

"Girls," she quietly said, her voice sounding exhausted. "What are you doing here?" she quietly asked, peeking toward the door, and making sure they had closed it.

Donna babbled excitedly. Mom's eyes brightened as she listened. She was doing better than we had thought. Excited, we spoke with her for two or three minutes until we heard someone yelling in the distance. Turning, we saw a nurse barreling around the corner of the building.

"You kids, git out of here," a nurse hollered, as she rounded the corner of the building. "Let your poor mother get some sleep," she demanded.

"Uh, oh," I said to Mom. "I think we're in trouble."

"You'd better go," Mom said, holding her tummy, as she laughed. "Quick! Run, girls! Run!"

Giggling, we raced to our bikes, hopped on, and pedaled as fast as we could toward home, constantly looking behind us to make sure the nurse did not tail us. It was a good thing we were moving fast. There was still much we needed to do by the time Dad arrived. Finally, safe at home, we locked the front door in case the nurse showed up. But, that night, we were in far better spirits than before, knowing Mom would be fine.

When Mom arrived home a week later, she was walking tenderly, and in pain. Dad helped her into the house and to bed. She appeared ragged yet assured us she would get better. We took turns caring for her, months elapsed, and Mom had yet to recover fully.

Appearing fine physically, but a deep depression had set in. Mom spent her days sleeping for days and wandering through the house at night. Instead of being her usual quiet and easy-going self, after an episode of irrationality, she would go to her room and sleep for days. Her actions were unpredictable. We never knew what would set her off, and we walked on tiptoes around her. Her physician had prescribed amphetamines, claiming they would lift her out of it, help her lose weight, and manage her hormonal changes. She referred to them as her "diet pills."

That summer, we spent our vacation fishing and camping with Grandpa, at Twin Lakes, up the road from where Mom and Dad owned property. She was still out of sorts and arguing with everyone, even Grandpa. While preparing dinner, Grandpa made an insensitive comment. Mom yelled at him, "As though you care enough about anyone to know."

Shrinking back to the table where he was cleaning fish, Grandpa appeared hurt and confused as she continued her rant, berating him for what had occurred during her childhood.

Dad touched her shoulder, saying, "Now, Darlene…"

"Don't Darlene me!" she ordered, pulling away from him. It was the first time we had ever seen Mom out of control and arguing with Dad or with anyone but us. The situation soon spun out of control.

"That's it! Kids pack up. We're going home," Mom ordered.

Upset, we dismantled the tent and loaded the truck while Dad tried to convince her to stay. "Darlene, it's our vacation."

"We are not staying," she insisted.

Mom hopped inside the cab and waited while Dad roped us into the bed of the truck. Pulling out of the campsite, we were devastated. Crying, while waving goodbye to Grandpa, our hearts broke as we saw him standing alone, next to his little stand, still cleaning fish.

Mom visited her physician more often after that episode. He ordered sleeping pills to stop the wandering at night and upped her dose of amphetamines. In the 1960s, physicians prescribed amphetamines for everything, women's hormone imbalances, depression, weight loss, pain, menopause, back pain, and all the other side-effects women that developed following a hysterectomy. The doctors felt it could fix all the women's health issues. It was the worst thing she could have done.

Considered a miracle drug, public consumption of amphetamines become a national epidemic. The United States had become a nation of amphetamines junkies with even President John Kennedy taking 15 mg of amphetamines a day, thanks to Max Jacobson, a German physician, known to Hollywood stars as "Dr. Feelgood."

During 1970, over nine million Americans consumed prescription amphetamines, one of every twelve people in the United States. In 1971, because of the addictive qualities, the federal government mandated drugs with an amphetamine ingredient required a prescription that a physician was to write for each time pharmacists filled it. The feds checked those prescriptions to prevent drug abuse and addiction. By then, it was too late. Our mother had become a junkie.

Grandmother's death, contracting cancer, and Mom's surgery, coupled with her addiction to amphetamines, imposed a severe, adverse effect upon her and our family. Her personality had dramatically changed. Mom was unhappy, seeking something she felt was missing from her life, though finding it was impossible due to her level of addiction.

Closing herself to everyone, but one close friend, one minute, she seemed happy and stable, and the next, she was down and depressed, riding up and down upon an emotional roller coaster. Peaks and valleys, highs and lows consumed her as she raced across Nevada highways in her 1955 T-Bird with the speedometer buried at 150 miles per hour. She engaged in excessive, impromptu spending sprees and would disappear for hours.

We consoled her while she wept. Mom did not know what was wrong. Nor did anyone else. Laughing one minute, she would become angrily explosive, then suddenly take a nosedive, landing into a severe depression. It became a pattern.

On Saturday mornings, Jim and I had a well-established ritual. While our parents slept, we escaped from home and headed downtown to visit the old security guard at the Capitol building. The poor old guy was missing a leg and had a patch over one eye, which occurred in the war, he said. We didn't ask which war, but considering his age, I figured it was either in the Civil War or World War I. We loved hanging out with him and fetching his lunch at Austin's Market.

One morning, we noticed Coca-Cola bottles scattered all over the floor next to the vending machine, spilling from several wooden boxes. Each of us picked one, tucked it into our waistbands, and cashed it in at Austin's Market to buy candy. The old guy was attentive. Noting the wooden was short two bottles, he awaited our arrival at our next visit.

That morning, when we arrived, our faces fell as we realized he had moved his chair from the front entrance to next to the vending machine. Laughing, he instructed us to sit on the floor next to him.

Realizing we were in deep trouble, we contritely sat beside his chair and confessed that we cashed the two empty bottles in and used the money for candy. Before leaving, he directed us to go to the Sheriff's Office.

Crossing the street and descending the steps into the old jail, we were two scared kids as we stood in front of the large counter in the Sheriff's Office. After a lecture from the deputy, relief filled through us after finding that wonderful old security guard had hooked us up with our first job instead of putting us in jail. He assigned us the task of fetching the weekly inmate canteen orders from Austin's Market and delivering them to him.

While we reviewed the latest FBI wanted posters, the deputy made up a list of items to take to the clerk at the market. We climbed up the short set of stairs from the basement of the courthouse where the jail was found and raced each other to the store two blocks away. Once there, the clerks filled the inmates' orders, and upon payment, we were thrilled to find a dime was designated for us to get what we wanted.

At a penny charged for two pieces of root beer barrels, we got a lot of candy that day. We loved that old man. He made sure we no longer had to resort to a life of crime to fulfill our sugar cravings.

In 1964, when I was in the seventh grade, our parents sold our home in the foothills. Dad wanted to buy an 1800s bungalow in the commercial part of town before beginning construction on the house they had saved for and planned to build in the foothills of Genoa.

Tired of waiting, tired of working, and tired of saving money, Mom rebelled. Weary of supporting Dad's dreams and always putting her own on hold, Mom could care less about the empty lands she and Dad had bought for investment, or anything else. She feared there would always be another house to build or to fix-up. Mom was feeling an intense sense of urgency. She wanted to live now. Mom had lost faith in "forever."

Depressed, she spent her days sitting alone in a ninety-year-old house that was dark and depressing. Longing to hang beautiful art upon her walls, and not strip wallpaper from them, she dreamed of holding a paintbrush in her hand and dabbing color upon canvas, not on ninety-year-old kitchen cabinets or crumbling plaster walls.

The sound of a ticking clock counting down the minutes of her life haunted her. She was eager to get out into the world and to experience every bit of living she could. Desiring to escape the stagnation of being caged in a house full of kids, all Mom wanted was to be left alone with her books, her art supplies, and a piano. All she wanted was to sing again.

To escape her surroundings, Mom volunteered to work for a political campaign. It only worsened her desire to be free. The experience of seeing a whole other side of life opened doors to one she had never known. It exposed her to an existence that extended far beyond the confines of Carson City. The spectacle of political campaigns left her awestruck.

Our parents had never argued in our presence except for that one time on vacation. As children, we never experienced conflict in our home. That evening, as they sat in the darkness and spoke for hours in the car, Jim, Donna, and I watched through the window, wondering what was occurring. We knew something was wrong.

"They're getting a divorce," I groaned.

As a child, I paid attention to details, noting the body language and the change in behaviors of others, more so after playing the card games with Mom. Seeing it coming, that winter, when I shared my concern with my teacher that our parents were getting divorced, I did not realize his wife was giving marital counseling to our mother.

"Then, where will we live?" Donna asked.

"I don't know, but no matter what, we stick together, right?" Jim suggested.

Our parents separated from one another a few days later. Jim remained with Dad, living in our home in Carson City while Mom, Donna, and I went apartment hunting. At first, we visited beautiful apartments, seeking a Ken and Barbie lifestyle. Mom dreamed of plush carpeting, a poolside apartment to suntan by, and pink princess telephones setting next to our beds. However, her budget only allowed for the same small, dismal court apartments where she grew up. Signing a month-to-month lease, she withdrew us from school, and we moved what little we had into the small brick fourplex in Sparks, Nevada.

None of us were wild about our new home. It was reflective of how Mom lived as a child, a two-bedroom apartment in a run-down court, with sparse furnishings, bedroom furniture, a small sofa, a kitchen table, two chairs, and Mom's stereo. Little had come from home since our parents did not intend the separation to be a permanent situation. Most of all, there was no one our age in the neighborhood.

Excited about her first full-time job at the Sparks Nugget, Mom had left for work by the time we arrived home from school in the afternoons and was fast asleep when Donna and I went for school in the mornings. We seldom saw her. Mom was living the life she chose not to pursue, to marry. But, the late-night parties and jam sessions with celebrities in Reno and Sparks never seemed as glamorous as they did when she awakened the next morning. She quickly wearied of it and realized the career she walked away from was not as she had imagined it to be. In revisiting her past, Mom was resolving regrets.

On Friday nights, Dad picked us up and took us to Carson City to stay with him, and my brother Jim. At thirteen, Jim was working a part-time job washing dishes at the Carson City Nugget Casino. I spent weekends with Dad, while our next-door neighbor cared for Donna.

Seeing Dad that first weekend, he hugged me tightly, reluctant to let go. Tears flooded his eyes. He missed us. The time he spent with us, we treasured. It meant the world to us. We grew to know Dad on an entirely different level, recognizing him as a man who was sensitive and filled with compassion. Emotionally wounded, he needed us in his life as much as we needed and wanted him in ours. We retained our loyalty to him.

One afternoon, while lazing beneath a cottonwood, silently watching the muddy waters of the Carson River passing over logs, and through stone and sand barriers, I asked Dad what he intended to do. Buried in grief, Dad shook his head and answered, "Lindy, I don't know. I just don't know."

His deflated response sounded reasonable. Life was uncertain for all of us. Uncertainty not only results from health issues as Mom experienced or hereditary predispositions to cancer, as Dad experienced, but it comes from many sources, including divorce.

"I guess I should come up with a plan," he said, as he stood, dusting himself off and offering me a hand up.

"I guess we all do, Dad," I added.

Dad had always been a planner. For years, I had watched as he drew up plans for his building projects on napkins at the coffee shop. I often created my own, which Dad reviewed, showing me how to make them better. Months earlier, if we had asked him what he wanted to do, he would reveal short-term, intermediate, and long-term plans, hopes, and dreams, encompassing dozens of years down the road. He faced difficulty envisioning a future after spending twenty years with Mom.

Meanwhile, Mom had planned for a new life. It did not include worrying about cancer, Dad, or even us. Despite the little apartment where we lived to be unaffordable, Mom spoke of picking up and taking off to Europe. She committed to living whatever time she had left, her way. Mom did not expect to live long. She was depressed with her circumstances. She wasn't happy being married and being single wasn't what she thought it would be.

Often, I arrived home from school to see Mom slurring words and unable to walk. Making coffee and sandwiches, and running cold baths to sober her up, we always got her to work. When Mom cried, I comforted her. "Your father promised me a piano."

When tears filled Dad's eyes, I comforted him. The situation proved difficult for both Mom and Dad. Each kept hearing the same ticking clock. Mom medicated herself to make it stop, and Dad worked through his pain.

One morning at a local coffee shop, after their separation, Dad was penciling a drawing on paper while drinking his coffee and, while I was sipping on root beer, I carefully watched.

"Lindy, what is the most important part of a home?" he quizzed me.

"The foundation, Dad," I answered.

"Right. Don't forget it. It is also the same for people. The foundation is everything. Always make certain yours stays strong," he said, almost in a way that seemed that he was preparing us to live without him. I wondered if he was considering moving, as Mom was doing.

In the summer of 1965, we spent six weeks in Southern California; it was an excellent place for three young kids to hang out while their parents were engaged in a contentious divorce. Our grandparents, aunts, and uncles cared for us, making it a wonderful time. Wearing pukka shell necklaces and surfer clothing, while listening to the Beach Boys and Jan and Dean wail songs over the radio about cars and ocean waves, we were having a fun time hanging out with relatives on the California beaches.

Before leaving, our parents were discussing reconciliation. They were making plans to build the Genoa home. Upon returning, Mom retrieved us from Dad's house, and as she drove toward Reno, she casually announced, "I have something to tell you, kids."

My eyes focused on Mom's hands. She wore gloves. Nobody did that in late July in Nevada when wearing capris and a blouse. Instantly, I knew why. Her dramatic game was disappointing. Gazing out the window, with little emotion, I sighed.

"You got married," I said, deflated.

Mom's new husband was a graduate student who had earned a master's degree in mathematics at the University of Nevada. At thirty-one years old, he now worked as a desk clerk in a Reno hotel. Upon meeting him, we were far from impressed. He seemed like a college kid. Something was amiss. Owning little, except for a half dozen vinyl records, a large ring he wore on his right hand, and having little clothing, he did not have much to show for himself, except an old used car. Moving from a fraternity house into Mom's apartment, everything about him screamed, "temporary."

The rest of our summer was spent with Dad, not wanting him to be alone. The four of us adapted to our circumstances, together, but it was only to be temporary. The mutual support we offered one another crumbled when school began that autumn. Dad distanced himself from Mom, and as a result, from us. It was unexpected. We did not hear much from him. Devastated, we needed him as an active part of our lives, but he always had something going on during his weekends.

Mom had always been the energy; Dad was the stabilizer. I especially missed that, and I missed him. He and I had shared a special bond. He taught me to play the ukulele and the banjo and shared his favorite books with me. Begging him to take me along when he fired up his Triumph motorcycle, we raced down country roads, with me hanging onto him for dear life, and unable to stop laughing. I loved the adrenaline rush of speed.

We saw less of Dad. He stopped calling and didn't see us on weekends as much as before. When we called him, he offered excuses for why he couldn't have us visit.

"Lindy, I have so much going on this weekend. Can we make it next weekend?" he would ask, but the next weekend, it was always the same. Disappointed, I would repeatedly call him at work. Something was always going on. But, in my heart, I knew Mom's remarriage had provided permission for him to move on. He wasn't even available during Christmas.

Then, one winter night, while visiting Dad, during the following January, we arrived at his house after a day skiing. That night, we met the twenty-year-old girl and her toddler that *he* had been dating the past several months, the reason he did not have time for us.

It was a lovely evening. Dad seemed happy. He had someone in his life, and we were pleased he was not alone. After, we did not see him during that spring. Dad continued to offer one excuse or another of why we could not come home on weekends.

Three months later, he stopped by for a "quick hello," before racing off to a business meeting. Looking entirely different, now wearing a mustache, Dad was dressed in a business suit and driving a newer El Camino truck instead of his old white flatbed. He had filled the back of it with our clothing and other personal items we had kept at our home. Having sold the house, he was now living in a small apartment and said he no longer had room for my sister and me, or our things.

"What about our pets?" I asked, devastated while unloading the truck.

"We had to give them away, Lindy. I couldn't keep them in an apartment, and your mother isn't allowed to have them here. Don't worry; they have good homes." Then he raced off to wherever he was going, leaving my sister and me, standing in a front-yard filled with our clothing and personal possessions, devastated.

Meanwhile, Mom was wheeling down the road to self-destruction, not having the time to notice how upset and depressed we were with our situation. She was busy, caring for a young husband who was dependent upon her to support him, while she placed her dependence upon the dozens of little pill bottles that cluttered the top of her dresser.

Living in Reno, a city filled with opportunism, everyone was seeking it, including physicians. Our mother was living in a candy land filled with mind-altering drugs. One doctor prescribed the pills that ramped her up during the day. Another wrote the order for the ones that put her to sleep at night. There were more than enough doctors to prescribe everything she needed, little capsules to lose weight, and bigger ones to reduce her level of anxiety and yet others to lift her moods out of depression. Finally, there were also the amphetamines, which kept her moving. When the pills did not work, a back-up existed in the liquor cabinet in the dining room, that she kept filled with alcohol. Drugs or alcohol, it didn't matter to Mom, anything to get her through the day, the night, or whatever.

A few weeks later, with Dad's encouragement, Jim came to live with us. Dad told him he no longer had the time to spend with him now, and it was best he lived with his mother. It would be too crowded with the addition of Dad's demanding, "insecure" young woman and her toddler. They were demanding constant attention, and there wasn't enough room for all of them.

Jim was stung and heartbroken. He felt as though he had become an inconvenience, and his presence intruded upon Dad's privacy with his girlfriend, who did not want him or any of us around.

That night, the three of us sat down and discussed it. Jim felt she influenced dad and questioned his feelings toward us. At night, while sitting in his room, he could hear her loud demands that Dad prove his love to her by telling Jim to leave.

With our father was in the wind, involved in a new living situation, we were lost, living between somewhere and nowhere. Dad's family, his mother, and our aunt and uncle were livid that he had abandoned us, knowingly leaving us with a mother who was always high and hiding out in her bedroom with her new husband.

Left to care for ourselves and one another, we adapted. It became clear to us that nothing was the same, nor would it ever be. It was a fact we accepted. Both parents had moved on and left us behind, as so many others did, with their children in the 1960s. We did what most children do.

We moved on, as well. Remaining close, our stability was soon reestablished in one another. That was when Mom decided my sister and I should attend a parochial school that offered more structure and security for us during that time of instability. I think Maizie helped her realize we were facing difficulty adapting.

She enrolled Donna and me into a tiny seven-room school in Reno, the Little Flower School run by Mother Catherine and her band of Irish Sisters of Mercy. It was the best thing our parents could have done, following their divorce and our displacement from our home.

It was a good thing that I was a rules follower. It was necessary for surviving Catholic school. We had a lot to learn. They had not baptized my sister or me, nor had we attended catechism during elementary school. We were far behind our classmates.

When our parents were married, they had wanted us to choose our religion, "someday." Within a year after our parents' separation, my sister and I were baptized, received our first holy communion, and I received confirmation into the Church. It was the best thing they could have done for us. We needed something to replace the loss of our family. I found it in my teacher.

"Lindy, please stay after class today," Sister Magdalene, whispered into my ear as she patrolled the small classroom, making sure we were diligently copying down the blackboard review of our catechism instruction.

"Okay," I said, my eyes wide with concern.

"Don't worry, dear," she said, patting my arm. "It is nothing bad."

I loved Sister Magdalene. Streetwise to the antics of twelve-year-old girls, the Irish nun moved fast and carried a big stick. If classmates were disrespectful, she would declare, "You are as bold as brass," in a thick Irish brogue. Demanding the perpetrator step up to the front, she shamed the child and smacked the top of the hand with "the cane." It was effective. The one time I forget my homework was the last.

Though staunch and strict, she was also loving. Sister Magdalene cared deeply about the children she taught. Always, she provided positive reinforcement for the good work we did. I needed to hear that, and I worked hard to please her.

As the afternoon wore on, my stomach grated. The only distraction from the mundane instruction was the intense anxiety I felt arising from the fear that I displeased Sister Magdalene, somehow. Worrying about what I had done to upset her, my mind raced to recall everything I could have done that could have offended her.

The bell rang. Students filed out of the classroom, while I sat in my chair, folding, and unfolding my hands. Some tossed questioning glances my way, while others offered glimpses of sympathy. After what seemed like hours for the room to empty, Sister Magdalene approached, arranging the loose flowing fabric of her black habit while settling into the chair next to mine.

Placing the pages of a story I had written upon my desk; I glanced upon it. It bore an enormous "A." I let out a deep sigh of relief.

"Lindy, I cried as I read this," Sister Magdalene said.

I'm sorry, Sister, I didn't mean…"

"You don't understand. It is very good. What inspired you to write this?"

I had drafted a story about a girl who feared she would die of cancer. That afternoon, I broke into tears as I sat with Sister Magdalene while we read it together. I felt so much pain as we spoke. Afterward, I felt better. It felt good to talk it out. For too long, I felt hurt for all of us, for our mother, our father, my brother, and my sister. I needed to share what I was feeling with someone. Like the girl in the story, I was dying too. I couldn't adapt to the loss of our father. The new life our mother was living had become unmanageable, especially with everything else that was occurring occurred in our lives. My way of dealing with it was writing it out.

Writing soon became a cathartic process allowing me to express my thoughts and emotions. Sister Magdalene always seemed to know when things were not right. Then, we would talk—about the day, the weekend, recent experiences, what was occurring at home, and of the future.

Sister Magdalene wrote that she had sent the story and others that I had written to a Catholic magazine, and they had accepted it for publication. I never saw it in print. It was only a matter of days before my eighth-grade graduation, Mom packed us up, and we moved to Wisconsin.

Chapter Seven

A MOVE TO WISCONSIN

The thing about life is that you must survive. Life is going to be difficult and dreadful things will happen. What you do is move along, get on with it and be tough. —Katharine Hepburn

In the spring of 1966, we packed up our house and were ready for yet another move. Our mother and father were battling, as usual. Hoping for a fresh beginning away from conflict, Mom asked Dad for his permission to take us out of state. He refused, though he had not had time to see us in several months. This move would be the fourth. As usual, none of us knew where. Mom had a significant amount of cash from her divorce settlement, and anywhere was okay with her if it was far from Dad.

Awakened by her just after midnight, she instructed us to take our beds apart and load them into the U-Haul trailers outside.

"Get up, Kids. We are moving to Wisconsin," Mom announced.

"But, Dad..."

"Quick, hurry up, kids. You can call or write to your father after you are there," she advised when we complained the telephone was disconnected. I felt bad. However, had Dad tried to see us during those three months of preparation to move or if he had even made a phone call, it might have been different. We may have stayed. If he had seen the owner's "For Sale" sign on the lawn or the packed boxes sitting inside the living room, something would have been different. But he hadn't done any of that. He was too involved with his situation with his girlfriend and her toddler daughter.

Even if our father had called, or dropped by, he could have asked us how we were doing, or if that were too difficult, Dad could have asked the private investigator he hired to background Mom's new husband, to find out how his children were. Had our father wanted my siblings and me around, we would have stayed. But he did none of those things.

His priorities had changed. We were merely an occasional thought. Angry with our mother, every bit as much as she was mad at him, we occupied little space in either of their lives. Dearly needing stability from at least one parent, we were entangled in the emotional upheaval of both, not receiving much from either.

Renting a vacation cabin on Lake Winnebago for a week, Mom and Chuck spent their days hunting for a temporary apartment where we would live. Those two weeks were like a vacation for us.

Within two weeks after leaving Nevada, we were living in a small two-bedroom apartment. With a phone installed, we called Dad at his work. He was happy to hear from us, though surprised we had moved to Wisconsin. He thought something was wrong when I wasn't at my eighth-grade graduation, though, he had come. He had called, and no one was home to answer the phone. Pleased to hear we were well, he promised to visit and promised he would call Grandma and let her know we were well. Within a week, she was returning our letters to her, also excited about our move. It was where she was born, and her mother had grown up.

Wisconsin was the perfect place in the 1960s for young, unsupervised adolescents. It offered a wholesome American experience. While California and Nevada were reeling with free love, drugs, and rock-and-roll, we were attending dances in the park, and after, boys were offering to walk us home. We lived as other teens, cheering on our football team, attending the regular weekly dances at our church, those at the park during summer, and across the street at the Blue Inn, a teen recreational center, during the school year. On Sunday afternoons, we strolled through autumn leaves and fresh snow. It was an idyllic place to live.

We didn't see Mom much after our move. The woman who never finished high school worked at night as a bank auditor. She wasn't happy with her job. Numbers meant nothing to her. Having become a 1960s "free spirit," Mom's passion was drugs, sunshine, auras, and colors. She was an artist, not an accountant. During the entire time that she lived in Wisconsin, I never once saw her paint or draw in her sketchbooks. Mom had stopped singing. Her passion for happiness was gone.

Every day, after returning home from work, she immediately disappeared into her bedroom. It was a blessing. We never knew what her reaction to any situation would be from one moment to the next. It was dependent upon her drug use. Fortunately, for us, Mom remained invisible when high.

The kitchen cupboards were full. We knew how to care for ourselves, as taught when younger. It had been two years since our life had been stable. We adapted and developed our sense of stability with one another. With childhood traditions deeply rooted in us, we had a permanent home where we lived, friends, and our routines, as we had when we were children in Carson City. There is one thing to be said about the young. They are resilient.

Mom bought our home on a land contract, paying a hefty down-payment with the proceeds from her divorce settlement with Dad. Years of saving to build their dream home had paid off. She was relying on her new husband to be able to meet the terms of refinancing and paying the mortgage payments.

Celebrating his new job, Mom bought him a Cadillac, expensive clothing to match his position of success. There was a set of golf clubs for those important golf course meetings that he kept in the car, and everything else he wanted so he would set up perfectly, and ready to live the life of a successful businessman.

With his starting date delayed, Mom was not worried until after a few weeks when there was no word of when he would begin his job. She began insisting that he go to the university and find out what was going on. The contract he claimed to have for the fall semester, he said. It was already July, and, already, two months had elapsed after moving there.

Chuck left, advising he would return home soon. He wasn't gone long. Entering the house, he was despondent, saying someone had accidentally filled his position. Mom sank onto the couch and began to sob inconsolably. Her fear suddenly turned into anger, as she rose and insisted, he immediately "get out and get a job, and don't bother coming back until you do."

Reluctantly, he packed some of his things and left. Within days he came home reporting that he had found a new position, an even better one. He had procured one as a vice-president of a paper company.

We were disappointed. We had hoped Chuck had left for good. With finances tight, Jim and I went job hunting. It didn't take long to find work. He worked part-time at a grocery store at night, stocking shelves, while I found a position for a wealthy family as an assistant to a housekeeper. That year, we paid for our school clothing and expenses. Donna was too young to work. We were the same size, so I shared my clothing with her.

Autumn rolled around. Jim and I quickly adapted to our new school and instantly fit in amongst the down to earth, Menasha High School kids. Choosing college prep classes, we readied ourselves to continue upward after high school.

Despite not having much parental direction, we watched as our friends lived and did the same. Most of the rules of their homes and their parents became ours. We studied at the dining room table after school. At night, we prepared our meals. As we had done as children, the three of us discussed our days as we ate. We kept the same routine as we had growing up on Martin Street in Carson City. Making good on that promise we made that night to remain together, the only difference between our lives and what occurred in homes of our friends were the two empty chairs at the dining room table.

That Easter, we flew to Reno for Easter vacation. It was a dearly needed trip, and we desperately wanted to see our father. We had missed him terribly. The breakdown of our family and the move to Wisconsin had torn us apart. At home, the situation was tense, and I was particularly susceptible to stress. Hospitalized for extensive testing for stress-related gastrointestinal issues, Mom faced difficulty accepting that we missed our father and our small house in Carson City. Keeping our sentiments and feelings between us, so Mom would not react to them personally, it eliminated the opportunity for her to make disparaging remarks about him. Her reaction hurt us equally as much, if not more than our stepmother's attempts to keep us from being a part of our father's life.

It was in my sophomore year of high school when I finally mustered the courage to stand up to Mom and to move back to Reno and live with Dad. We had told him what was occurring at home. He knew I was facing difficulties adapting, and he was worried about me. Assuring we always had a home with him, I felt comfortable leaving Wisconsin.

Then, living with him was his now twenty-year-old girlfriend and her two-year-old daughter. At night, I could hear them argue. "I told you I do not want your children here," she would insist loudly.

She was particularly angry with me after opening a letter that I had written to my mother that she had failed to mail, as promised. I had written that I was lonely and uncomfortable in the enormous school I attended. For some reason, she took those feelings as a personal rejection of her and turned the situation around to focus on her, making herself the victim.

Dad took me to breakfast the next morning and apologized. I told him I felt I should leave. He begged me to stay, saying, "She has a severe problem with insecurity, Lindy. She is working on it. Try to understand that, okay? We can get through this."

Conflicted, I sought direction from Sister Magdalene. After extensive discussion, we decided I should go back home, suspecting that the situation was far more complicated than Dad realized. That night, I hopped on a flight back to Wisconsin.

In the years to follow, my brother and sister experienced the same. My brother experienced the same after moving in with Dad during his senior year of high school. He did not last long in their home either, also facing the brunt of her "insecurity." She knew he had no other possibility of living elsewhere but continually insisted Dad to make him leave. With Donna, she created a scene at Grandma's house, calling Donna names because she was Donna was dating a black student at her college. She targeted all of us with some sort of abuse to keep us away from Dad.

Resulting from those uncertain times with the negative situations we experienced with our stepmother *every time* we saw Dad, we were leery of having any contact with him when she was around. Having lived with a drug addict, we learned to protect ourselves and to get out of uncomfortable situations that were not good for us as soon as possible. But, with Dad's girlfriend, it was difficult to tell what would set her off. It was impossible to trust her. As a result of both became fearful of close relationships and ended most of them within days of their beginning.

Wisconsin was the perfect place in the 1960s for young, unsupervised adolescents, offering a wholesome Americana experience. While California and Nevada were reeling with free love, drugs, and rock-and-roll, we were attending dances in the park, and after, boys were offering to walk us home. We lived as other teens, cheering on our football team, attending the regular weekly dances at our church, those at the park during summer, and across the street at the Blue Inn, a teen recreational center, during the school year. On Sunday afternoons, we strolled through autumn leaves and fresh snow. It was an idyllic place to live.

We didn't see Mom much after moving into our home. The woman who never finished high school worked at night as a bank auditor. She wasn't happy with her job. Numbers meant nothing to her. Having transitioned into a 1960s "free spirit," Mom's passion was drugs, sunshine, auras, and colors. She was an artist, not an accountant. During the entire time she lived in Wisconsin, I never once saw her paint or draw in her sketchbooks. Mom had stopped singing. The drugs had taken away her passion for happiness.

Each day, after returning home from work, she disappeared into her bedroom for the evening. It was a blessing. We never knew what her reaction to any situation would be from one moment to the next. It depended upon her drug use. Mom remained invisible when high.

The kitchen cupboards were full. We knew how to care for ourselves, as taught when younger. It had been two years since our life had been stable. We adapted to it, developing a renewed sense of stability. With childhood traditions deeply rooted in us, we were grateful for a permanent home, friends, and the routines we had developed as children in Carson City. There is one thing to be said about the young. Most are resilient during times of crisis.

Mom had bought our home on a land contract, paying a hefty down-payment with the proceeds from her divorce settlement with Dad. Years of saving to build their dream home had paid off. Mom was relying on her new husband to be able to meet the terms of eventually refinancing and promising to pay the mortgage payments. With him now having as important a position as before, she was once again looking forward to becoming a homemaker.

Our home was large enough to allow us to steer clear of our stepfather. He was abusive when angered, something we learned early on, after moving to Wisconsin. Shortly after arrival, an incident occurred one evening while Mom was working. He would not allow me to leave the house to meet with friends and go to a dance. I picked up the phone to call Mom and ask her to confirm to him that I had her permission to go.

Snatching the receiver from me, he hung it back up on the wall and grabbed me by the arm, spinning me around. Jim confronted him, telling him to stop. He pushed Jim away; I tried to intervene, racing forward, and pushing him back. The massive ring he wore struck my face, leaving a bruise below my eye.

Realizing he had hurt me, Chuck stomped off to his room. Jim and I went to the home of Jim's girlfriend, the daughter of a police detective. Viewing my swollen and bruised face, and upon hearing Jim's rendition of what occurred, her father sat Chuck down and had a "discussion" with him. He never tried to touch me again, at least not in that town.

Moving to our new home, in Menasha, another incident occurred, again while Mom was at work, I awakened from napping on the sofa to find my mother's husband bending over me, trying to kiss me.

"What are you doing?" I demanded, pushing him away in disgust.

"I thought you were your mother," Chuck stuttered, his eyes wide.

"If you ever touch me again. I will tell Mom *and* Dad," I threatened, as I readied to fight him off if I had to.

He left the room. Avoiding me for weeks was a welcome change. Donna and I took preventative measures to protect ourselves. We hung bells on the interior doorknob of our bedroom, hoping they would awaken us if anyone were to enter while we slept.

Keeping our doors locked, even during summer, I made it a habit to cover the keyhole of the bathroom door with a towel when in use. Jim watched over us as we slept. His room was twenty feet from ours. He left his door open if we needed him. It was comforting to know he was nearby. With Jim, the bells on the doors, and having a light on all night, we were finally able to sleep.

Ignoring Chuck during the day, we viewed him as nothing more to us than the creepy stepfather who was part of Mom's baggage. It frustrated us that Mom refused to recognize his inadequacies. He contributed little toward the family, the household care, and the maintenance. We took care of that. Often, he disappeared at night. We later found out he was smoking dope with kids who attended our high school.

Autumn rolled around. Jim and I quickly adapted to our new school and instantly fit in amongst the down to earth, Menasha High School kids. Choosing college prep classes, we readied ourselves to continue upward after high school.

In 1968, my peers elected me the sophomore-class secretary and the president of the Menasha Youth Council. Being involved with the debate team, taking part in plays, and active in the Catholic Youth Organization, Jim and I were always busy with after-school activities. He played football, wrestled on the varsity wrestling team, argued issues on the debate team, and held the leads in several school plays.

We quickly adapted to the move and met most of the kids in the neighborhood. Walking home with us from the park, was a boy who gave us the rundown of the neighbors, telling us who was "cool" and who was not. Upon revealing information about himself and his family, we had something in common. Our fathers were both vice-presidents of the same company.

"Your stepfather does what?" he asked, with surprise.

"He's a vice-president," I repeated to him.

"That is what I thought you said." He paused, appearing uncomfortable, but he continued, "Well, I don't know how to tell you this, but so is my father."

"And?" I asked.

"There's only one. Cross my heart."

Why would Chuck lie about that?

Embarrassment swept over me. I made some weak excuse about having to leave, pretending to be late getting home. The next afternoon, while walking home, I heard him calling out to me and rushing to catch up with where I was. Stopping, I waited for him.

"I need to tell you something," he mumbled, out of breath.

"What?" I asked.

"Your stepfather is a shipping clerk."

"A shipping clerk?" I asked, in disbelief.

"Yes," he confirmed.

"Oh, my God. This will kill Mom. Please don't tell anyone," I begged.

"I won't say anything, I promise," he assured. "I am sorry. I thought you needed to know."

"I *do* need to know," I said, my voice breaking. Tears filled my eyes as I thanked him. We spoke a few minutes and parted ways at the corner.

"I'll call you," he said, before continuing his way.

Within days, Chuck lost his job, along with his imaginary golf dates with other executives every Wednesday afternoon at the golf club. After, my friend never called. It was a relief as I had hoped he would not. I was sure he was as embarrassed as I was. Though, his father often smiled and waved as he drove to and from work. It made me feel better.

Again, being resilient, we continued to live as ordinary kids, hosting dinner parties before formal events and socializing with friends who came by to study or to visit. If anyone knew of the problems in our family, they were kind enough not to mention it. As far as we knew, they considered us as the kids with the cool, hippy parents who were never around.

While Mom and our Chuck continued their cloistered existence, we had no complaint. The patterns we learned and practiced growing up as young children in Carson City continued, creating our sense of stability.

The two best things about living in Wisconsin and a big part of my stability were my two closest friends, Sandee and Pat. Like most adolescents, we supported one another through teenage heartbreaks and adolescent dramas.

Sandee lived around the corner from our home. She was my dearest friend in high school. Vibrant and outgoing, she was a natural athlete, a cheerleader, a student leader, and an incredible hunter and angler. I admired her strength, determination, and fearlessness.

A teacher at heart, Sandee was a positive influence. She excelled in gymnastics; I was not near as good as her. My skills were in trying to get out of class. She did not allow me to give up.

"You can do this," she said, insisting I leave the locker room where I had been hiding to get out into the gym. "Now, come on!"

She created a gymnastics routine using equipment that better suited my physical abilities — the horse, the bars, and floor exercises. With her training and motivational lectures, I not only perfected doing a "fish flop," I ended up with a B in the class. I loved her for it.

A few months later, she encouraged me to take part in synchronized swimming and to join her in performing in the annual water pageant. Not good at swimming, I was less than enthused. Sandee cared less as she dragged me to the pool to sign up.

When Sandee decided senior lifesaving would be useful for both of us, I really balked. It was for the best of swimmers. Again, she said, "Come on. You can do this! We'll get certified as lifeguards, and we can get jobs during the summer." Whispering silent prayers that I would not drown, I again signed up alongside her. The certifications we received were a highlight of our high school years.

That summer, Sandee and I spent time at her father's hunting cabin on the Fox River. Young, bored, and desirous of experiencing something new, we laid upon the water on our backs. Each of us held onto a ski rope, while the other drove, taking turns dragging each other up and down the river behind her father's fishing boat. Flying above the wake at high speeds, and hanging onto that rope for dear life, we were experiencing one of the most exhilarating, adrenaline rushes, ever. Not once did we ever think about what would happen should the rope break or something else occur. Fearless and emboldened, water was our turf.

"What's the matter with you?" my mother asked when I told her about it. "Do you have a death wish or something?"

"Not at all, Mom. I just want to live as much of life as I can while I'm young," I answered.

She gazed at me for a few seconds, then pulling me close, she hugged me. Stepping back, she said, "That's what I want to hear."

It was that year that I confided my fear of cancer to Sandee and revealed to her the cancer syndrome existing in our family. She remembers it well, far better than me. She understood better than anyone. Though she came from a home with her parents intact, she also lived with uncertainty.

Sandee has experienced the same, not knowing why the women in her mother's family were dying from breast cancer. Like many in Wisconsin, her family lives with the BRCA 1 gene, which creates a high predisposition for hereditary breast cancer. Tragically, she has lost two sisters and a mother to it. Sandee is resilient, far more so than me. She realized "someday" and "forever."

When Sandee first saw Tom, in the ninth grade, she told her mother, "That's the guy I am going to marry." Sandee was confident and did not fear the future as I did. They hooked up in high school, the football quarterback, and the cheerleader.

Sharing a love of the outdoors, he taught her how to become a better fisherman, and she taught him how to hunt. Today, they have celebrated over forty years of marriage and live an active life, filled with two sons, a daughter-in-law, and two beautiful grandchildren.

Sandee always smiles and is positive. I don't know how she copes with the losses, as she does. She is strong, loving, and still noticeably confident, looking the same as she did in high school, despite everything she and her sister, Sue, have experienced.

Strong and decisive, Pat, has an immense capability of caring for others. Intuitive and compassionate, she was my redeeming grace. Always ready to listen, Pat offered a perspective of balance when times became difficult. One of those rare persons who find the good in everything, Pat tunes into people and reads what they are not saying.

With Pat, what is, is. Like Sandee, Pat is practical. She adapts to any situation. Pat also met her husband in high school. The first time she saw Scott, Pat realized he was the one *she* would marry. Teenage matchmakers went to work. It only took minutes and one slow dance. They married a year after graduation and have been together for over forty- seven years.

Pat also faces similar challenges. Some of her loved ones live with a hereditary rare disease condition. As a caretaker, she is a symbol of strength. An influential matriarchal figure, Pat is supportive of others, positively embracing life and living outside herself. Not only involved with her church and its youth ministry, but she is a master mom and a grandmother who still bakes pies from scratch.

I was different in that I socialized and dated. However, any interest I felt in anyone waned within a few weeks. Through my teen years and well into early adulthood, I dated guys who lived out of town, and who were not around much. Any time someone got too close, I hit the road. I found close relationships to be terrifying.

Once risk-takers, the three of us are now doers. Pat and Sandee have spent decades teaching and working with children. Sandee is getting ready for her fiftieth anniversary in working with the children in her city. No matter what needs doing, the two always get it done. Life is more fulfilling when living outside themselves and caring for others.

Despite what they live with, and what we live with doesn't make us any different from anyone else. Everyone's DNA is different, and many are living with the effects of the genetic situations that affect our health and our loved ones in many ways. Everyone is born with several genetic mutations. They just do not know it.

Chapter Eight

LEAVING HOME

Music is very spiritual; it has the power
to bring people together. — Edgar Winter

Late one winter evening, Jim left home, fleeing out into sub-zero temperatures, and disappearing behind the snowbanks without so much as wearing a coat. If anyone wants to escape from where they are, there is always a way. At least it was so for Jim. Not owning a car or even cash, he hitchhiked from Wisconsin to California.

Though preparing to graduate from high school in six months, he left home following one of the regular conflicts that occurred every time Mom and Chuck stepped out of their bedroom. The disputes ordinarily arose from nothing of importance but always ended with Chuck losing self-discipline during a quarrel and taking a swing at Jim.

Jim had enough of his bullying and verbal attacks. This time, he swung back. The fight was on. Taking the hit, Chuck staggered backward, and regaining balance, charged at the much smaller and younger Jim. Falling to the floor, the two engaged in a knock-down, drag-out battle, Chuck found himself at the losing end, even though he was much bigger.

Yelling, "Get out," he pulled a drawer out of a cabinet and threw it at Jim, hitting him in the side.

Looking expectantly at Mom, Jim waited for her to intervene on his behalf. Instead of protecting her son, she stood silent, her eyes moving back and forth between the two. A sting of betrayal waved across Jim's face. He ran outside and disappeared behind a snowbank.

"Mom, how could you let him do that to Jim?" I confronted her. "He's seventeen years old! What is wrong with you?"

Tears filled her eyes as she fled to her bedroom. Chuck followed closely behind, his head dropping like a chastised child. Jim didn't come home. Weeks passed without hearing from him. Donna and I were sick with worry. We had difficulty eating and sleeping, not knowing where he was and how he was doing.

At last, he called. We were relieved to hear that he had made it to California and was with Dad, who was building a room for him in his downstairs garage. Not wanting to intrude on Dad's Christmas, Jim had spent the Christmas holiday in Carson City with friends. Doing everything possible to stay out of Dad's way and not be a problem; he was looking forward to his graduation that June.

Dad was riding on the fast track at work. Since his recent promotion to the executive offices of Pacific Telephone in San Francisco, he had been living with his girlfriend and her daughter in Orinda, California, a suburban town on the outskirts of the city. He was remodeling an older home he had brought in a beautiful suburban area.

Jim liked it there. Enjoying school and looking forward to college, he developed an interest in a girl—adapting well, making friends, and adjusting to the Bay area lifestyle everything was working out fine if he kept a distance from Dad's girlfriend.

Despite his efforts, from his downstairs garage quarters, he could hear Dad and his girlfriend arguing at night. "I don't want your children in my house," she demanded, insisting he make Jim leave. Realizing it was the same that had occurred with me the year before, it not only alerted Jim to be more careful around her but also upset Dad. Despite everything, with three months left until graduation and no chance of any permanent residence with a stable parent, Jim moved out, following a conflict involving Dad's now twenty-two-year-old girlfriend.

At seventeen years old, he dropped out of school, and at Dad's insistence, enlisted in the Army, as Dad had done at his age. By the time he was nineteen, Jim was carrying an M16 in Vietnam. Strapped across his chest were bandoleers filled with ammo, with grenades hung from his flak jacket. He was a walking armory.

Assigned as one of two cryptology trained electronic communication technicians to a specialized intelligence position, Jim volunteered for a special mission to the DMZ. His job entailed supporting an enormous effort to disrupt traffic through the Ho Chi Minh trail through Laos and to interrupt the flow and delivery of Chinese and Soviet weapons to the enemy, shortly before the 1971 Tet Offensive.

Initially hopping into Hughey helicopters and flying clandestinely into darkened landing zones at night, Jim spent the first few months of his deployment repairing battlefield communication systems.

After an assessment, he was offered an assignment as a radio operator at a semi-secret command bunker of the Vietnamese Armed Forces Command, located at LZ Leatherneck, overlooking Highway 9 near Khe Sahn.

During much of that time, Jim was emotionally numb as he took risks while working within one of the hotbeds of the war. At that camp, while top-level brass from the South Vietnamese forces strategized battle positions, Jim spent his days and nights radioing to helicopters that were running sorties in support of the Vietnamese Marines in Laos.

Staffed by mostly officers, they remained inside the bunker while experiencing enemy fire, huddled under the long table. Instead of joining them, Jim chose to frequent outside, between barrages, to identify and relay the type of incoming fire hitting around them. A few of the officers were new. They had yet to gain the experience to identify the specific artillery rounds that were targeting their positions.

One afternoon, as Jim fixated upon watching the mortars strike the hill below where he was sitting, he began to worry as he noted they were "walking up the mountain," with each coming closer. The next hit could take them down.

Leaning against the outer doorway, he overheard an officer calling to the United States Air Force F4 Phantom fighter jets flying overhead. "We're being barraged with incoming rockets," he reported

Jim immediately called out to him from the doorway, "It's mortars. They're firing mortars, and they're walking straight for us."

"Correction," the Air Force officer said, nodding toward Jim while speaking on the radio. "They're firing mortars, and they're hitting close."

"Copy," came the voice of a pilot. "We'll attempt to locate."

Silence filled the room, as most ducked under the table and awaited their fate, praying the F-4 Phantoms that conducted fly-bys of the area would arrive in time.

At last, a voice broke through the silence, reporting, "The incoming fire is coming from a mortar system setting on the mountainside, in front of you." A few seconds of silence followed. "We are seeing rail tracks leading inside the cave. We're going in."

Jim at once exited the command center, watching as the F-4 Phantoms worked in pairs, racing against time to annihilate the source of the fire before the Viet Cong could hit the bunker.

His eyes caught upon the first Phantom as it flew by, firing its missiles at the mountain, with a second one, following behind, providing backup. With the first pulling off, the second took its place, firing at the interior of the cave. As explosions sounded, the long line of jets continued flying in the same circular manner, repeatedly taking turns performing fly-bys and obliterating the cave and everything around it.

Finally, a voice sounded from the radio. "A sizable number of secondary explosions are coming from the inside," a pilot reported. "Whatever's in there, it's exploding."

Cheers, filled with excitement, and mixed with sighs of relief, filled the bunker. With the cave destroyed, the lives of thirty high-ranking Vietnamese officers and the five Americans, one from each branch of the U.S. military who were working as advisors, were saved.

By now, Jim had perfected his risk-taking tendencies. His experiences in Vietnam offered a good sense of confidence and accomplishment in doing something important for others, interplaying with the night sweats and the intrusive dreams imposed by post-traumatic stress disorder. Jim had saved lives and played a crucial role in protecting the Vietnamese people against the insurgency of Chinese and Russian-style communism; at the same time, paying for it with the development of his own demons, that he has since spent a lifetime battling.

Vietnam was a long-lasting tragedy for most young soldiers engaged in battle, but for Jim, it was a blessing, except for the ongoing effects of PTSD. Fortunately, most of his symptoms occurred at night. Like many who came home from Vietnam, he is still living with the results of battle.

Jim's level of willingness to take on risky assignments was as strong as his acceptance of taking on responsibility. With his intense level of determination to complete his mission, at any odds, his commanding officers respected Jim's keen sense of survival.

Once, after returning from a mission, Jim reported to the rear with all his explosives, hanging from his flak vest, appearing as battlefield regalia. his First Sergeant was quick to help confiscate the grenades, ammunition, and other various non-issued weapons that Jim and others, in his rank and type of assignment carried upon them.

The soldiers assigned to the inner confines of the Long Bien military base, where Jim's command headquartered, were referred to as the STRAC... the ones who were perfectly dressed all the time, with polished shoes and safer assignments. Operating within the relative comfort and safety of the base, most had never seen battle. Not used to seeing soldiers who worked in the outback, returning from the front, and walking around with grenades hanging from their vests, it created a significant amount of alarm for them, realizing the reality of war that was going on outside their compound.

There had been some fragging incidents that had occurred recently, at which point enlisted soldiers had killed their officers with grenades. The extra care taken by the officer was more than reasonable. However, their concerns were not necessary when it came to Jim. They were simply exercising caution with everyone returning from the front.

Jim's battle experience enhanced his level of confidence and expanded the independent nature he developed as a child in Carson City. The skills he learned then not only proved of value while fighting for survival in Vietnam but also at a later age when he found himself battling hereditary cancer and heart disease.

Like other veterans, Jim arrived home detached from everybody and everything, trying to figure out where he best fit in within the scheme of everyday life that had evolved without him. With no parent in a position to offer support, he worked on the PTSD issues while completing college.

While Jim adapted to his circumstances on the battlefield, we were going through changes of our own, at home. I missed him, our long talks at night, his laughter, and his support. Now, it was only my younger sister and me who sat at the dinner table. Mom stopped working and tried to serve as a buffer between Chuck and us to make sure his actions toward us did not escalate. I suspect she knew we feared him.

I avoided being at home. Involvement in the Catholic Youth Organization and Sing Out, a local organization of Up with People! helped me cope with the problems at home. The uplifting music and the messages that Sing Out sent to a demoralized society was refreshing. It focused on improving one's self and reaching out to others. The encouragement we received from the lyrics in the music, encouraging us to "do the best we can with what we've got," and to care about others proved invaluable.

It resonated with me and supported the same message Dad instilled in us as children. During my teen years and after, whenever I was down, there was always a song to lift my spirits. Singing was therapeutic. I had done it all my life. When dealing with uncomfortable situations, I learned to walk away from conflict, to view it from the outside looking in, rather than something creating an immediate problem that was threatening me.

Spending considerable time with Father Eagan and Father Paul, our local priests at St. Patrick's Church, both offered positive coping methods with demanding situations. Between song, the support and counseling they provided, and my faith never wavering, the Pollyanna type sense of hope that existed when young, got me by. During times when choice did not exist, I forced myself to adapt. In doing so, I learned I did not need to accept what was happening. I only needed to recognize its occurrence, realize what is, is, and what was, was. Not wishing to look back, I made myself move forward. I had to keep active, for me and everyone else in our family.

Family dysfunction is not unusual, especially while growing up in the 1960s. Half of America's children received care from a single parent during some part of their life. Often, one parent was not capable of solely fulfilling their needs. Some had no parents to care for them. Those children grew up with the responsibilities of adults, caring for parents who refuse to accept adulthood.

My forty-something father had regressed to twenty-two years old, the age of his girlfriend. He drove a fast truck, had a mustache, and was "looking cool" in his trendy new clothing. Hitting the scene with his hot, young babe, he didn't have the time for his adolescent children.

Filling his role was Grandma, our Aunt Marcella, and our Uncle Hassan. They were deeply concerned about us and called often. They kept us balanced, helping us to realize the primary root cause of our family circumstances were not a result of anything we did, but a result of our parents.

Hereditary and family cancers played an enormous role in all of this. They are a part of what we are, of what our parents were, and what our ancestors once were. Nothing can change that. It does not help to get angry. It is merely sad. There is no one to blame. It is the luck of the draw, a matter of circumstance, a part of our family, and a major element of what we are.

Learning to accept was that none of us could choose our parents or change them or the way *they* react to us; I finally decided only the addict can resolve his or her issues with drugs. It took a long time and distance to realize the only person who can control the number of prescription bottles lining the top of Mom's dresser is Mom. The only persons who can resolve the issues with Dad's actions and those of his spouse are Dad and his wife. And they were the only ones who could make changes in their lives as Dad finally did, later in life, when he realized his end was near.

The only person who can effect a change in me is me. Only I can make a difference in how I react to circumstances, whether it be the response to abandonment by a loved one or how I adapt to living with an unknown hereditary cancer syndrome, or to a diagnosis of cancer. I have never stopped wishing things were different. But wishes mean little. Actions are everything, and we have far more options when we accept the responsibilities to form our futures than we realize.

Life was never as much of an adventure for our parents as it has been for us. Exposed to the gritty, heartbreaking tragedy in living through the Great Depression, the days of eugenics, World War II, Korea, sending a child to Vietnam, both had lost parents to cancer, with each experiencing turbulent times due to discrimination. It was too much for Mom to manage. She was unable to adapt.

Many genetic counselors face difficulty understanding why the fear of diagnostic testing exists. Some cannot understand why a code of silence prevailed within some families with hereditary cancers. Growing up under the conditions detailed above disallowed our parents and us, as their children, to confront adversity. Silence equated to survival. The eugenics movement imposed a lifelong negative effect upon the grandparents of those diagnosed today. Most people don't realize it was *still* in existence until the mid-1960s, just two generations ago. I was a teenager when it ended.

Today, those of us who are younger and did not have the experiences of our parents may or may not be able to discuss personal issues and concerns, ask questions, and confront those working with us, to make our own decisions with our lives. My father was never comfortable discussing the pressure he felt from physicians that wanted him to become sterilized, nor was my mother when she underwent a hysterectomy. She opted for the surgery to remove her female organs only because she feared cancer, not because she was an "imperfect" person who may bring "imperfect children" into the world.

Those born in the 1940s and the 1950s existed during a time when families could not speak openly about it. People who came from "cancer houses" and "cancer families" did not discuss cancer or any other illness that was considered a severe defect in human quality. It was not due to denial. Some of us and our parents grew up fearing it and others, as did we and our aunt. It was real, as were the actions of others who held control over us and our bodies.

Many from our generation and that of our parents, mostly male, faced sterilization because they were born diabetic, or they had a family history of some other hereditary risk of disease. Doctors strongly recommended vasectomies for them in the 1960s and 1970s.

Opportunities did not exist for the children of those affected by a hereditary disease to trust their medical professionals during the era of eugenics and for some time after. While ill with cancer or some other "unacceptable" defect, physicians badgered many to become sterilized because they were "defective." Hearts broke when ministers demeaned them in front of their neighbors and others because "something was wrong with them."

The generation before mine and those who came before them still face difficulty trusting health care professionals, as do some of us. The actions of society and the eugenics movement forced silence. Placing trust in those involved in the medical profession was risky.

We lived during a time when those who were "different" had little choice and control over the health care procedures offered them. Before 1940, many chose not to seek medical treatment when they became ill, preferring to die than to subject their families to the abuses of those involved in the eugenics movement. They did not want paternalistic medical professionals, genetics experts, and judges to control their lives and deny them their right of reproduction.

The eugenics movement ended in the mid-1960s when I was twelve years old, about twenty years after cancer centers, such as the City of Hope, began development. Growing up, our parents always reminded us, "Don't discuss your personals with anyone."

The medical profession, circumstances, and society prohibited Americans from living on their terms. Paternalism was rampant. The solutions they offered were not those of benefit to patients; they only served as a tool for those who felt we were a burden. They viewed us as far too incompetent to make "appropriate decisions for our children and ourselves. Many still do. I cannot count the number of times I have heard the words, "You don't know..." from some genetic counselors when discussing social and family issues involving the genetic testing of our children.

Naturally, there was and still is distrust as the same attitude exists with the policies of genetic counselors, specifically to their firm stance that children should not test genetically for Lynch syndrome until adulthood. As in the days of eugenics, many are still making the decisions for families, based upon their own beliefs, rather than allowing parents to do what they feel is best for their child.

What occurred in 1965 was only sixty-five years ago, and many of us, who were children, still remember it like yesterday. In today's radicalized circles of some involved in genetics, there is considerable fear of them that is justifiable, despite the changes that occurred during the past decades. There are some in the genetics professions that regressed backward. For us, it is genuinely frightening.

The stark reality, however, is Mom and Dad experienced more challenges and problems than most could ever realize today. Mom did not have the skills or the strength to protect herself, nor did she have the support from others to resolve her fears.

Dad lived walking on eggshells, not wanting to go through a divorce or any situation where he again felt like a lesser person, ever. It was a bold, painful reminder of his childhood. He had serious decisions to make after

Mom underwent her hysterectomy, and he wondered if he should follow suit with his own sterilization. After their divorce, he often contemplated whether he should have made a different choice.

Not as fortunate as us to experience an early stable childhood, there were no public service organizations to help Mom with addiction or to supply the counseling for her family's unknown hereditary cancer. Nor were there support groups to deal with familial diseases as those existing today.

There was and still is no name for the cancer syndrome affecting Mom's family. Until 1993, when tests were finally developed for Lynch syndrome, there was no name for it either, and we did not find out what it was until fourteen years later, in 2007, after Dad had died and three more of us had contracted cancer. Until then, Dad was simply part of a "cancer family." For the families of both, there were few treatments, no preventative measures, no dedicated cancer centers in Los Angeles County until after 1940, and no cures. Life, for many, was hopeless.

For me, it took years before I felt comfortable discussing family matters with anyone, without fear, especially with those I loved. Today, we can, knowing there are hundreds of thousands of others, like us. Any stigma, today, is almost nonexistent. It is nothing like that faced by those who came before us, despite what any doctor or genetic counselor may write with their own beliefs of how we may feel.

Then, when my parents were young, the only reprieve for Mom was the considerable number of physicians handing out pills, and the many television shows and movies normalizing unhappy, conflicted women with perfectly styled hair, staying home, popping pills, or "little dolls" as they used to call them, and sipping on cocktails.

Dad limited his focus upon achieving success doing only that which he did well. He set his priorities and allowed it to distract him from uncertainty. Facing the same pressures his father confronted, Dad worked hard to provide for his family, should he die.

In the 1960s, when our parents divorced, the male responsibility was paying child support, and providing a home for his family, while a wife remained in the house, caring for the children. Today, male responsibility is taking an equal role with the mother and the father holding the same obligation of involvement in their children's lives. Today, we accentuate that quality of life with both parents and grandparents who actively participate in the lives of children. At the same time, we define"success" differently. It focuses on achieving happiness and the relationships we share with others.

In the summer of 1969, before my senior year of high school, I deliberated future options while attending an "Up With People!" Sing Out conference in Gambier, Ohio. I joined the international cast and its traveling high school.

At sixteen, I left Menasha, Wisconsin, for Pittsburgh, Pennsylvania, to spend my first night with them. The compelling drama of that evening became a strong influence on my life. Surrounded by hundreds of others who also sought something greater than themselves, we heard Neil Armstrong's voice sound upon the giant television screen setting upon an enormous stage. "Houston, Tranquility Base here. The Eagle has landed."

Everyone in the room cheered as we watched men doing what we thought to be impossible. They had traveled through space to a different world. Later, we saw Armstrong step down from his space capsule and become the first human to walk upon the moon. As he climbed down the ladder, he said, "That's one small step for a man, one giant leap for mankind."

Being amongst so many others while viewing Earth from space, I realized my place in a world of billions. Apart from so many others, we do not count for much. I am just one small person. However, when we reach out and extend ourselves out to others to join us, we can become a powerful force. Glancing about the lecture hall and upon the others, I knew I was at the right place at the right time... where I was meant to be.

The youngest of us set out for a month of intensive preparation before hitting the road, in Ardmore, Oklahoma, while those of college-age traveled in a different direction. Four casts, totaling five hundred young men and women, headed out into the deep throes of life to share positive messages within a troubled world.

The 1960s were a turbulent time. A war raged in Vietnam and Cambodia. Protests rocked the country while communism threatened to small countries, and National Guard troops shot Kent State students taking part in antiwar demonstrations.

Police beat civil rights demonstrators with batons. The assassinations of President Kennedy and Martin Luther King devastated a nation already rocking with violence. Five days of rioting stormed in New York after the New York City police raided the Stonewall Inn, a gay establishment, and struggles existed between communistic and democratic governments in the smaller, weaker countries in Africa, Asia, and South America.

Armed with a semi-truck filled with thirteen tons of stage, sound, and lighting equipment, sound vans; three commercial buses; one hundred kids, twenty-four teachers, and administrative staff members worked to prepare for a year on the road, educating students and performing an upbeat, musical experience.

Our high school was definitely "non-traditional." We traveled through the country and performed in a professional musical production, met political leaders, learned about legislative policies, and experienced cultures different from our own. Having completed the classes needed for graduation, except for senior English, I had five more credits than the sixteen required by the State of Oklahoma. Therefore, a few others and I traveled ahead of the rest, performing media and advanced logistical work to prepare for their arrival.

We took on the challenging tasks of filling a house that often held up to thousands of ticket holders each night that we performed. We set out to find a site for cast members to study and attend classes, to find 120 beds in the homes of local families where cast members would stay, and schedule assemblies and smaller presentations throughout the city.

Working with the local media and other nonprofit organizations, we arranged for the donation of a week's worth of meals for the one hundred and fifty people in the cast. The experience in learning to encourage others to respond to the calls for action I was able to use several non-profit organizations we founded.

Staying in the homes of families, different from mine, had a profound effect on how I viewed my home and my family. It was then I began pulling apart my tightly woven emotional past, thread by thread. It left me vulnerable, realizing my battered, blue suitcase was my only sense of stability. Everything I treasured existed inside of it. It had become my home.

Jim and I went back to Wisconsin for Christmas. Our home was in foreclosure; Mom was in a depression. Everything around her was falling apart. With Jim preparing to leave for war and me traveling with Up With People! Mom commented she felt like she was stepping backward while her children were moving forward. It was the one reality she acknowledged.

We spent an evening at the local bowling alley visiting with old friends. It was a bittersweet experience. Though good to see them, we realized we were at different points in our lives. While they were still in school, Jim was preparing to deploy to Vietnam, and I was trying to change a world in crisis. Our only sources of stability were the military and "Up With People! Theirs were their families, schools, and their hometown.

On the way home, Jim asked, "Lindy, do you feel different?"

"Yes," I answered. "Very much so."

Our house no longer felt like home, and both of us felt lost. Dark and empty, it seemed it was mourning the loss of us. I grieved with it. There was not much left that reflected genuine emotion or happiness. Dad's words haunted me as they echoed in my mind. "Once you leave home, you can't go back. Nothing is ever the same."

Later, upon reading Thomas Wolfe's work, You Can't Go Home Again, my heart winced as his words stabbed deeply. I think Wolfe's book must have reminded Dad of the loss of his father the same as it brought back to life the memories of mine.

Both Wolfe and Dad prophesied what was to come into our lives. They served as a warning to be ready to accept loss. "You can't go back home to your family, back home to your childhood… back home to the father you have lost and have been looking for, back home to someone who can help you, save you, ease the burden for you, back home to the old forms and systems of things which once seemed everlasting, but which are changing all the time."

Chapter Nine

FLOUNDERING

The fear of drugs running out is manageable,
the fear of time running down isn't. —Ann Marlowe

A month had hardly passed when I received a call from my mother while traveling on the road. Distressed, she begged me to return. Between some unknown time between my being a child and my senior year of high school, we had traded roles. I had become her parent, and Mom was my child."

"Things are bad," she cried. "Chuck has cancer, tumors in his arms. He can't work. Please come home, Lindy; I need you."

"Linda, don't go," Mary, our cast director begged while trying to convince me to stay.

"But you don't understand," I said. "My mother needs me."

"Please stay. Think of yourself. Nothing will change."

Agonizing between staying or returning to the responsibilities of caring for family needs, I could not sleep or think of anything else.

Though never speaking of the circumstances at home, I suspect Mary, one of our cast directors, realized the dysfunction. Dad had called cast directors the previous October, on my birthday, wanting to know who paid the costs for my travel. They told him a Wisconsin corporation sponsored my tuition, and I had the opportunity to sell records at the show to pay for my personal needs.

Dad explained he had just married. His bride was expecting a child in the next month. No longer having to pay child support for Jim and me would ease his financial burden, especially since he now had two more dependents with a third coming. Once again, supporting a second young family, money was tight.

It embarrassed me that he had called. Like it or not, the sins of the parents often fall upon the children. It was something I had to accept and adapt to, the same as our mother's drug addiction. His living situation with his girlfriend, an unwed mother for a second time, was still unacceptable in many parts of the country.

Our cast directors encouraged Dad to spend time with me while we were performing in Northern California and to tell me he was now married. Dad followed their advice. He invited me to spend a day with him and his new family. It was Thanksgiving. I accepted. I had not seen him in two years.

Picking me up in Santa Rosa, where we were performing, we spent the morning at a San Francisco beach. Without distraction, we spoke for hours, while his now three-year-old stepdaughter played in the sand.

"We married last summer, Lindy," Dad confided as we watched the toddler play upon the beach. "She's expecting a baby any day."

My heart stopped. My voice breaking, I wished Dad the best.

"Wouldn't it be nice to be children again, with few worries?" Dad asked as he watched the little girl laugh as she poured sand upon herself. "To change the past and do things differently?"

"Yeah, it would, Dad," I said. "What would you change?"

"Nothing, Lindy. So, don't you go thinking I don't love you. I do not regret anything." Dad said. "I am very proud of you and what you have accomplished."

"Thanks, Dad." Tears filled my eyes as he spoke. It was only half of what I needed to hear. Regrets are painful to admit. Then, he said what I dearly needed to hear.

"I am so sorry, Lindy… about everything. Some things are just out of our control."

I nodded, tears filling my eyes. Dad acknowledged our pain. Unable to hold in my emotions, I cried while he held me. I felt guilty for having been angry with him in the past, despite feeling violated when I found that Dad had spoken with my cast directors and confided his situation to them.

Working hard at compensating for our childhood, I had found a haven with the cast and was able to leave all the family problems and everyone's secrets behind me. It was where I could be an "everyday kid" and forget about the difficulties existing in my family. That haven no longer existed for me.

Dad's call was an embarrassment. It had nothing to do with concern for me and my wellbeing, but everything to do with him and his new wife. But I didn't tell him any of that.

Instead, I said, "We have missed you, Dad. All of us."

After dinner, he drove me to the home of my host family in Santa Rosa.

"Will you let me know when you are ready to enroll in college? I will help," Dad said. "I love you, baby doll. Visit this summer. Things will get better. I promise."

That one morning on the beach with my father and the drive back was memorable. I no longer felt so alone, with the chance to sit next to him and talk, once again, as we had done when I was younger.

Receiving Mom's telephone call two months later was painful. It overwhelmed me. My best interest would be to remain with the cast, but I could not live with myself if I weren't available for my mother.

It was time to be practical and let adolescent desires remain just that. Without the resources to pay for my expenses, I could not stay even if I could handle the knowledge of others knowing about my problems. With no one available, I didn't feel comfortable asking for help. Knowing I couldn't sell records when I was in another city preparing for the arrival of the cast, options to remain were nonexistent.

But none of that mattered. The deciding consideration was my mother was a part of me, and I was a part of her. I couldn't walk away, knowing how it felt to be alone and needing someone who cared. Despite her self-destructive qualities, I had to stand by her. There was no one else she could rely on to be there for her.

A lure dangled before me as I swam in my safe pond of "Up With People!" Hungering for our mother's love and acceptance, I was reliving the fear from my childhood of everything falling apart again. The situation was not good for either of us. I couldn't afford to lose Mom after losing our father. She was the only sense of security I had. I was not going to be the daughter she was to her mother. Starved for anyone's approval, at that point in my life, and not having other alternatives, I faced the situation and took the risk. There would be other opportunities, I thought. I went home.

Though less than a month had elapsed since being back with the cast after Christmas, when I arrived, the living situation for Mom and my sister had changed dramatically. It was dismal.

After Dad ceased paying child support, Mom had lost her home. She moved into a small, rundown apartment in the commercial part of Appleton, Wisconsin, above a pet shop they had bought. Mom was having difficulty adapting to it.

Chuck lost yet another job and was feigning having cancer as an excuse. It was the only way he could gain Mom's support. During their entire marriage, he had never kept a job for longer than four months. The family had no money, and the cupboards were bare. Donna was not attending high school and was doing what she had done when living in Menasha, spending her days sleeping. Since I had left, she had missed an entire semester of high school. Both Mom and Donna were depressed.

Mom's hands trembled as she was experiencing the symptoms of withdrawal from drugs. Having a bronchial infection, she coughed constantly. Her little pet shop was not making money. Debts were mounting, and she could no longer afford the drugs that kept her flying high in her sphere of existence. She hid out in the basement during the day, refusing to come out. It was her way of avoiding the bill collectors who were always calling, insisting upon payment. When I arrived home, she came back upstairs. Stone-cold sober and required to face reality, she underwent a significant self-assessment. It was hard for her to face the fact that she had reached "rock bottom."

Finding a job, any job, became my priority. The first place I interviewed was at a Kentucky Fried Children, a block from their home. Within hours, I was wearing a red and white apron and was busy taking food orders. Making enough cash to pay the rent by working nights, I was also able to bring unsold food home. It helped resolve the immediate issue of having nothing to eat.

A week later, I found a job as a long-distance operator at Wisconsin Telephone Company, following in the tradition of my father, his father, his father, and all his uncles. Basic, straightforward work, it paid sixty-four dollars a week. For eight hours a day, five days a week, I placed and pulled cords from a large switchboard filled with dozens of bulbs, lighting up in front of me.

"How may I help you?" I asked callers several hundred times a day, taking down their billing information and placing the call for them.

With two jobs nailed down and living expenses paid, I explored opportunities for attending college. Peering into a classroom of the local community college, I viewed former classmates inside, working on a project. My heart longed to be with them.

Entering the admissions office, I didn't expect the boatload of obstacles awaiting me, all involving how I would pay for it. I did not even get past the counselor to register.

Mom's poor credit rating did not qualify her to co-sign loans, and that of Dad was far too high to be eligible for grants. The information I received was devastating. Remembering what Dad said on Thanksgiving, I called him from the admissions office to see if he could help.

Our stepmother reported that Dad had provided for college funding in the divorce settlement with Mom, and nothing more would be available for my brother, sister, or me. She said what Mom received in their agreement was to cover everything. The admissions counselor put her hand on my shoulder as I broke into tears. I had put a lot of faith in Dad's promise.

Anger swept over Mom as she dialed the number of her attorney. He confirmed *both* Mom and Dad had agreed to share the costs of our college expenses. They had written nothing in their divorce settlement about college for us. It was not part of Mom's divorce agreement.

Later that afternoon, Dad telephoned, apologizing for the earlier call. He had found building his new home was more expensive than he thought and unexpectedly, was strapped for cash. Dad had to use the money tucked away for our educations to build their new home and to provide for their household expenses while doing so. With a growing family, he was no longer able to help as he had promised on Thanksgiving. He vowed he would find a way to make up for it. I didn't know how, and at that point, it didn't matter.

"Lindy, if you need anything, call me at work, okay?" he asked. Dad was trying to insulate himself due to his difficulties at home. I didn't blame him. Dad faced trouble dealing with conflict with his wife. She disallowed him to have contact with us. He shied away whenever possible.

My brother and sister had distanced themselves from him because of her. I wondered if I should do the same. I still could not allow myself to do it. I always held that bit of Pollyannaish hope that things would get better.

"It's okay, Dad. Don't worry," I told him as Mom angrily stomped out of the room upset with both him and me. "I'll find a way," I said.

As a child, I learned to be resourceful. With the help of the counselor, we decided I should enroll part-time. It proved to be a positive alternative, allowing me an opportunity to ease into becoming a full-time student and still be able to work a full and part-time job until I could apply for financial help on my own. I had enough of everyday stress trying to keep my mother balanced while helping to support my family. If there were a way, I would be able to find it.

June rolled around. The cast to hold our high school graduation in Chicago. I didn't intend to go, but after speaking with Dad, he said he would try his best to be there. Mom could not even consider the thought of traveling across town, let alone go to Chicago. I hopped on the train and traveled the one hundred and ninety miles, anxious to see Dad again.

After arriving, and speaking with the cast members I dearly missed, I searched for him in the crowd, fearing he did not know where to come. He had never traveled outside Nevada and California, had never gotten upon a plane, and knew little of large cities except for Los Angeles and San Francisco. It concerned me. During the entire ceremony, I continued searching for him. As the closing speech was ending, my heart ached as I finally accepted that he was not coming.

Watching classmates standing beside their parents and memorializing the day with family photographs, I noted their mothers were prim and proper. Holding silent gratitude that Mom did not attend, I knew she would have felt uncomfortable. She had gone through much during the past years. Her white skin was blotched, and Mom appeared ragged, not as she had once been when our family was intact. Looking and acting like Cher, right down to the same blank stare, she would have felt out of place.

At day's end, I had time to contemplate where I had been and where I was going as I waited to board a train back to Wisconsin. Dad, Mom, Jim, and I had all moved in different directions. Now, I was heading in a different direction from my classmates. They were college-bound, while I was heading back to where I had tried to escape from a year earlier. Worse yet, I realized it was on me. I was the only person who could change that and gluing myself to a relationship with a stranger I didn't know. Our mother had become to us years earlier.

Arriving home, later that evening, I saw Mom sitting outside and socializing with neighbors. It was good to see her break out of her self-imposed isolation. Home on leave for a few weeks, he was staying with friends before deploying to Vietnam. His short visit had warmed her heart. Mom had not seen him since Christmas. She was the happiest she had been in a long time. Approaching, I pulled my high school diploma out of my tote.

"Look, Mom, here…" I handed my diploma to her. She took it into her hands and scrutinized it. Then, she lovingly stretched out her arms, pulled me close, and hugged me tight, kissing the top of my head. For a few short minutes, the mother I once knew had returned.

"I'm so proud of you... the first to graduate high school in my family," she said with tears in her eyes as she tightly grasped it, studying it one more time. Stunned, I could not speak. Mom always said that she loved me. With that, there was no doubt, but I cannot remember a time when she ever said that she was proud of me, no matter how hard I tried or how well I had done. Handing it back, I was beaming as I tucked it into my bag.

Chapter Ten
A GOOD TIME TO GO

"We'll take the best, forget the rest, and someday will find that these are the best of times." —Styx

I moved out of my mother's home during the summer of 1970, four months before turning eighteen years old. Having reached an impasse with Chuck, I stayed as far from him as possible, but when living in close quarters was difficult. He was not easy to avoid.

The tension came to a head on a sunny day, one of the rare days he had been around. As I opened the door to leave the house, he was coming up the stairs. Stepping aside to allow Chuck to enter, he crossed the threshold, then slammed it closed, hitting me as I was sliding out.

Raising my hand to deflect from the impact, my palm connected with a windowpane. The fragile, old glass shattered, cutting into my wrist, and severing an artery with its jagged edges. Mom cried as I left for the hospital.

"I'm not coming back, Mom. Why do you let Chuck hurt us like this?" I asked her, grabbing my purse and wrapping my bloody hand with a towel he had thrown at me.

"I don't know why he does that. Please don't go," Mom sobbed.

"Do something about it, Mom. Come with me," I begged.

"I can't," she cried. "He's my husband. I need him. What if I get sick?"

"But, Mom, he is not responsible. He can't even keep a job or make more than a minimum wage. You have been the one taking care of him. Look how hard you are working."

"Lindy, Someday, you will marry and be gone, and I will be alone. Who will want me like this?" she asked, looking down upon herself.

I understood what she was saying, more than she realized. We were not so different. Like me, Mom needed to have some sense of certainty in a life that had none. She had created a false sense of hope in Chuck and was hanging onto it and to him, while I had created a similar false sense of confidence in Dad and Mom's eventual recovery. We were a family of Pollyannas. Though I knew it was time for me to let go of impossible dreams, I was never able to let go of the last bit of hope.

Receiving twenty-one stitches, the emergency room physician, and dear friends helped galvanize the tough decisions I had to make. The situation was escalating. Mom would never leave, and I could no longer stay to protect her.

Home became a tiny, two-bedroom cottage, shared with a good friend. It was one of those little white Great Depression-era houses often seen in Menasha. Set back from the street, the small white cottage set within a long-established neighborhood. In autumn, colorful leaves dripped from the several grand trees, standing in the oversized yard. As the air cooled and the days became shorter, a tapestry of vibrant hues of golds, rusts, and browns covers the autumn ground. Then, as the season succumbs to winter, snow blanketed the yard, and a peaceful silence fell upon the neighborhood. It was the perfect place to live.

Our little yellow kitchen beamed with happiness as a constant stream of friends flooded in and out, bringing themselves, others, and a lot of laughter. We designed the interior in 1960s décor, with tall wall shelves crafted from beer cases. The kitchen cabinets bulged with Top Ramen and little else. With the refrigerator filled with beer and Nehi soda, all we needed was some good music to help us through the winter of 1970. We spent it lazing in our living room upon garage sale sofas and chairs and sleeping on mattresses lying on the floor.

Once again, living with the vibrancy one feels when one is finally free from conflict, and within a buffer of distance, my relationship with Mom was comfortable. I visited often. Determined not to make the same mistakes she made with her mother, I made sure to always be there for her.

That year, I baked Christmas cookies. In between college classes, shifts at KFC, and the phone company, I stopped to drop them off. Mom's house was dark. There were no vehicles in the driveway. No one answered the door when I knocked. Mom seemed fine a few days before and had not mentioned her plans to go anywhere. Something was wrong. She never left home.

I peered through the windows, and my heart dropped as I viewed the vacant rooms beyond—the dark emptiness of their house and a devastating sense of the heartbreak of abandonment filled inside me. Stunned, I sat on the steps in the snow. Our mother had disappeared without telling us.

Why would she do that to Jim and me?

Neighbors reported they had fled in the middle of the night, with Donna, who was then a senior in high school. They were moments ahead of the repossession agents, the bill collectors, and everyone else who wanted a piece of them. Mom did not bother to tell anyone. I presumed Chuck had been involved in something serious since they were deep in hiding.

I needed an explanation. I spent weeks searching for them. It took over a month to find their unlisted phone number. They were living in an apartment in Beaverton, Oregon.

"Mom, I'm calling to see if you're all right," I said, masking the relief flooding through me upon finding her alive.

A few seconds of uncomfortable silence passed. Mom asked, "How did you find us?" There was no "How are you doing?" or "Are you okay?" Only "How did you find us?"

She spoke as if it were natural for parents to disappear without telling their children. The realization hit she was high again and unable to understand the emotional implications that her irresponsibility imposed upon Jim and me. It broke my heart. Then, she said, "I love you, Lindy. Come to Portland. Please, I think you'd like it here."

For weeks, deciding what to do weighed heavily upon me. One day, for no apparent reason except nothing glued me to remain in Wisconsin, I left. Giving whatever furniture and household items I accumulated to my roommate and packing what little I had left into my old, battered blue suitcase, I hitched a ride with a friend to O'Hare International in Chicago.

In exchange for a twenty-dollar bill, he dropped me off at the front door of United Airlines. Uncertainty filled deep inside as I watched him drive away. Second thoughts raced through my mind as I was standing on the sidewalk, deliberating what to do next. It was the desire for warmth, out of the icy Chicago wind, which begged for action. Gathering my things, I stepped inside.

Approaching the ticket counter, an enormous wave of anxiety hit. Frozen, I was unable to answer the agent when she asked my destination. A lump had developed in my throat. Needing time to think, I backed out of the line, and sat upon a chair, weighing, and balancing my options.

I could go to Portland, though nothing had changed. Same situation, different place. Mom still acted as bizarre and crazy as ever. That was not going to change. I could return to Menasha or stay with Jim, but it would not be fair to him. He was adapting back to civilian life after returning from his year in hell.

What I wanted was to be with the mother I once knew. It was an impossibility. Mom had again relapsed and had begun using drugs. All the grieving in the world could not change an addict or help me feel any better. The final possibility available was I could move forward and start anew. It presented itself as the riskiest choice, but it was more desirable than returning to my little house and all the other options I considered.

Needing commitment, starting anew was my rite of passage, a way to move forward and begin to take responsibility. I had to break from the pattern of bouncing back and forth with Mom. I did not know where to go.

No matter where I ended up, I was standing in the airport and already partway there. My bags packed, all I had to do was buy a ticket. I approached the counter.

"Where's a good place this time of year?" I asked the ticket agent.

"Miami, of course," he answered, looking at me carefully.

"Sounds good. May I get a ticket, please," I asked as I pulled my wallet out of my purse.

"You sure?" he asked, his eyes wrinkling with concern.

"As good a place as any," I answered.

I handed him a wad of money. Straightening it and putting it into the till he passed me back a few bills, I counted them. Six one-dollar bills. Enough for twenty to thirty eighteen cent fast-food hamburgers or several dozen cans of soup at a quarter each. Deciding if I found immediate work in a restaurant, I could get by.

Those first few weeks in the land of palm trees and sunshine, I spent many nights sleeping on hard floors, sofas, and patios of some good friends. I did not mind. As a child, we camped during our vacations. I learned young to sleep anywhere.

In the past, if there was one thing I cherished, it was the belief I had always held that if we keep faith in ourselves and believe that anything is possible, it is. Our parents constantly reinforced that thought. Both Jim and I subscribed to it, doggedly trying to master every challenge before us. No matter the past, offering me strength was the thought that Miami would be a suitable place to settle if the trend continued, and if I could make it so.

After a few weeks, I found a respectable job, sitting at a desk at the Miami Herald, working in their advertising department. Renting a room from a family who lived off the MacArthur Causeway, in a beautiful mansion on Palm Island, everything was working out beautifully.

Believing the only certainty we have is our will to live, and our ability to protect and care for those we love and ourselves requires that we accept ourselves for who and what we are. I realized I had to make my own choices for my life while still being available for those I loved during times of need. For me, it was an essential element of emotional survival.

One night, while sitting under a palm tree, with moonbeams kissing my shoulders and warm sand sifting through my toes, I gazed up at the moon. Reflecting on the past while gazing at the quiet waters, suddenly, an immense sense of gratitude struck. I realized how fortunate I was to have a safe place to live and a job I liked. For the first time in years, I felt comfortable, secure, and happy. Then an even bigger realization struck. There were not too many places in the country I could have chosen that were further from Portland, Oregon, and Carson City, Nevada, than Miami, Florida. I was learning to protect myself.

During the summer of 1971, I visited Mom in Oregon for a few weeks and then headed down to Central California with a friend. We had planned to get an apartment and work there that summer. There were no jobs. I spent a brief stint with "Up With People!" It wasn't the same. I had outgrown it.

Leaving the cast in Denver, I remained living there for a while and attended a semester of college before deciding to move to Boston, Massachusetts. In Boston, I worked for a stock brokerage firm in one of their back offices, processing trades.

Weekends offered me time to explore the museums and the living history of the city. A sense of familiarity existed everywhere in that part of Massachusetts, where my ancestors once lived. Everything I had learned from Grandma's history teachings about Boston, Salem, Haverhill, Marblehead, Ipswich, and Boxford came back. It was fresh in my mind, prompted by family names lettered on street signs, buildings, and upon the headstones in the ancient cemeteries, where they once lived. I felt a sudden sense of being rooted in who I was and where I was.

In Oregon, Mom was going through a reality check. Looking for something in Chuck's wallet, she glanced at his driver's license. Her heart stopped as she read that his birthdate reflected that he was fourteen years younger than her. Realizing he was only a few years older than her children, his long-termed deception sent her reeling.

Jim and I called it right. He was not a college graduate or a veteran. He did not even have a bachelor's degree, let alone a master's. There was never an academic or executive job offered or ever held in Wisconsin. An ex-wife and a child lived in Central California. The man's entire life was nothing more than an elaborate fabrication.

Devastated, Mom cried. "Oh my God, I married a kid," she grieved while trying to resolve why it occurred. Focusing on a single issue, his age, Mom remained in denial of his compulsive lying and deceit. It did not matter to her, nor did the fact that she married a stranger, someone who fabricated a life, a work history, and who possessed little motivation. Being forty-two-years-old, and dependent upon pharmaceutical drugs, Mom found herself handicapped, unable to manage the uncertainty she felt, and captured by the fear of contracting the cancers of her mother and grandmother.

Our mother saw few options for herself. She carried a lot of baggage that was too heavy for her to move, let alone to allow herself to have the confidence to seek someone else who would accept her as she was. Changing was not worth the effort.

Jim and I allowed Mom her dignity. We left her alone to wrestle with her decision. We never once mentioned our knowledge of it. Fortunately, good things happened during that first year they lived in the Pacific Northwest. Receiving a sudden windfall of cash, they rebuilt what they lost of Mom's divorce settlement. After buying two tracts of undeveloped land and an oceanfront home in Gleneden Beach, Oregon, Mom slipped right out of her depression.

She designed her homes with contemporary furniture and beautiful art, including an original Degas. Beneath coastal fog, a fleet of six Jaguars lined the driveway, rusting in the ever-constant rain. It was odd that Chuck seldom drove them but allowed them to waste away. He always hopped behind the wheel of his hideous little powder-blue Volkswagen convertible. My bet was the cars belonged to someone other than him.

Mom and Chuck were busy adopting a family of their own, four adorable children from Korea: Bill, Stephanie, David, and Amy. Often staying at their home, I cared for the children. Mom was not enthusiastic about parenting them. Chuck left her alone. He disappeared for days at a time. Neither were psychologically or physically equipped to care for a young family.

To please Mom, I had recently married, at her insistence, to someone she chose, not someone I loved. Giving up on any hope of a long-term relationship and someone coming to rescue me, I did the same as she did to please her mother. It was an endless pattern of tradition throughout the generations of women in our family, for the daughters to marry young, to satisfy their parents. Besides helping them, it was the only expectation of me. And, anxious to please my mother, I settled for who and what she felt was best for me.

In Mom's youth, marriage was often impulsive, offering security for the woman and convenience for the man, who, more than likely, had returned from military service. Not so for me. Neither the man my mother accepted for me nor getting married was attractive. I had been waiting for someone to come and rescue me. But it never happened. We lived in the real world, and not as characters in a fairy tale.

Opting for her approval, which I desperately needed, I did what she felt was best. For years, she insisted I marry, ever since graduating from high school. She expected little more than that from me. The three months of marriage was a nightmare. The same as Mom, her mother, and others, it didn't last.

We had lived for only a few weeks in Salem when my husband went to the beach to work. Seeing him seldom, I continued living in my apartment and working there, paying the bills. Returning two months later, and during a night of anger, I made an insensitive comment that offended him. He slammed his fist into my face. Fleeing outside, but not fast enough while descending the stairs, he slammed his hands into my back. I lost my balance and tumbled down the concrete steps onto the sidewalk.

The next day, instead of coming directly home from work, I tenderly stepped upon a bus that took me downtown and rented a room at the YWCA. That evening, I met with an attorney. We filed a police report. Sheriff's officers served my husband with annulment documents and a restraining order within forty-eight hours.

In my follow-up appointment with my physician, through the bruises were healing, nausea hadn't gone away.

Circumstances, those pesky matters in life which crop up, that we have little control over, but we must face and resolve, are sometimes difficult to confront. Sometimes we need to revisit those situations in retrospect to obtain a view of what occurred through different eyes. Studying them carefully and looking at the positive that comes from tragedy and devastation, we can pick ourselves up and find a gold lining somewhere, especially during a later period of crisis.

Doing so is the foundation of survival, extracting the good from something that initially seems dark and impossible to conquer. I didn't realize it until a few days later, when sitting alone, in a semi-bare apartment with the empty cupboards my ex left behind.

Monumental was the realization to come that leaving was the best thing I could have ever done. It imposed an enormous impact on my life. While sleeping in the only thing left in that room, a big orange, vinyl bean bag chair, the telephone rang.

It was my doctor, announcing I was seven or eight weeks pregnant, and, fortunately, my unborn child was unaffected by what occurred that night. As I looked around the room, I noted it was no longer empty. The news I received had filled it with the hope of new life.

I helped Mom and Chuck for over six months, moving in during the last month of my pregnancy. One night, Mom and I battled over her abusive treatment of the second oldest. She was high and extremely harsh. I stepped in, grabbing the leather belt she was using to spank her. Mom attacked me. That night, I left with my three-month-old daughter, only seeing Mom seldom.

The savings I had collected during the prior two years, I had lent to Mom for the down payment for her house. Leaving, I knew I would never see it again. In the grander scheme of everything happening, it didn't matter. I didn't feel it was the right place for my infant to stay.

The next day, I spoke to a social worker about the situation where our mother and the kids lived. They contacted the kids' schools and arranged for the teachers to watch over them. It was one less worry.

Judi and I moved into a little apartment in Gresham, Oregon. Close to everything, it was comfortable and allowed a renewed sense of independence. I spent my spare time with my daughter in the wilds of Oregon. They were exhilarating. There, the stress of living with Mom had dissipated. I was again free to hike in the hills as I had done as a child. I was still captured with the same magical enchantment the mountains offered, as I was when younger.

Trekking for miles, without meeting another person, it was peaceful to hear only my feet crunching over pine needle-covered earth in the silence of the ancient forests. With the appearance of dawn, the mountains transformed into a sanctuary, filled with magic as the morning fog rolled in and out of the towering trees. There, one's sense of strength and empowerment becomes refueled, merely by standing amid a cedar grove that has endured a millennium, leading back to hundreds of years before the Age of Enlightenment. Realizing my place in this world where life has existed "forever," it was clear "forever" lasted longer than a second. The forest was a place where I could get lost in it and wander through my mind without feeling any discomfort.

Chapter Eleven

LOSS

The most beautiful people I've known are those who have known trials, have known struggles, have known loss, and have found their way out of the depths. —Elizabeth Kübler-Ross

Jim and I remained in contact with Dad over the years, mostly calling him at work. Donna, not so much. It was on and off. On with us staying connected with him several times a month by telephone, and off when we wanted to see him, him due to the tenuous situation that existed at his home with his wife.

At forty-four years old, when most fathers are seeing their children off to college and preparing to retire in the next decade or two, Dad was again raising a young family, working at a demanding job, and trying to achieve recognition as an accomplished builder, while living on a single income. It was far more complicated than when he was younger.

Dad had now worked on the construction and improvement of several homes, three in Carson City, one in Orinda, and a more substantial home overlooking Carson Valley. In the seven years prior, the efforts required a significant financial and personal investment of time and labor, on top of his commitment to working fulltime in an executive management position at Pacific Telephone. The stress was beginning to take its toll. Exhausted, he often slept during his lunch hour with his head resting in his arms on top of his desk.

In November of 1973, we received a call reporting that Dad's physicians hospitalized him after suffering a heart attack. Jim, Donna, and I at once responded, converging upon Carson City, and meeting in the hospital's lobby. Assuring him of our love and concern, we were there to support him any way we could. Amazingly, Dad was doing well and seemed in good spirits. Making his rounds that morning, the doctor asked how he was feeling. Dad responded solemnly, as he answered.

"Whenever I get up, I teeter forward, then I reel backward, then I sway forward…

Concerned, Dad's doctor asked, "Why do you think that's happening?"

"My pajama bottoms are too long," was Dad's forlorn answer.

Accustomed to being active, when he was bored, Dad thought of ways to keep those around him, amused. As children, when adversity hit, it was

Dad's sense of humor that always got us through the challenging times. We learned to do the same as we aged.

"Sometimes all you can do is laugh, Lindy. It's good medicine," he said.

That night, we chipped in to buy a bucket of fried chicken for dinner. Dad's spouse insisted on paying for it. "Your father plans to leave everything to me in a trust when he dies. I'll have it all spent by the time you ever see it. So, why don't you just let me pay for this, huh?" she stated.

Her icy, self-absorbed comment placed a damper upon the evening. We did not understand why *she* decided to tell us what she did, when she did. For some reason, it was important to her, and she needed to take over control of our relationship with our father. It wasn't anything intended to offer comfort. It upset us to hear her cold comment while Dad was recovering from heart problems. His wife was contemplating what she would receive from his death, while we were praying for his recovery and fearing his loss.

We were now young adults that were once children who never asked or expected anything from our parents. That night, we still paid for our meal, continuing our longstanding practice of paying our way. Fortunately, Dad didn't die. It was all we wanted. He lived another twenty-three years with more vitality than ever before. Even retiring from his work, he did not slow down.

When Dad called early one morning, in February of 1974, three months following his heart attack, and a few weeks after my daughter was born, I intuitively knew something was wrong. He had not called in months and had never done so, that early.

"Lindy, I have some sad news," he said, pausing for a few seconds. Detecting something was wrong, my heart began to race.

Oh, my gosh, Grandma.

Dad sputtered, "Lindy, Danny died."

The devastation and heartbreak his voice revealed, along with the anguish and grief of words, shattered my heart. He spoke for a few moments while I listened until there was a lengthy period of uncomfortable silence.

"Would you like me to come, Dad?" I asked, breaking the quiet.

"Please. I need you," Dad said instantly.

Our father had always said he loved us. With that, he never wavered. I held no doubt of his love. However, I do not recall him ever saying we were he needed, until that day.

Later, I pondered the question as I contemplated how different our family was from other others. We asked for permission to support our parents during times of crisis. Most do not.

Upon my arrival, I noted Dad appeared in control. It was easy for me to tell he was experiencing immense grief, as he had once taught me to do, I realized he was compartmentalizing emotions and working hard at being the glue holding everybody together. Dad was consoling and supplying support for the surrounding people, but he was not receiving anything from anywhere, for himself. His wife was unable to concentrate on anything but herself.

Comfort is something often evasive when one becomes buried in grief. Dad and I spoke quietly in the backyard. While grieving the loss of his son, I could hear the constant ring of the telephone. Embroiled in a local political campaign for public office, people were calling Dad to ask for information on his platform. He was unable to speak with them.

"Need help with it?"

"I don't know. None of that matters anymore, Lindy," he stated despondently. "Right now, I just don't want to go back in there," he said, nodding toward the house. "I'm just trying to get through today, baby doll," he said. "I can't think any further than that."

"That's okay, Dad. You don't have to. All you have to do is what you feel you need to do to get past this, no matter how hard it is." His tear-filled eyes tugged at my heart. Dad was finally letting out the agonizing pain of loss that was tearing him up. We remained in the yard for a good forty-five minutes that afternoon until he could get himself together.

"That hug and getting away from in there for a while is what I needed most, Lindy," he said. "Thank you for being here, even after everything that has happened."

"I love you, Dad," I told him. "That's what families do. They look after one another."

He looked upon me for a moment and, with his eyes flooded with tears, nodded.

"Yes, it is," he agreed.

Jim and I sat beside one another in the same pews of the rear of St. Teresa's Church, where we attended as children, behind Dad, his wife, her parents, and her daughter. It was dark and quiet. The priests crossed the threshold into the church, wearing long, white robes. Stepping aside, they made way for Danny's tiny white casket to pass. Trailing it, the procession headed toward the altar, the priests chanting prayers and swinging bowls of incense as they walked behind it.

Afterward, we met at a saloon in the historic town of Genoa, where our parents had once planned to live. Our table was quiet. There was not much to say. Sitting in silence, we tightly gripped our wine glasses and mostly gazed out the window.

It is hard to find the right words to bring comfort when one's four-year-old child dies of an undiagnosed swelling to the brain. What can one do to help one's parents who are in immense grief, besides merely being there?

Words are not enough. Little eases the pain, even the passage of time doesn't work. The most loving thing anyone can do to be there and listen, and that is what Jim and I did.

In the days following, Dad would go to Danny's grave and work on its landscaping, sobbing the entire time. He worked through his grief privately, by keeping busy and often speaking with us on the telephone. It was difficult for Dad to hold everyone up and not be able to express his agony. Though he seldom saw us, Jim and I became his sounding boards.

Everyone, at some point in their life, experiences loss. Each of us handles it differently. Some of us are blessed with resilience, bouncing back, while others remain frozen in place and are not capable of movement in any direction. And, sometimes, those we love are gone from us, long before they die, like Mom. We never stopped grieving the loss of her, and we never gave up hope that she would get better and come back, "someday."

Dad managed his problems by putting everything behind him with distraction and fighting off the demons whenever they attacked, while Mom fled reality. I still don't know how we handled it if we ever did. We were young and used to hopping from one crisis to the next.

In later years, my thoughts reflected upon Danny's death, every time I worked with a parent who had lost a child who was affected by Constitutional Mismatch Repair Deficiency (CMMRD), also known as Biallelic Mismatch Repair Deficiency (BMMRD).

A subset of Lynch syndrome, CMMRD, is a predisposition to cancer that sometimes affects the children of two parents who are affected by Lynch syndrome. In the past several years, physicians have diagnosed 270 children, and a lesser number of adults, as suffering from it.

This subset of Lynch syndrome presents with aggressive brain cancers, hematological cancers, colorectal cancers, and the other cancers of Lynch syndrome. A hallmark may include the appearance of café au lait marks.

Being born with café au lait marks is not unusual. Many, like me, have been born with them. Sometimes they appear at birth and sometimes at a later age. The tan or brown colored spots on the skin are ordinarily oval.

Born with one that was sizeable, mine shrunk to the size of the head of a finishing nail, following chemotherapy. Most are harmless, yet a rare few may show a hereditary condition. Being born with one does not mean a child is affected by CMMRD. Nonetheless, if there is a history of cancer on both sides of the family, the parents should consult with their physician and request an appointment with a genetics specialist to assess the risk of their child.

Until further research occurs, no one knows for sure what patterns of symptoms exist in children with a history of cancer in both parents. It is not likely robust research that can detect childhood hereditary cancers predispositions will occur any time soon until the provision of more funding reaches child cancer research centers, and until more children are tested for hereditary cancers.

The key organization researching CMMRD and conducting research is "Sick Kids" in Toronto, Canada. Being the top global center for CMMRD research, treatment, and care, their website is comprehensive. In the past few years, they have developed an international consortium on CMMRD and are learning more about it to keep affected children healthy.

LovealwaysBeccaJean.org is a Georgia-based nonprofit organization that supports the research efforts of "Sick Kids" and families affected by CMMRD and Lynch syndrome.

Most of the diagnoses of children with CMMRD occur *after* contracting cancer. Doesn't it make sense to practice prevention, rather than allow a child to contract cancer, especially when childhood hereditary cancer can be prevented? Doesn't it make sense to allow parents to have the knowledge of their child's condition and to enable them to make that choice so they may protect their children?

During the past twelve years, I have met dozens of parents who have lost their minor children to Lynch syndrome cancers. I know many more who are practicing preventative measures to keep their children healthy and alive, especially since most were not aware that they, themselves, had a mutated gene until their child received their diagnosis with cancer.

The social factors affecting individuals and families with hereditary cancers have yet to be recognized by genetic experts. Most genetic counselors have only seen a handful of patients. Seldom do they meet the members of the families of the patients, unless it is to test them. Primarily trained as scientific research assistants, they are brilliant scientists and genetic educators. They are not psychological counselors. They have not been provided the social science backgrounds or the educations and learned skills to provide psychological counseling to patients.

It is an undeniable fact that individuals with cancer seek one another out for support. Many cancer survivors marry other survivors and bear children, as our parents did during the eugenics era. If both have a mutated mismatch repair gene and have little or no knowledge of CMMRD, it could present in their children. It is crucial for everyone with Lynch syndrome, who wants to marry, to learn the family history of cancer of their loved one, and for both to obtain genetic testing.

The estimated numbers of children affected with CMMRD are questionable because of the professional standards of genetic counselors that discourage the genetic testing of children. Many have died from their cancers. But today, some are living longer, with diagnosis, screenings, and prompt treatment. There are middle-aged adults, today, who are now known to be living, diagnosed with CMMRD.

Since many genetic counselors frown upon the genetic testing of children, nobody knows the actual number of children under the age of eighteen that are affected by Lynch syndrome. We are more than likely speaking of thousands globally.

Every one of us with Lynch syndrome was a child at one time. Most of us grew up in a family affected by some "family cancer thing." It is almost impossible to hide the existence of cancer in a family from children, especially when a high prevalence of the disease is present. It is naïve to think children would not realize something different in their family than that in the families of others. Many of us grew up not knowing a grandparent. Many of us cared for a parent, or other loved one affected by cancer. When one contracts cancer, it affects an entire family, and that is when children gain strength and empowerment, being part of a team. When the knowledge is not provided, and cancer in a family is kept secret, it can be devastating. In families, it is a complicated secret to keep with the regular screenings, the testing in laboratories, and the appointments with various specialists that patients must keep. It is even more complicated when a family member is ill.

A recent guideline published by the ACCR (American Association for Cancer Research) developed by genetic counselors, states, "Referral for genetic counseling should be made at the time of tumor diagnosis so that genetic testing can be completed promptly."

This one statement is an enormous barrier for Lynch syndrome families, having to wait for the diagnosis of cancer in their children to allow them to test. If a parent is allowed the opportunity of knowing if their child is at risk, they can protect the life of that child and take preventative measures to detect cancer at an early stage, in the same manner, they protect everyone else.

The guideline continues, stating, "Genetic testing for adult-onset conditions in children should not be undertaken without medical or psychosocial justification and a discussion with family members, although pathogenic variants in adult-onset cancer genes may be revealed by large panels, tumor-based testing or whole exome/genome analysis as an incidental finding."

It is an unrealistic policy. As said earlier, many genetic counselors do not have a background in psychological counseling or even training in crisis or conflict resolution counseling. The three credit units involving psychosocial issues required by most of the genetic counseling masters' programs are not actual psychological training courses used to obtain licensure to perform psychological counseling to determine "psychosocial justification," or to make a qualified psychological assessment of others, in most states.

The guidelines of the AAP (American Academy of Pediatrics) and the ACMG, (American College of Medical Genetics) initiated in 2018 conflict with that of the genetic counselors. They read, "The *AAP/ACMG guidance gives parents wide leeway for conditions that present at any point in childhood because parents are the presumptive decision-makers for their minor children.* Genetic counseling can *help* parents decide when this testing is appropriate for their child, and the decision to test the child in this scenario at either age should be respected." These two determinations, one by genetic counselors, the second by medical professionals involved with the American Association of Pediatricians, and the American College of Genetics, sit at polar ends of one another.

Some parents have relayed their genetic counselors have told them it would be "immoral" to for them to test their children genetically. Reports of these occurrences had come from all parts of the country. There is a united thought, despite the guidelines of the ACMG and the ACP, not to test children until they have reached the age of eighteen. This informal policy leads to a presumption that parents of those with Lynch syndrome are incapable of making sound decisions for their children. It reflects the same attitudes of paternalism seen during the eugenics movement.

Paternalism in counseling occurs when counselors interfere with the right of self-determination of individuals to protect themselves from self-harm, or harm to their children. To assess the parent as immoral because their beliefs are different is a paternalistic practice. No person should judge the morality of a person based upon a difference in opinion regarding the management of their children's health.

One child dying is far too many when genetic testing to prevent cancer is available and is key to our survival. Knowing who and what we are and having an excellent medical team, robust health coverage, and with the grace of God, we can live like anyone else, *and* we can protect our families.

Chapter Twelve

WALKING AWAY

"Have the courage to walk away, those that value you will want you back, and those that do not won't hold you back."
—Trevor Driggers

During February 1975, my daughter and I moved back to Carson City. Since Danny's death, I had seen Dad often. He even visited me once in my Oregon home. After, Dad suggested I move back to Carson City. He wanted to be a part of our lives.

I was living with my daughter in Oregon. Donna was going to college in Forest Grove, eighty-five miles away. Mom and Chuck had pulled another quiet middle of the night disappearance act, following an unexpected visit from some unsavory characters bearing weapons. Again, I only discovered their absence upon finding their home vacant when stopping by to check in with Mom.

This time, it was not as devastating as the last. During the past few years, Mom had become more unpredictable and, during times of anger, had become volatile. After two decades of prescription drug abuse, her actions resulted in our desensitization to them. I did worry about the children, though. Every time I saw them, they seemed happy and well.

Donna reported they moved to Spain. Their exact whereabouts were unknown, but it did not matter where they lived anymore. It might as well have been to the Arctic. My mother had become a stranger to us.

Leery of uprooting myself from our cozy apartment in Oregon, deciding to move was not easy. Though Dad had spent years without active involvement with us, he had readily embraced the role of being a grandfather to my daughter. He remembered her at Christmas and on her first birthday. It was a dramatic change since he had only remembered our birthdays sporadically.

Not much had changed with his living circumstances. "Hap, don't you give those ungrateful kids anything!" his wife would still berate him in a reminder, loud enough to us to hear, as he spoke with us on the telephone.

Moving to Carson City was a risk, but if in doing it, the risk should be on someone that one has known for a lifetime. Everyone deserves second chances. During that visit with them, I decided to do it. It was best if we lived closer to family members.

I worked hard at keeping a relationship with Dad and with those in his second family, trying to remain close after the loss of their child. Facilitating the adoption of their youngest daughter, I made it a point to stay in constant touch with Dad. I was there if they were in need, making sure not to ask for anything for my daughter or me.

I drove into Carson City, down the icy roads, and through mountain snowstorms, in early February, with furniture tied to the top of my fourteen-year-old 1961 Chevy Bel Air, with the rusted holes in the floorboards. All the essentials I needed were with me, selling all else before moving.

Upon arrival, I rented a large, furnished room for my daughter and me, on the second floor of an old, rundown Victorian mansion. It was perfect. The house offered kitchen privileges, and I did not need much to start again. It was a great temporary fix until I could find a job, settle into an apartment, and find reliable daycare for my daughter. As it had been for my parents and my grandparents, at that age, a humble life was good enough. Preferring to keep some distance and to continue exercising independence, doing it myself offered a layer of insulation from any conflict from his wife, that I dearly desired to avoid.

Dad's efforts at trying to make my life easier, in any way he could, didn't go unnoticed. After breathing in gas fumes while driving my fourteen-year-old Chevy, he offered me his old, blue station wagon that he was unable to trade-in due to the cost of repair of some of its mechanical issues. Having bought a new car, he wanted the old one out of his driveway.

"Here's your Christmas gift for the last ten years," he said, laughing as he handed me the car keys. "I've been saving it for you. Unfortunately, it is worth a little less than the cost of repairing and registering it."

"It's great, Dad," I laughed, hugging him. "Thank you!"

Though the cost of vehicle registration and mechanical repairs *did* exceed its value and almost wiped out all my savings, the thought that came with the sad looking, massive, old blue station wagon warmed my heart. It came from my father.

"Once you get it fixed, you should be able to drive it... for a while," he laughed. "I know it's not much, but at least you won't be asphyxiated."

A "while" was precisely how long it lasted; about six months later, I needed to buy another vehicle. Its transmission was slipping, and I didn't have the money to pay for it. The cost of those initial repairs was far more than a down-payment for a newer, more reliable vehicle. I was conflicted because the sentiment that came with the old car was priceless.

With a heavy heart, I traded it in for a little, older green Toyota, once I had gotten the mechanical issues Dad had experienced with it, resolved. Dad thought it was a great trade. His wife, of course, complained that I was "ungrateful." I didn't have a driveway to warehouse a nonoperative vehicle.

Following the death of a loved one, we often realize the value of relationships and the attempts to compensate for not prioritizing them. A transformation had occurred within Dad. Time was healing the effects of the emotional roller coaster ride he had experienced. It encouraged him to invest more effort into his relationships with us.

Lord knows how much I had longed to return to bask in the comfort of living where I had as a child. Awakening beneath the towering mountains was heavenly, taking in deep breaths of fresh air. I missed wearing Levi's and T-shirts, smelling the sweetness of the sagebrush following a spring rain and camping amidst the big pines.

Here, once again, living underneath an endless sky where I could see forever, the priority was to find work. In Carson City, jobs were rare—at least in the positions that I had previously held, working for corporate presidents or in the trading rooms of securities firms.

Having worked in offices, full time, since the age of seventeen, it was where I felt comfortable. Edging my way up, holding excellent recommendations from former employers, it was clear I would be starting back at the bottom. "Any port in a storm" was the way I looked at it. I was willing to do anything to support my child.

The positions I once held were nonexistent in Carson City for someone my age. The State of Nevada was the city's largest employer. Most of their jobs either required a degree or were entry-level typing positions that barely covered living expenses. Promotions came from within the agency.

Hoping to find work as a waitress on the graveyard shift, my thought was I could spend my days attending college classes and being a mom to my one-year-old daughter during the day when she was awake. It only took a few days to find one as a food server. Solely supporting a child, I was not fussy about how I made a living. Caring for my daughter came before my ego. Again, any port in a storm.

Within a few months, this led to cocktail waitressing, from six o'clock in the evening, after dropping Judi off at her daycare providers' home until two in the morning. After catching a few hours of sleep, I arose, picked up Judi by seven in the morning, and caught up on my sleep by napping with her in the afternoon. Not only did I work nights, but I adapted to sleeping on a split shift. It was easier than I thought it might be.

Within a few weeks, Judi and I moved into a furnished apartment in an older complex, the same where Dad lived when he and Mom divorced ten years earlier. Far from glamorous, it was clean, affordable, and "mine." I was proud to do it alone. I felt an incredible sense of pride.

With our living situation and Judi's daycare needs resolved, the next priority was to challenge thirty general education units at the community college through the CLEP process. It reduced a year of the four-year average time to get a degree. Added to the other units I had collected, and by combining credits, I was a few credits shy of being able to attain an associate degree. My biggest dilemma was deciding upon a major at whatever university I decided to attend. I still did not know where I would be in the future, let alone what I would do as a fulltime career. Living one day at a time, it was easier for me to "go with the flow."

Since leaving Carson City, I had traveled full circle, returning to where the happiest moments of childhood occurred. If I learned anything, it is to measure the quality of life through the relationships we share with those we love. Old friendships became renewed, and I cultivated new ones. Returning to the simple Nevada lifestyle and feeling the comfort of driving down familiar streets, I focused on the dreams of my child attending the same schools as me.

I ran into that red-headed, kid again, the one I insisted I would marry when I was three years old. Working as a cocktail server at a local casino, I glanced up from the table I was clearing and noticed him leaning against the bar. He seemed familiar.

Hanging around until I was off work, he introduced himself to me as I was getting off-shift. We drank coffee and talked in the restaurant until dawn. Walking toward my car, the sun was rising in the east, casting a pink and golden glow upon the clouds. There would be little sleep before picking up my daughter from her care provider, but I did not mind.

He and I shared much in common, a passion for autumn, being outdoors, and our attachment to the small town where we were both raised in a down to earth and humble family. Each of us held lofty wishes for "someday." That one night developed into an almost two-year relationship.

Despite all our similarities, we were vastly different people. I was coming up on my twenty-second birthday; he had turned twenty-eight. Though growing up in the same neighborhood in our younger years, our experiences differed.

Graduating from Carson City schools, he entered the military. Returning from service in Vietnam, and attending college in Reno, he moved back and began working in the career he desired. In age and maturity, he was light years ahead of me. He had already embarked upon the career that he had always wanted.

Bouncing around from state to state, and job to job, later becoming a single mom supporting a child, and trying to catch a college class, here and there, when possible, I was more of a free spirit. Having no clue what my future may hold, I was not worried about it. Like my mother, my biggest issue was facing difficulty with imagining "forever." I was living "today" with an insatiable sense of urgency.

Relationships often bring complications for those raised in a cancer family. Questions and self-doubts about my worthiness always flew through my mind, not just with him but with every man I met. Would he be concerned about how my health situation would affect us? Would he be alone with children, "someday?"

Could he afford me and the medical costs if I inherited the cancers of my parents? Would he leave me if I were to be like my aunt and my grandfather and contract cancers as they did? The unknowns in my life were many. My desire to be comfortable in a relationship resulted more from a need to be secure than anything else. Like Mom and Dad, I, too, kept hearing a ticking clock.

Carrying too much baggage for anyone to manage, especially me, I was needy. Realizing the pressure, I had always placed upon the men with whom I chose to be involved; I no longer felt it was fair to them. There was not much I could do about my circumstances. Most of it was out of my control. Statistics showed marriages with individuals who face chronic diseases were not successful. Seventy-five percent end up in divorce. Fearing that, I sabotaged potential relationships before they left me upon finding out how much baggage I carried around.

It was my mistaken belief that few people place bets upon persons with unknown hereditary health conditions, especially one as serious as cancer. Life is not a fairy tale. Reality has shown, "happily, ever after" is rare with those involved with my circumstance, at least it was in our family.

When young, I would lose myself in the adventures of Alice as she journeyed through the looking glass in *Alice in Wonderland*. I shared her concerns when she once asked the White Rabbit, "How long *is* forever?"

He provided her with an opaque answer. "Sometimes, just one second."

It all comes down to time and timing. Many affected by chronic, life-threatening conditions cherish time. A second can sometimes seem like "forever" one day, and like nothing, the next. Those two and one-half years spent in Carson City filled me with some of the most memorable and some of the most painful seconds of self-awareness I had been through, including acknowledging my fear and feelings of inadequacy.

Much of what I experienced in Carson City filled me with confidence, a reinforced spirit of independence, and the ability to make better decisions as a young, single parent. I learned how to walk away from people and relationships. The consequences of allowing myself to get close to someone supplied me with some of the best experiences I could ever have in learning how to protect myself and my child.

"Lindy, don't ever postpone your life for anyone, especially for a man. Learn to protect yourself and put yourself first," Dad consoled as I agonized. He admired how hard I worked to be independent and understood the magnitude of what I tried to do on my own without asking for his help.

The level of confusion I underwent while dealing with personal matters caused Dad's concern. "Please promise you will never do this again. And whatever you do, do not speak with your stepmother about it. You can always call me. All she does afterward is harp on me and complain about you guys."

"Dad, she has no right to judge *me*, not after what this family has been through because of her," I snapped at him.

Immediately, I regretted my comment, wishing that I had been a little more cautious and sensitive with my words.

"I didn't mean…" he stammered.

"I know what you meant, Dad," I said, more gently. "Don't worry about it. It's nothing new. You do what you must do, and if the relationship between you and me creates difficulties for your wife, then you and she need to do something about it. It has nothing to do with me. I'm a big girl who can care for myself and Judi without anyone's help. I've proven that. The only ones who can resolve this are you and her. It's doubtful that she is interested in making life easier for any of us."

"She's just insecure, Lindy," Dad again commented.

"That is her problem and shouldn't be mine. I'm not a part of it. Then, she needs to get help."

Her issue was far more extensive than that of being "insecure." It was obvious. "Dad, It has been going on for ten years, and nothing's going to change. *That* is the reality," I said. "Her 'insecurity thing,' which we both know minimizes her problems, doesn't justify what she does, and I'm tired of it.

"Oh, Lindy," he begged.

"My relationship is with you, and it is not on her terms, or their terms, or when anyone allows it, but on yours and mine. I'm tired of her control over our relationship, Dad."

"I am too, Lindy," he softly admitted.

Suddenly, I felt guilty. My father was in a tight spot. He had violated his own rule and "had gotten himself into something he couldn't get himself out of."

Softening up, I said, "Dad, my concern is what's best for you. I can't even imagine what you go through."

Suddenly, it hit me. Dad knew I was preparing to leave Carson City. For a long time, I had felt the situation was far too dysfunctional, and after a decade of hurt, it was not a good place for us to be.

The tension was heavy in Dad's truck, as it became clear to him that the submissive daughter he had always known, no longer existed. I was now the independent woman he raised.

"Aren't I the one who should be saying that?" Dad asked. "I don't want to lose you again, Lindy."

He was, but it was not necessary. There was no need to beat him up. Instead, I threw my hands up into the air and looked toward the heavens to hold back the tears, as I nervously laughed. "I'm not even going to go there. You are never going to lose me, Dad. No matter where I am, I will always love you."

Circumstances weighed heavily upon my siblings and me, after the ending of our family. Like a ghost, Dad floated in of our lives and out while we three spent ours trying to resolve why he never stayed. We grew up believing we would never know.

Dad's words broke my heart. It saddened me that he felt pressured to choose between his wife and his children. People who love someone don't put them in that situation. I decided to keep working at it, for him, and me, despite the dwindling hope for any opportunity to revitalize that positive, ongoing relationship we once had during my childhood.

The two of us put a lot of effort into our relationship. Dad realized as I did that nothing would change unless he also made some meaningful changes in his life. After our conversation, he dropped by work and my apartment more often. On one occasion, Judi had become ill, facing difficulty breathing. Admitted into the hospital, they fitted her with breathing apparatuses to help with respiration issues.

The days spent sitting in the drafty hallway, while they worked on her, were difficult. Without being asked, Dad arrived and sat with me during those tense hours, making sure I did not have to be alone.

Later, he would stop by when I got off shift from work. Drinking coffee, we shared a few minutes discussing our week. One afternoon, glancing up at the enormous mirror of the back-bar in front of me, I spotted Dad's wife angrily marching toward us.

"Uh, oh. You've been busted," I alerted him. "Didn't you get permission to have coffee with me?"

Dad peered up at the mirror. "Oh, no," he groaned. "What in the hell is she doing here?"

As his wife angrily approached, he spun around on his stool to meet her hostile glare, that was drilling through him.

"I knew you were with another woman," she confronted, her voice raised.

The bartenders stopped working, captured by the confrontation, as did my friends and co-workers. Confused, I glanced up at her and groaned in embarrassment, burying my head in my arms, on the counter, as she continued her outburst.

Another woman?

"How could you do this to me?" she demanded. Dad sat silently on his barstool, his hands tightly cupping his coffee cup, and his eyes filled with confusion. The expressions on the faces of my co-workers were priceless as they sat silent, their eyes rolling back and forth, watching the show.

What is she talking about?

My facial expression had turned to one of sheer horror by the time I watched her turn and stomp away. Dad's expression had transformed into one of amusement. He broke out into a burst of hearty laughter.

Now, what is wrong with him?

"I'm sorry, Lindy. I am so embarrassed. I never thought she would do this here, not here at your work," he offered, still laughing.

"No big deal, Dad. It is not like it is the first time."

"Ah, come on, Lindy," he begged.

"Every single time you are with any of us, she does this," I said. "We weren't even allowed to speak with you on the phone when we were younger."

"I don't think she recognized you," he answered, chuckling.

"Dad, she is possessive and flipping jealous of any attention you give to anyone other than her and her kids."

Silence overcame him for a moment.

"Well, aren't you even going to go talk to her?" I confronted.

"Uh-uh, not right now," he answered, beginning to laugh again. "It's best to wait until things calm down. And, Lindy, before you ask me again, I will tell you this, right now, I *am* getting tired of this."

There was not anything he could do except give her time to cool down. Dad was as desensitized to her actions as we were. The out of control, angry public exhibitions had become a pattern.

Dad was a man of commitment to the women he loved. He was the kind of guy who chipped away at the problems until there was nothing left of himself. Men like him are the ones who die with memories of conflict and dreams unfulfilled. It was hell for him when she forced him to choose between his wife and the children of his former marriage.

Regardless of what *he* was willing to accept, I was questioning what I could continue to take since it had now affected my work. For a while, I took a lot of teasing about being "the other woman" in my father's life. The problems he and I had with her were no longer a private matter.

My fear of a repeat performance contributed to distancing from Dad. It was what she wanted. Dad didn't come around after work anymore to avoid another public confrontation. The demands upon him, when at home, did not allow time to spend with my daughter and me.

Unable to get past the embarrassment, I finally quit my job and chose to work in an office. My goal had surpassed that of being able to attend college part-time while working fewer hours, to that of becoming someone who would be viewed by others as being more socially acceptable. The priority had changed to the quest for gaining the approval of others. Somewhere along the way, my sense of self-esteem had been severely damaged.

Working in an office fulltime, as a hostess in a restaurant on weekends, and participating in my Nevada National Guard drills, didn't allow for much time for anything else. I lived with urgency, racing time to put into my life, everything I needed.

It is interesting how time plays a significant part in the lives of those who walk on a tightrope. We pour as much of our hearts and souls into the spaces of silence between the ever-constant ticking of a clock. Sensitive to the fact "forever" and "someday" are not guaranteed, for anyone, let alone those like us, many of us realize living offers risks, not guarantees. Life is all about people and the relationships we have with one another. They take risk and effort. Without reciprocation, there is no respect, no trust, and, without either, there is no relationship.

Jim and I never played into the conflict in the manner Dad and his wife did. We did not have an appetite for it or for the drama she continuously created to get what she wanted. We each managed our one life with a wild sense of urgency, trying to squeeze every second of experiences we could from it. We hungered for distractions and the sense of empowerment we gained from them. Donna, not so much. She lived a different lifestyle, like that of Mom. We all sought out partners who felt little emotion and who were distant, not allowing the ability to grow close. If relationships didn't work, due to the circumstances, it was meant to be.

I decided to take a step back, to move on and work on my original goals. If Plan A was not enough, Plan B was in the wings. Dad taught us well to cover our bases. I did not always know what Plan B was, but I wasn't worried. Things always worked out for the better.

Moving to Steamboat Springs fifteen miles away, I quit my jobs and again worked three days a week cocktail waitressing, in Reno, making far more than I did working in an office and my other two jobs. I felt happier than I had in a long time. Getting my carefree life back and being able to be with my daughter more, created a safe and distant place from the past. Finally, it allowed me to take my time to decide my next course of action was to be who and what I was or thought I was, with a focus on who and what I wanted to be.

That Thanksgiving, Judi contracted the chickenpox. Dad called and asked if she could come to their house for dinner. I advised she would love to, but she was sick.

The next call was from his wife, screaming on the telephone, accusing me of lying. "You're just trying to keep her away from us."

I invited her over to see my extremely ill toddler, who was burning up with a fever and infested with red dots and brown scabs. She declined and hung up on me. It was the final straw in my dealings with them. Considering Dad's advice, I put into motion Plan B, after Judi got better, I acted. Packing what I owned and tossing my towheaded youngster into the back seat of my little Toyota, I quit my job and headed west to join my siblings.

It was late afternoon in early December 1976 when Jim arrived at the tiny, seventy-year-old Altadena, California Craftsman cottage, where our father grew up. He laughed as he found Judi, and I slumped upon the sofa, our arms crossed behind our heads, and our feet kicked up on Grandma's coffee table.

"Hey, Jim!" Leaping up and giving him a big hug, I stepped back, adding, "You need to do something about the security in this place, a*nybody* can get in."

Jim laughed. "You're staying here for a while, right?

"Until I can find one of my own; if it's still okay."

"Take your time, Sis."

"Thanks. It shouldn't be long. Judi should graduate from high school in about, uh, let's see, maybe fifteen years, unless she is like me," I said with a straight face. "Then, well, maybe a little longer."

"Okay…" he uttered with feigned uncertainty, softened by his windswept Nevada drawl. In a more quiet, serious tone, he added, "It's about time all of us had some stability; don't you think?"

"Yes," I answered.

The one-word response said it all. The Nevada experience still hurt. Being close with my brother again, and, later, with my sister, Donna, in the warmth and comfort of Grandma's little cottage, eased the sting.

After enrolling Judi into a nearby Montessori school, I set out in search of a job. In a matter of days, I accepted a position in downtown L.A. as the assistant to the vice-president of Wedbush, Noble, Cooke, Inc., one of the largest securities trading and clearing firms in the country. With the transition completed, time stopped. I was back to who I had once been, and doing what I had once done, before going home to Carson City.

Judi and I moved into a lovely, little apartment in the foothills. The balcony connected with that of the one next door. Our neighbor, also a single mom, had a son the age of my daughter. At night, we shared the cost of a babysitter while we went out. The feeling of sweet freedom and awaking to sunshine pouring through the window was wonderful.

Away from the stresses existing in Carson City, I felt more comfortable. I missed Dad, but I loved being close to my grandparents, my aunts, and my uncles. I loved living in the land of sunshine, where I had a fantastic job and a terrific boss. Not only did he support my efforts, but on Thursday afternoons, he bought lunch—always Red's juicy hamburgers, greasy French fries, and a chocolate milkshake.

My siblings and I had shared memorable times living near one another. Six of us would pile into Jim's VW bug. Jim and Mary sat in the front seats, with his Irish setter, Simon, on the floor, and Donna, eighty-eight-year-old Grandma, and I sat in the back with Judi on my lap. Our weekends we went to the beach, out to dinner and played frisbee in the park.

Grandma was a good sport. Jim had rescued her from an assisted living home, where she sat depressed. He was afraid she would die if he didn't. Her home eventually sold, and Jim and Mary had bought their own. Now having a place for Grandma, Jim picked her up and took her to his house, where she lived with them for a few years.

We hauled Grandma everywhere. She loved hanging out with us. While we played board and card games, she listened to rock-and-roll and would laugh at our jokes. Grandma gravitated toward the simpler things in life, particularly her grandchildren and enjoying autumn walks. Her attention always focused upon the beautiful stones that she would find lying around or the leaves that drifted to the ground.

"Isn't this beautiful?" she would utter as she would pick up a leaf and gently tuck it into her pocket to take home. One of her dresser drawers was full of her treasured rocks and leaves. She wouldn't allow us to clean it out for her. Like me, she, too, was attached to the vibrant, colorful colors of the earth during those magical months of autumn.

At night dementia would strike. Sitting in her rocking chair, in front of the fire, she would chant in the Ho-Chunk-Winnebago language, then suddenly stopping and looking at me, in a confused manner, saying, "I know you from somewhere."

"Yes, Grandma. I'm Lindy, your granddaughter." I would say.

"Oh, yes. Oh, yes, I remember. Lindy."

Satisfied, she would continue rocking and again chanting in Winnebago. When she was three, and living in Wisconsin, the Winnebago would approach and speak to her in Winnebago.

"Hello Daughter of Long, how are you?" they always greeted. She always answered back in their language.

That next year, Dad invited us to spend Christmas in Carson City. He wanted us to see the beautiful home he had finished building with what he received from Grandma's gift of half her estate.

We were excited, looking forward to the first Christmas we would spend together since seventh grade. Jim and Mary rented a car. We drove up together, with Grandma and Judi, and converged upon Carson City. Donna and her husband, Jon, met us there. It was Dad's way of apologizing for not being more involved in our lives.

On Christmas Eve, 1977, I ran into that guy who turned my heart upside down when I lived in Carson City. It was one of those déjà vu moments that turned into reality. Again, he was standing at the bar with his best friend. Our eyes met. This time, I turned down the invitation to coffee, but saw him on Christmas Day, catching up on one another's lives.

Since I had moved, I was becoming adept at correcting mistakes immediately after being made. After leaving Carson City two years earlier, we had moved a few times, and I had become involved with others, made some terrible choices, and found myself seeking security rather than a relationship. When it didn't work, I at once detached myself.

As I gained more confidence in myself, I quit looking for one. The security I now realized was I was no longer tethered to a relationship based upon dependency. It was within myself and my work. As the marketing manager with a sporting goods import company in San Diego, I was far more mature than I was in Carson City. He asked for my phone number and promised to be in touch.

That Christmas, with our family finally together, was perfect. We appreciated the efforts of our stepmother in making it a wonderful day. Grandma was thrilled to see the beautiful house that Dad had built with her early gift of the liquidation of her estate. It was filled with second chances to resolve old issues with family members, the opportunity to unravel and view a former relationship from a different perspective.

During the ten-hour drive home, my mind raced, trying to sort it all out. Upon arrival, I changed my telephone number. Not ready for any instant replays from the past and still intoxicated with the beautiful feeling of spending the first Christmas in thirteen years as an intact family, it was time to let go and move on. I wasn't ready for a call to come, or worse yet, for a call to never come. I was no longer emotionally frozen in time, as I once was. I could move forward. Those who were once special in our lives were so because of a reason. They will always be dear to us, along with the memories that would last "forever."

Chapter Thirteen

MOVING FORWARD

No doubt exists that all women are crazy;
it's only a question of degree. — W. C. Fields

Y ou want to do what?" Phil's voice boomed, his intense brown eyes widening as they stared through me. I had told my friend I was considering working for the California Department of Corrections (CDC) at the Correctional Training Facility at Soledad, a level three prison, warehousing violent, young gang members from Southern and Central California.

I was looking forward to hearing his thoughts about working inside one of the most notorious prisons in the world. At twenty-six years old, restlessness was again stirring inside.

I didn't need a new job. I liked where I worked Good at what I did, sitting at the right hand of one of America's most respected entrepreneurs, my boss was great. Nothing topped his generous gifts of bonuses and cars.

However, the allure was gone. Fielding executive problems were no longer challenging, and even taking the regular calls to him from the White House had become predictable. Already sitting as high as I could imagine, little room for advancement existed. The only other position upward was occupied by a happy career employee.

The daily challenges were routine. Wanting more than I could tackle, something gritty, risky, down to earth, and in line with my active, independent lifestyle, I was ready to move on. A strong urge was gnawing inside, insistent I defy fear and its control.

A few weeks earlier, I read an article about affirmative action and how women were now working in non-traditional positions. Since, I had been researching the new opportunities in the field of Corrections and asking friends for their thoughts on whether I should consider it as a career change. Phil's response was the same received from others. They felt I was crazy to consider it.

In retrospect, I realized he was not the best person to ask. Most men viewed women working in an institution filled with young, violent offenders, pure lunacy. In the mid-1970s, women did not go to work in all-male, medium-security prisons. They became homemakers, secretaries, nurses, or teachers.

"Hush," I whispered as I noted other diners were glancing in our direction.

"You want to do what?" he reiterated.

Laughing, I realized my speculation was right. Phil *had* thought I lost it. Realizing he was a man of the late 1970s, I was ready for it.

"Come on. It can't be all that bad," I bantered.

"What fairy tale world is that that coming from?" he asked.

"Great opportunities exist for women. They only have seventeen working at Soledad and over six hundred men."

He shook his head in disbelief, muttering, "Plus, thousands of violent male inmates. Please tell me you will not do it."

Whirling in my mind, was the conflict between what he was saying and what the recruiter promised. Confusion was beginning to take over the near certainty I felt about moving on.

"We are required by law to hire thirty-seven percent women and minorities to meet federal goals and recent laws. Having already completed your background, I can assure you it will be worth your while if you would come and interview tomorrow," he had said.

It was the era of affirmative action. Government agencies were seeking out qualified women and minorities to recruit into professions currently filled with white males. The government regulations intended to ease the enormous numbers of hiring and advancement disparities that existed in public employment.

Television shows and movies featuring women working in non-traditional roles had become commonplace, with the characters in the series Cagney and Lacey, Get Christy Love, and Policewoman, working as detectives. The Mod Squad, T.J. Hooker, and Hill Street Blues featured women police officers on the streets, and Private Benjamin, bless her heart, was recruited into the Army, expecting condominiums to live in and sailboats as promised by the military recruiter. Sitcoms featuring single moms holding male-dominated occupations and taking positions of power flooded television screens. Everyday life was changing.

After reading the advertisement placed by the CDC in the Chronicle, I was intrigued. My thought was, why not work in a prison?

We, the women of the seventies, were asserting our newly found freedom, and the prisons were responding with encouragement for us to apply as peace officers. The lure of the money was a tremendous draw, and the opportunities seemed endless, especially for a single mom. It would reduce the stress I had once felt with working two or three jobs to pay for my daughter's expenses when visiting Dad or when playing catch-up with the unanticipated costs of medical bills.

The next day, I drove the eighty-six miles to the institution. Completing a written test, passing a physical examination, clearing a background check, and interviewing at one time, was exhausting.

Pulling out of the parking lot, I held a more than a decent job offer in my hand. It included twenty-five percent more than my current salary in wages, excellent health benefits, paid sick and vacation leave, life insurance, dental insurance, and a pension. Coupled with as much overtime as I wished, it was tough to turn down. The overall package was twice the salary of the average male wage in California. It offered opportunities for advancement. As a single mom, I could comfortably support my daughter.

The California prison system was growing in leaps and bounds. With fifty thousand gang members engaging in drug sales and violence on Southern California streets, a massive prison overcrowding was occurring. Plans for the construction of fifteen new prisons were "in the works" at a time when federal regulations were mandating public agencies to practice affirmative action policies.

"What's with you?" Phil confronted me. "Soledad is not a playground or a camp for troubled children. And it's not juvenile hall. You could get stabbed or raped, or God knows what else."

"Trust me; there are worse ways to die," I said.

Settling back in his chair, his eyes began to lose their paternalistic flare. His voice softening, he said. "Okay. Now I get it. So, this is your answer?"

After a period of uncomfortable silence, I added, "No. I don't see it that way. It is an opportunity to prove myself. Listen, It is only an hour and a half down the highway, and if it gets to be too much, I can always come back to my old job here or transfer to San Quentin."

He dropped his head and banged it a few times on the table. Glancing up, he said, "Oh my God! San Quentin? Oh, my God!"

Unable to think straight, my heart and my mind were engaged in a bout of tug-of-war. Whether I could do the job was not at issue. I always held this strong belief I could do anything I wanted to do. All I had to do was try. Embedded in me by our parents and stepmother, what plagued me was the deep-rooted fear of what others thought.

After a few hours with Phil, I was wallowing in uncertainty and questioning my capabilities. Finally, setting self-doubts aside and weighing the pros and the cons to decide what was best for my daughter and me was a starting point at making any decision.

I should call Dad.

Speaking with my father was the first thought that came to mind. I had not seen him in a while. Wondering what he would think and not wanting to upset him if it was something he may not approve of, I decided to shoot him a call. He would want to know what I was considering and if I had weighed the pros and cons.

My greatest fear was he would tell me to continue along my socially acceptable path as the women in our family had always done. Fortunately, his sister, our Aunt Marcella, was not in sync with that thought. She was a feminist long before they coined the term. She was the first person to which I presented my dilemma. She was cheering me on.

Marcella understood that I was not trying to move upward because I was unhappy with where I was working. I was in a much better position than many I knew, though I still did not have a telephone at my home. For a single mom, it was as unaffordable then, as a cellphone is today.

Work offered stability and a comfortable living. The one thing I would miss would be the little hillside apartment where we lived, with the soothing comfort of strolling through thick billows of the San Francisco Bay fog and feeling the morning dew kissing my face. There, our evenings were peaceful. After darkness arrived and the outside world fell silent, I would tuck Judi into bed and take a deep breath. It was my time to escape from reality, and to relax, read, play guitar, and sing to my heart's content.

Adjusting to change is difficult; for some, it takes effort. Uncertainty had become a conditioned part of my everyday life. It dictated over everything. Unable to commit to relationships, a lifetime career, or even to keep a stable living situation, I struggled with a relentless urge to move forward. The biggest fear I had was stopping what I was doing. I was dependent upon that drive that pushed me to experience life. It kept me distracted from anything creating a sense of not being "normal" and feeling different because of who and what I was and what I may someday be.

Working against it was the ever-constant anxiety churning inside. It was as though I was continually waiting for something to happen that would trigger an implosion. I feared a backfire turning my world upside down just when everything was going great. Needing a constant stream of challenges that I could overcome, the resulting rush of confidence to keep me going kept relaying a message back that I was capable and worthy of doing whatever I wished.

Making the call, I reflected upon how I was still working at keeping a relationship with him. Judi and I visited their home every few months. During the last five years that I lived in Southern California, he visited once, to drop in for a few hours for my sister's wedding.

It was important to me that my daughter get to know her grandfather, and I made sure he saw her whenever he wished, even during several Christmas holidays. On two occasions, we postponed our family celebrations to accommodate that of his family. But some things didn't change.

"I told you I do not want your children calling this house," our stepmother's voice would assail Dad as he answered the phone.

"Can you call me at work tomorrow?" Dad whispered. I could hear his wife haranguing him in the background.

"No problem, Dad," I laughed. "She still hasn't gotten a handle on that 'insecurity thing' yet, huh?"

Dad returned an uncomfortable laugh. It was clear he was not able to talk. She was again upset with him about something and projected her anger upon my contact with him. We were responsible for everything that caused her discomfort. Desensitized to it after a twelve years pattern of existence, I let it go.

The next morning, Dad and I discussed my dilemma. "Lindy, did you assess the pros and the cons?" he asked.

"Got 'em right here, Dad."

"Good girl."

The list ready, I read it to him.

"That is an awful lot of opportunity to walk away from, Lindy. It's more than I make," Dad determined.

My heart stopped. I had not expected that statement or his support. Apprehensively, I kept waiting to hear, "But, Lindy…"

It never came. My father approved of my plan. I felt the tears well in my eyes. Spending a lifetime trying to please him, all he had ever wanted from me was to "settle" for what women of his time did… to get married, buy a home, and live in Carson City. He finally recognized me for my capabilities.

"Dad, that's entry-level," I told him excitedly. "They are adding twenty more institutions to the existing fifteen. The sky is the limit for women who get involved, and as young as I am, the opportunities are enormous."

"It sounds great, Lindy. Especially health insurance for you two."

I silently groaned. That one issue alone had become the main reason to accept the position, above all other considerations.

What if I contracted cancer? The anxiety that raised always got my gut rocking. Dad's repeated references to health insurance meant health insurance was a necessity in our family, but most of my life, it was out of my control. I had worked for large corporations that passed out benefits only to the men. Positions women held seldom came with them. Employers expected husbands to provide it for their families. We had prayer to get us by, and, hopefully, an ex-husband somewhere who had health benefits. It was the one subject I did not wish to discuss it with anyone.

Dad had experienced events and heartbreaks I never had. He spent months sitting by his father's side, watching him die a devastatingly painful death. While growing up, he heard the stories of how cancer ravaged aunts, uncles, and grandparents. As a child, he, too, had been shown where they once lived and where they died.

Contracting cancer was a rite of passage for everyone in our family. We were more fortunate than those who were older. We had not yet experienced any losses from the death of our parents. Dad was fifteen when his father died. He did not wish to experience another loss, whether it be the result of divorce or someone he loved contracting cancer. He thought about it often, while I avoided it.

It did not make sense to worry about "someday," since nobody knew if or when it would hit. I had decided to live now, putting "maybe" aside to worry about later.

"You're right, Dad," I said.

"Oh, and Lindy…"

"Yeah?"

"You don't need my approval or anyone else's. I love you."

"I love you, too," I responded. As I hung up the phone, I cried. After composing myself, I called and accepted the job offer and prepared to move to the Salinas Valley.

Surrounded by agricultural fields, the savory aromas of herbs wafted through the air. About twenty-five cadets attended the correctional academy, seven of us women. Most of the men were young Vietnam veterans, stationed at nearby Fort Ord. The few women, other than me, came from local communities.

I viewed my new position as most everyone did in the beginning, a temporary stomping ground and a base to springboard into something involving cultural diversity before diving deeper into a career somewhere else into the criminal justice system. For most of my tenured male peers, it was merely another job. They were far from happy about the wave of women they referred to as "females," invading the institution. Some were downright hostile toward us.

A respectable number of officers were big, beefy war veterans who had served in Korea, Vietnam, and elsewhere. For years, they had worked at one of the toughest prisons in California, supervising the most dangerous people in the state. They lived through some tight situations in the battlefields and later when working in the prison.

I understood their sentiments. It would be difficult for me if I saw myself as a rugged guy who worked in a dangerous and challenging job. I would not be wild about an attractive, five-foot-three-inch, twenty-seven-year-old woman, weighing 120 pounds and wearing lipstick, diamond earrings, and tailored uniforms doing the same work I did. It would do a number on my ego, especially if it were a big part of my identity.

Letting their comments roll off me, I ignored them. Whenever someone hurled discriminatory statements about women, I laughed while a protective little voice inside me reinforced, "Let it go. Someday, you will be their boss." The word "Someday" had taken on a whole new meaning at a perfect time in my life. In the context it arrived, it was welcome. I dearly needed it and the empowerment it offered.

Early on, spending a few rare moments in the training area, and casually combing through the pages of a magazine, by an article written about the numbers of women who were merging into the ranks of correctional and law enforcement agencies captured my attention. The quote of one, "Because I am a woman, I am a different type of officer, and because I am an officer, I'm a different type of woman," struck at my heart.

It defined me. I never experienced the luxury of being involved in the trivialities of being a young mother or a wife or sat in on the neighbor's morning coffee klatches, discussing recipes, and various brands of diapers. Pushing a stroller with other young moms on morning walks was not my style. Neither was wearing makeup or clothes shopping. Away from work, I embraced a comfortable, casual lifestyle I could afford, while sporting faded Levis and worn t-shirts.

The weeks at the academy flew by. At night and on weekends, while classmates hit the bars and guzzled beer, I was hitting the books or torturing myself with excruciatingly painful tae kwon do classes.

Hobbling on sore feet from walking up and down a corridor and trying to conceal the painful muscle strains in my abdomen, arms, and legs, from tae kwon do, the first few weeks I spent in misery.

Being the only woman in the BOQ and assigned to a position where I was isolated from others, I often felt alone. Religiously, every six hours, I tossed down two painkillers to keep the pain and the stiffness in check, sucking it up for weeks, while hoping no one would notice. I was not going to complain or admit my discomfort, even if confronted. In a prison setting, any injury is a weakness, especially when working amid thousands of male predators. At night, feeling battered and wretched and alone with my thoughts, I often wondered what I was doing there.

Resolving that issue *was* within my control. Quitting was not an option. However, not within my power was the lack of preparation to accommodate me or any of the other women. That sent a message. It was not a priority. Little thought into integrating women correctional officers into the system occurred. The first I noted when we stood in line to order our uniforms.

"A size six petite, please," I asked of the tailor as he slid women's slacks across the rack, toward him. Taking one look at me from across the table, he began to laugh.

"No can do," he said after he finished.

"Oh, good Lord, what can I do?" Being the first in line is sometimes not the best place to be, but there was some comfort in knowing it was not solely my problem. It affected a few of us, who were standing behind me and edging in close to listen.

"You can gain weight and grow a few inches in the next couple of days, or we can tailor them," he offered with a chuckle. The cost of the tailored uniforms was three times more than what men paid for theirs, but ours did look classier and more polished on us.

On the shooting range, lack of thought in the differences between men and women again occurred. The heavy leather belts designed to carry the weight of the firearms and other equipment we were all to wear sent another strong message. They came in one size, to fit men. Big men. Wrapping mine around my waist twice, I managed to get it to fit. Resolving the issue of the intense pain from the kick of the shotgun was trickier. Making myself not fear its kick and tightly tucking into it, helped, as did some bubble wrap tucked over my clavicle.

Graduation came and went. I banked another fifteen college credits after completing the academy. Enrolling in three more courses at the college, gaining nine more, started the process to put me into an advantageous position for future promotion within the Department.

On our first day of working inside, we women walked together into the institution for our first shift. A weary, sad-sack appearing, older officer shuffled toward us, on his way to the parking lot.

Stopping directly in front of us, with his metal lunch-bucket clutched tightly in his hand, he pretended to inspect us and laughed.

"Welcome, ladies. Now, yellow be sure to find someone weaker than you and go for them," he offered with a wink, laughing louder.

We could still hear him cackling in the parking lot, as we headed toward a tiny shack constructed underneath a large tower. Ahead, behind the enormous granite walls and barred windows of the central facility, we could hear a nightmare unfolding. Through the myriad of little windows looking out upon us, scores of caged men screamed obscenities.

"Bitch! Let me see that ass."

"Aha, chica. How about a little play, huh?"

Great, chortling officers and screaming caged men.

As we advanced, the volume increased after passing through a chain-linked gate leading into the guard shack. I started, and my heart dropped as the gate slammed behind us. Caged between the two gates, an alien feeling of being overwhelmed surged through me as we submitted to a search.

"Bitch, get my money." "Hey, look at you, you tramp." "Whore!" the yelling of the inmates continued from the building beyond. I found the name-calling to be offensive though I was sure their intent was for it to be intimidating.

A woman officer, staffing the main tower overhead, stuck her head out the window, as we huddled close to one another.

"Hey, sisters. Welcome. You all be sure to come to see me if you need anything," she hollered.

"Ladies, pay attention," a surly officer ordered as others, with potbellies and big mustaches, grabbed our IDs from our hands and growled at us to lock our purses up.

"Come on, no time to dawdle, girls. Let's go. Get moving," one of them reminded, clapping his hands like an animal handler when we weren't quick enough for him.

"Leave this crap in the car," another ordered in a hostile tone as he tossed a purse to one of the women.

"Oh my God, I feel like Alice in Wonderland," I groaned to the rest as we gawked toward the stone building ahead, trying to build the confidence to pass. The female officer again stuck her head out of the tower window, pointing toward the screaming inmates. "Don't pay them no mind. I called. They're gonna get a visit. Don't let none of them see it's getting to you."

Just before passing, the yelling from inside the building suddenly ceased. A quiet suddenly fell. Sighing in relief, it was clear to me the visitor, or visitors, whoever he, she, or they were, had arrived.

At day's end, I pulled off my shoes, and on tender, aching feet carefully stepped down the hall of the bachelor officers' quarters (BOQ). A bouquet of roses sat outside my door. A note tucked inside revealed a room number where the sender, a correctional sergeant, lived. I had never met him. The warning received from the tower officer flashed through my mind.

Don't pay them no mind.

Placing the flowers in the general living area of the BOQ, and scribbling a quick, polite thank-you note, saying how thoughtful it was and that everyone was enjoying them, I slid it under his door.

During the few weeks that I stayed at the BOQ, sleep evaded me. Quickly, I learned that the "bonus of overtime" was mandatory. The first place they filled those vacant slots was from those temporary quarters. It was a test of endurance. Every night, around 11:30 p.m., a tapping sounded upon my door, followed by a male voice informing me the watch commander was ordering me to work a second shift.

"He likes looking at you," the Sergeant remarked. I quickly learned to hit the rack after my day shift, falling asleep by four each afternoon. Allowing a little less than eight hours of sleep and little else, in the end, it was well worth it. On the first of the month, I laughed all the way to the bank. After depositing my paycheck and my overtime check in my account, I felt great.

"Being tested," as the male officers called it, was not easy to accept. It was like being hazed, only uglier. Going through it was one of the most demeaning experiences I had ever encountered.

One morning, upon being beckoned into the Watch Sergeant's office, I was instructed, "Go to North Facility and help with the cell feeding."

Complying, I took a shuttle to another facility. Passing through the gates and approaching the heavy iron door leading into the cell block, the officer who let me in asked, "You're the one helping us out today, huh?"

"Sure am," I answered enthusiastically.

"Well, aren't you the lucky one? You don't have to help cell feed. We got you a special assignment," the officer advised, smiling as he handed me a bucket, a mop, some rags, a broom, industrial cleaner, and bleach. "I hear you females are good at this cleaning stuff," he tossed over his shoulder as he walked ahead of me.

Really now?

A problem was sure to occur whenever an officer referred to women officers as "females." A red flag furiously waved, with that one term that alerted us to be ready for anything.

Dummying up, I smiled at him as I nodded, clutching the supplies ever so tightly and trying to figure out the best way to respond.

"We sure are," I finally said.

Following him up the stairs to the second tier, he directed me to a specific section of three cells and instructed to clean them. Entering, I suppressed the urge to vomit. Mottled with blood and other bodily fluids upon which maggots feasted, the floors and walls were filthy with blood splatter. My heart stopped, and my stomach turned.

Hold it in. Don't let him see it is getting to you.

"Gross, huh?" the officer asked, leaning against the doorway, his arms folded across his chest.

Responding to him took all I had. I merely answered, "Yep," to his question, as he handed me the rest of the cleaning materials.

"Some inmates were killed up here a few weeks ago. The DA just released the crime scene this morning," he stated.

Ignoring him, I wrapped a clean towel around my face, bandit style. Pulling on a pair of old gloves, I hummed to myself silently, blocking out his instructions on how to clean, while concentrating on not becoming ill.

Let it go. You have a child to support.

It was best not to say anything. Straight talk was not something occurring with women when the "old guard" wanted to get rid of us.

They were not interested in what we had to say or what we felt. Replies to our comments or questions, if any, were ordinarily one or two words if we were lucky, but mostly it was just a groan or a grunt. We were women. They seldom spoke to us. Communication passed through veiled messages. I began cleaning and worked hard not to reveal the disgust over how demeaned I felt. There was no way I was going to allow them any satisfaction out of it. Once finished, I handed it all back to the officer.

"Here," I offered, with a smile, hoping the officer and the others watching received my message. No matter how hard they tried, they could not intimidate me. If I left, it would be on my terms, not theirs. They would never have the satisfaction of "getting to me."

When I returned to my institution, one of my male partners whispered, "I heard what happened. It's jacked up. I'm gonna say something."

"Please don't. Someone here had to have approved it. It will just make things worse for both of us," I begged.

"Are you sure? Because I will."

"Yes, trust me on this, okay? There are better ways to deal with it."

Waiting until I was off the institution's grounds before I released the immense amount of anger pent up inside, relief flooded as I drove the country roads for hours before returning to my BOQ room. Fuming, I worked through the rage I felt inside. I sang every anti-man song I knew that evening. Helen Reddy's music got me through it all.

Shortly after returning to the BOQ, a tap sounded at my door. I first considered ignoring it, in the event it was the watch sergeant ordering me to work another mandatory overtime shift. My conscience and my work ethic disallowed me to do it. Peering out the door, I saw a middle-aged woman with wild, curly hair and wearing wire-framed glasses standing in the doorway.

"Hi! I'm Judy," she said with a big smile. "You're Linda, right?"

"That I am," I answered cautiously.

"I heard what happened today," she said firmly." And I'm here because we take care of our own. But first, important matters."

Watching her make herself comfortable and sank onto a wooden desk chair, she pulled out an already opened bottle of wine from her purse, holding it up for me to see. "See? Important matters!"

Laughing, I decided I liked her.

"Thought you could use some after today," she said as she struggled to pull out the cork.

"You don't know how much," I said, feeling a flood of relief surge through me, resulting in wanting to sit down and cry for joy. At last, a form of support.

Pausing, she stopped struggling to remove the cork and focused upon the only personal item in the room, an oil painting of a blooming white rose.

"I like it," she announced, again trying to open the bottle.

"My aunt was the artist," I informed her as she finally pulled it out.

"Got some glasses?" she asked, holding the bottle up, ready to pour.

"Sure do," I answered, stepping toward my desk to grab a couple of plastic cups from my stash.

"You know, it's pristine," she finally decided, standing in front of the painting, and getting a close look.

I laughed. "Close. It represents the loss of trust, innocence, and vulnerability."

She let out a hearty laugh. "Whoa, okay, well, at least it was close enough for government work, right?

Depicting a white rose, it's petals were trimmed in soft pink, and the color red dripped down their sides. The oil painting held special significance.

Created while I was contemplating the job offer, Aunt Marcella intended it to help me to be ready to acknowledge the expected changes in myself that I would soon be experiencing. What they were, we would not know until it happened. But having been born in the 1920s, and being a young woman during World War II, when the expectations of women were especially strong, she did.

"Don't worry, Auntie. I'm not going to allow myself to become hardened. I *will* leave before that happens," I had promised her.

"Wow, heavy. Steinbeck and Buck too?" Judy asked, looking through my books on the desk.

Smiling at her, I answered, "I'm kind of into the early California sense of social consciousness."

"Big words, but it sounds like it is needed here. So, what do you think of this place so far?" Judy asked, sitting back down.

"Not bad... the neighborhood isn't the best. It's full of criminals, and the cops keep knocking at my door every night, wanting to take me in."

She laughed. "Yep, they do that here. The baptism is brutal, performed by a bunch of idiots who can't even spell."

"I just signed papers on a place in town."

"Smart girl. Just make sure you don't get a phone, a pager, or an answering machine. They won't stop calling."

"Gotcha," I said. "Didn't think about that."

And, you're keeping a book on everything that happens, aren't you?"

"Yes, M'am," I answered, patting my shirt pocket.

"Good. I documented it too." She patted her own, tucked in the pocket of her slacks. "You did good."

"Thanks, but on days like today, I question that," I said with a smile.

"You passed the test and didn't let those jerks see that they were getting to you. Here's to you," Judy said, with one hand holding her glass, sipping it, and handing me the other.

"Ahh, this is good." The first sip set off my tongue with a gentle tingling sensation. Good wine, I had missed it. Finally, I had a glimpse of the first promising sign of the existence of an advanced civilization at Soledad.

"Mondavi... Reserve. Anyway, now that you've shown them that they can't get to you, they're all gonna want to start hitting on you."

"Ah, so that's what that 'Don't pay attention to none of them is all about?"

"Yep. They talk."

"Ooh, I see," I paused for a moment. "Well, that's no problem for me. Right now, I can't stomach anything that looks or smells like a man."

"Oh, Linda," she said softly. "That'll go away in time."

"You think?"

"After a while."

"Well, I kind of doubt it. I have trouble seeing that far ahead."

"That's probably a good thing. We all find our ways of getting past what happens here. Now, getting down to work, I need to fill you in on who's who. What I don't tell you, Gladys will. You are supposed to ask for an appointment with her."

Gladys was Glady's Crawford, the Deputy Superintendent at North Facility, one of the seven women who were the first to work in California's male prisons. We looked up to her as a role model.

Things were looking up. I had a mentor and a women's underground support system that was in operation. No longer alone, and now that I had support, I knew I could get through anything.

Chapter Fourteen

TAKING RISKS

*There can be no life without change, and to be afraid of what is
different or unfamiliar is to be afraid of life.*
— Theodore Roosevelt

A dapting to working inside an all-male prison more rapidly than the
male officers and the inmates adjusted to the women who were
"invading their territory," it was merely an extension of dealing
with the uncertainty I had always endured. Exposed to my mother's
addiction and Chuck's con games, while growing up, I found working with
inmates to be familiar, which was discomforting. Most of my peers were
familiar with being around people who were different from them. Many,
like me, had a story to tell, that they kept to themselves. Each situation I
faced reinforced that I could survive better than imagined.

In our housing unit, we took turns delivering lunches to the newly
arriving inmates placed upon "confined to quarters" (CTQ) status. Locked
inside their cells until their past histories were known, and their enemies
and gang ties named, the behavior of inmates was often unpredictable
when confined in unfamiliar environments.

Today was my day to distribute the lunches. Fortunately, there was only
one inmate to feed. With a sack lunch in one hand keys in the other, I
approached, announced, "Room Service," and unlocked the door to his
cell.

Leaping off the bed, he raced to the cell bars and began pushing against
the door. "Let me out of here," he yelled, his eyes raging with anger.

"Move away from the door," I firmly instructed, propping my foot
between the door and the wall, disallowing it to open.

"I said, let me out," the inmate growled, pushing harder.

"Step back," I ordered more firmly, keeping the weight of my body
against the door's edge, praying I would be strong enough to keep it closed
until help arrived or until I could get to my whistle, safely.

"Lady, I told myself I'd throw the next officer off the tier if I didn't get
out of here, and that's what I'm gonna do. I mean it. I want out."

"It's not going to happen. Get back on your bunk, and we'll talk."

"There's nothing to say. I want out," the inmate snarled. Contradicting his words, I could feel the pressure of his weight lighten up. He was listening. Continuing to struggle with him to keep the door closed, he angrily threatened, "I swear you're going off the tier, lady."

The guy was serious. Fortunately, the anger brewing inside masked my fear.

"Listen, slick; you've got three options here."

"Yeah?" he replied.

"Yeah," I answered. Drastic times call for extreme measures. If there was ever a right time to pull out my "girl card," it was now. It was *my* superpower.

"You can try, but you're gonna end up in PC (protective custody) because you'll be nothing more than a sniveling wimp for beating up on a chick, or you are going to end up there because I just may get mad enough to beat the living hell out of you," I continued.

"Huh? What?" he interrupted, suddenly confused. Then falling silent, he thought for a minute and asked, "Or what?"

"Or you can go sit on your bunk and let me deal with your counselor to figure this thing out, because I am frigging tired of this, too."

As his weight lightened against the door, an opportunity opened to pull my whistle from my shirt pocket. The inmate's eyes widened, then narrowed with concern as he saw me raise it to my mouth. One blast would call for backup from throughout the institution. His body tensed, and fear crossed his face as he weighed his odds.

"Wait, wait. All right. All right," the inmate begged as I lifted it upward. "But if something ain't done, I will do it. I mean it."

Ordering, "Then, step back!" he moved a few steps. "All the way…"

His sigh signaling surrender, tears of frustration formed in his eyes as he flopped onto his bunk. I tossed the bag containing his lunch to him and keyed the door locked. Walking down the tier, toward the stairs, I heard him yell.

"Make sure you are good for your word, lady."

Continuing, I ignored him.

"Hey!" a voice hissed from behind me, just as I reached the landing.

Turning, I approached a cell where I noted an old inmate. His reddened, watery eyes connected with mine as he tightly gripped the cell bars with yellowed, tobacco-stained fingers.

"Yeah?"

"Pull out a cigarette and light it."

"Why?"

"Your hands are shaking. If these guys see it, they'll eat you alive." I glanced down. My hands were trembling uncontrollably. I didn't even notice, but the inmate did. The years he spent living behind bars, looking out his little window upon the world, and watching others live free gave him the ability to see details in behavior many never notice.

"That guy was serious," he said. "You were lucky."

Gazing down upon the concrete deck below, I decided he was right. It was doubtful I would have survived the forty-foot fall. Suddenly, overcome by the most intense sensation of physical fear I had ever felt, a thought flashed through my mind. What if the inmate had not been selling wolf tickets and had made good with his threats?

Emotional fear was a constant sensation I had realized since childhood. Then, plaguing Jim and I was the fear of rejection, of angering our mother, of not receiving approval, and that our parents did not love us any longer. We feared, because of the constant abuse of our stepmother, that we were not good enough for our father. We spent a lifetime living with it. We learned to adapt and to deal with each situation as it occurred. Physical fear was something new, as was the adrenaline rush that came with the everyday fight for survival.

When dealing with others, in stressful situations or during crises, I learned that offering options is essential. Not only do they give a person a sense of empowerment and control over their fates, but places the responsibility of actions falls from the person offering the choices to the person who must decide which alternative is acceptable.

It took a while to learn for me to adapt to the hostility the men extended toward women, and to be able to communicate effectively with inmates and my co-workers. While working at Soledad, I was fortunate that Captain Sam Brown, a gruff, but compassionate black man, who had learned to deal with the issues of bigotry and racism in the institutions, himself, had decided to make me one of his projects.

It began the day I stormed into his office, angry as all hell that I was forced to send the same request for a job change, three separate times, by a sergeant. I marched into the Captain's office and dumped all my frustrations upon him.

"They're making me go through changes," I advised. It was an everyday activity at Soledad. To modify behavior, rather than resolve issues, requests, and actions often had to be submitted several times until the person requesting something gave up.

As my eyes filled with restrained tears, he looked upon me and firmly stated, "My officers don't cry."

Marked with anger, I haughtily responded, "I'm not crying because I'm weak or scared. I am crying because I am so mad at you right now; I could just spit!"

His eyes widened, and he urged me to sit down. He spoke softly, trying to calm me down while telling me about his daughters, who were also strong and independent young women. We discussed the problems that women faced working inside the institutions. Telling me if the guys in my unit didn't accept me as a woman, I needed to find a way to become one of the guys. "Get crazy with them, challenge them," he recommended.

I *was* working in a man's world with less than two dozen other women at Soledad, and over four hundred guys who didn't adapt well to women doing "their jobs." What he said made a lot of sense. I realized a need to create a balance in staying genuine with whom and what I was, but I also had to communicate with them in their language. It was difficult for me.

I practiced all night on how I would become engaged with them. The next day, while sitting in the office where the guys were discussing football, I seized the opportunity by joining in when someone mentioned that the pro-team that was playing the Green Bay Packers that weekend had "more heart."

Their comment was far from a politically correct thing to say in front of someone who had lived in Wisconsin. Those were fighting words. In fact, in some circles, they could be a declaration of war. I decided to try out Captain Brown's suggestion. I knew a bit about football and had been reading the newspaper daily, keeping up with it.

"What? Are you crazy, homeboy?" I confronted him. "The Pack *is* the only team with heart," I interjected my eyes drilling through him, like the spinning steel bit of a drill. Trying hard not to laugh as all three of the guys I worked with looked up and stared at me as though I was an alien, I continued. I was on a roll.

"Geez, you guys. What's wrong with you? They've got Bart Starr as a coach, the best quarterback ever, and right now, they're second in the NFC Division. Seriously, what do you think your team's *really* going to do against them? Come on, boys, lay your money down," I said, patting the desktop. "Put your money where your mouths are. I'll take bets right now."

"Whoa, check *her* out," one of the guys commented to the others.

"Listen, homeboy; I come from the land of the Packers and Rocky Bleier. Do you want to talk about heart? Football is a way of life there, a passion. Nobody raised there *ever* gives up," I added as I walked out of the office with an attitude.

Impressed, they got both my messages. I knew about football, and I could keep up with their "guy talk." I was not the blob occupying space in the corner of the room, and I was also not going to give up, so they may as well just get used to me being one of them.

What they didn't realize was most of it was "just talk." But the "wolf tickets" I was selling sounded good, and that is all that mattered. It is all it took for *my* message to be transmitted effectively. Taking a risk, I found myself accepted as one of the guys, though I still suspect Captain Brown may have had a secret discussion with them. What I learned from him was life-lasting. It worked equally as effective with co-workers, inmates, parolees, recalcitrant teens, and husbands, at least with mine, who is a sports junkie. Sometimes, to be effective, we need to communicate in a different language, one understood by others, especially in survival situations. It was there that I also learned to swear to get my point across.

During our lifetime, we will deal with many people who speak far different languages than us. Live involves the ability to communicate with others in a straightforward manner, even if you have to talk like a guy.

Eventually, the work at Soledad had become routine. The allure of the challenge had faded. Like having an addiction, it was not enough for me. I found myself hungering for more. I needed something that presented a bit more risk.

During the winter of 1981, I left the California prison system to work at a rural Wyoming Sheriff's Office. Recently married to a young, aspiring police officer, we decided the small western town where we would be was the perfect place for the two of us to begin our careers in law enforcement and to start a family.

Driving through the quaint, old western frontier town, I was at once seduced by it. Flanked by an open prairie with a winding river running through the middle, the surrounding countryside was wildly beautiful. Reminiscent of Carson City, I was more than ready for it. Tucking in during the snowy winters, baking bread, cooking from scratch, and drying venison jerky was appealing.

Picking up a few items at the local pharmacy, we passed a couple of old geezers silently rocking back and forth in their chairs, on the sidewalk, in front of the radio station. The old guys were talking small talk while watching the vehicles and the big rigs cruise along Main Street.

As we stepped past them, one said, "Californiyans… bet you they even got some of that 'marijooana' stuffed in their back pockets." The two of us chuckled. It *was* funny.

Neither of us had ever smoked marijuana or used drugs of any sort. We were drug-naive. Besides an interest in law enforcement, it was about the only other thing my new husband and I had in common. I was a perfected codependent, learning to settle and to have someone need me, rather than take a chance on waiting and never finding anyone who would accept me, for me, as an equal, despite all my baggage.

One of the few times I was exposed to marijuana was years earlier, in a social situation at a party hosted by some college students living in our apartment complex in Oregon. I quietly left. Another was the breaking point of a San Diego relationship. On our way to Lake Powell to waterski, we stopped by a party.

Later that evening, after a long discussion with friends, I searched for him, finding him in the backyard, smoking a joint with others. Repulsed, I went to the camper of the truck we owned and slept there until he was ready to leave. Our relationship ended the moment we arrived home from our vacation. Just the thought of him smoking dope was disgusting to me.

Abhorring drug use, I refused to associate with people who used drugs. It accompanied the rule I made for myself that I did not date anyone whose hair was longer than mine. Living with a drug-addicted mother encouraged me to think seriously about my personal choices. The last rule I set for myself was one I learned young. I swore I would never live with a drug user again, not after what I saw occur with our mother and the harm drug addiction inflicts upon those who love them.

The Wyoming conservative culture was more than the Sonoma County, California boy I married, expected. The police chief where he worked wanted his troops clean-cut, instructing him to get his hair styled short. Not California style short, but Marine Corps style short.

The barbershop was not open. We went to the Pamida store and bought a pair of hair-cutting scissors. Standing over him, I recommended I cut it in a military-type "flat-top" like all the other cops I had earlier met at the sheriff's office where I had begun working.

He scoffed at the suggestion and instructed me just how he wanted it done. Rolling my eyes and chuckling, I cut it precisely the way he wished.

"Now, don't forget to get that haircut." the Chief reminded him as they crossed paths the next morning.

My husband returned home after his first shift, feeling despondent. Again, he showed me how short he thought it should be.

"Are you certain?" I asked. "How about like the others at…"

"Just cut it this short," he instructed impatiently, again showing the length of hair he wanted to keep. The next morning, he headed back to work, feeling confident with his collar-length, Starsky and Hutch type, California hairstyle.

"Didn't I tell you to get a haircut?" the rugged former marine again asked, this time more firmly.

"What does he want?" my husband cried out in frustration as he flopped into the "barber chair" for the third night of wearing a towel around his neck.

"This, like he and everyone else has," I answered as I picked up the clippers, I had bought that morning, predicting he would need help to adapt to rural Wyoming hairstyles.

"Oh, no," he whined, looking apprehensively toward it as I flipped the switch. Closing his eyes, he got "the buzz."

"A word of wisdom, grasshopper," I whispered into his ear. "When in Rome, do as the Romans do," repeating the words of Captain Brown.

The following morning, my husband went to work, this time extremely confident that his new hairstyle would meet the approval of his police chief. That morning, I reassured him, "What could anyone say about a buzz?"

"You're looking good, there." the Chief said to my then-husband who was learning to survive in the real world, far from that of academia and the California police academy he had attended. The Chief wanted everyone to look alike, to be identifiable. If the young officer felt uncomfortable, all he had to do was wear his Smokey, the Bear hat to conceal his head. Hair grows back.

It was the first of my ex's many experiences that contributed toward his disenchantment with western, rural criminal justice traditions. The challenges of rounding up and investigating the identities of the various chickens and cattle that fled from their barnyards, pastures, and hen houses did not fulfill what he wanted in a law enforcement career. His vision was chasing down drug dealers and solving urban crime, not apprehending antisocial fowl, or coaxing reluctant bovine back into their pastures. He wanted to solve urban homicides, not remove roadkill from the highway. Everything he wished for was not possible in a town of six thousand, found in the heart of an enormous, barren prairie. But he had to start somewhere.

My husband and I existed at extreme opposite ends when it came to dreams of a future. Loving my job, and the small, rural town lifestyle, I no longer felt a need for risk and excitement. I bonded with the town folk and my daughter's school, where teachers instructed children around a fireplace. I wanted to live there forever.

While attempting to adapt to rural life, my husband had not. After months of hearing whining and complaining, finally, in mid-autumn, I sighed as we put the two homes we owned up for sale, packed up what we owned, and headed back to California.

Chapter Fifteen

HELLO, SAN QUENTIN

Life for him was an adventure, perilous indeed, but men are not made
for safe havens-the fullness of life is in the hazards of life.
— Edith Hamilton

After moving into a small patio home amid the Napa Valley vineyards in November 1981, I returned to the Department of Corrections at San Quentin, a maximum-security facility that, along with Folsom prison, housed the most violent offenders in the state.

On my first day of work, I felt a chill run through me as I looked at the monstrous stone structure and its surrounding gun towers that were shrouded in a November fog. A ghostly aura emanated from the ominous structure as it stood defiantly upon the tranquil banks of San Francisco Bay.

Institutional security was tight. To reach the belly of the maximum-security institution, I had to pass several checkpoints, beginning at the front gate. Walking through a discomforting stillness, I climbed the stairway up the hill from the parking lot and crossed the street, entering a darkened tunnel drilled through a massive granite wall.

Suddenly the loud crash of metal sounded from behind me. Startling, I spun around and watched as the enormous iron gate crashed closed. As I turned to step forward, my stomach plummeted upon viewing the other massive gate closed. The desolate sense of being caged swept within me. The anxiety existing inside me awakened, beginning to whirl deep in my gut. I didn't like the feeling of being trapped.

Approaching a small bulletproof window where an officer sat, I handed her my I.D. Comparing it with the dozens of names upon a list that she had, she checked it off and offered a smile, saying, "Welcome."

The second gate slid open. Exiting, I found myself amid a peaceful courtyard filled with tropical plants. Surrounding it were massive stone walls, topped with a series of intermittently placed peaked towers connected by catwalks. Gunmen slowly strolled, cradling their rifles in their arms as they patrolled back and forth. My eyes searched for the various buildings for the Captain's Porch, a small group of offices set off one side.

After meeting with Captain Art Calderon, he turned me over to Larry Poole, the sergeant of the upper yard, where they had assigned me to work the day watch, Tuesday through Saturday. I was grateful to be able to spend time with my family from Saturday afternoons through the weekend's end.

Knowing Larry from Soledad, where he had worked for a brief period, a familiar face was great to see. Casually chatting about old times, we crossed the "upper yard," an asphalted area surrounded by tall granite walled housing units.

"We average over a thousand inmates here each day," the sergeant said as the resounding boom of a shotgun pierced through the otherwise calm of the morning. More shots followed, my heart leaping with each. Officers raced past us, weaving through the sea hundreds of tattooed men, dressed in blue. Their batons wildly swung at their sides as they ran across the yard, while others leisurely strolled by, unaffected by what was occurring around them.

"If you hear the gunman rack in a round, turn your back. Get as close to the wall as you can so you don't catch the ricochets and be sure to protect your eyes and face," Pool instructed.

"Gotcha," I said.

"And you are aware there is a no-hostage policy, right? Like Soledad?" he asked.

I again nodded, a lump forming in my throat. A no hostage policy meant the prison would not consider a hostage's status in negotiations, nor would they consider the exchange of a hostage for any action intended to control the situation. I glanced toward the interior of the yard, at the hundreds of inmates milling around. Looking up, I realized the gunman standing over us would be holding my life in his hands. My mind was flying with thoughts of how I would protect myself.

An officer approached. "Sarge, it was a stabbing on the C-Section yard. It's under control."

"Thank you," Pool offered respectfully.

"It gets active here, especially in the lockups," the sergeant explained. "Different from Soledad, huh?"

"Very much so," I answered. Only on three occasions during the year and a half I worked there did I respond to an alarm. It had been less than an hour that I was on the San Quentin upper yard, and there was already an altercation that had occurred.

"Yeah, we fired a few thousand shots last year, most of them up here on the yard, or in the seg units," he quietly advised.

Spring was late that year while I was assigned to work outside. The four months of the icy winds and the freezing rain of winter ripping across San Francisco Bay and slamming against us, and penetrating through our jackets, was intense. However, I did not mind. I loved the freedom of working outdoors with the yard crew, who were a great group of guys.

In my twenty-nine years of life, I contracted colds or the flu on only two or three occasions. A picture of health, I seldom wore a jacket, even when it was freezing outside. But within months of working there, I suffered through the most prolonged bout of the flu I had ever experienced. When it did not go away, I became concerned, and I consulted my doctor.

"No fever?" he asked while assessing my symptoms.

"No, sir," I said.

"Muscle aches?"

"Uh-uh."

"How about congestion, runny nose?"

"Nope, just nausea," I answered.

"I think I'm going to order you a pregnancy test," he said as he sat back down on his small black stool.

"Oh, no! No! Not now!" I groaned.

"Come on. It's not all that bad," the young doctor laughed.

"My God. You do not know. It's my job. They'll never understand."

"They may not have much choice, you know?" he said as he arose and walked out the door.

Prayer and wishes didn't work. Fate had other plans. Being pregnant was another problem that was well beyond my control. I was learning how to work my way each matter, one by one. The next step was a visit to the office of the personnel lieutenant for an intimate heart to heart conversation.

I wasn't comfortable having to see him. It was the second time, in two years, in working within the prison setting, that fear flooded through me. I liked the people at San Quentin, the good old boys at the top with the beer bellies folded over the edge of their belts, who worked hard at keeping their images as the "baddest asses in the joint." Their rough talk and other methods of communication were entertaining. Most were marshmallows with big hearts.

But he was different.

Climbing to the top of the stairs, I softly tapped on Personnel Lieutenant's door.

"Come in," a voice growled.

Opening it, I poked my head inside.

"Lieutenant?" I softly asked.

"What do you want?"

"May I speak with you for a moment?"

"Is it important?"

"I feel it is," I said, glancing at all the guy stuff pasted upon his wall. Notably, a poster stood out. It read: "Marines. We're looking for a few good men." On the bottom, written boldly in magic marker, was, "San Quentin will take all the rest."

It *was* funny, but the message was not particularly friendly toward women, especially those in my situation. Confident there would not be much love coming my way, I prepared myself for the worst.

"Okay. What's up?" the lieutenant groaned, tossing his papers onto the top of his metal desk.

"Great," I thought, realizing I *was* disturbing him. Deciding to get it done, I stood in front of his desk, sputtering, "Lieutenant, I'm nine weeks pregnant."

"What?" he spewed as he leaned back in his chair and glared at me. "How in the hell did that happen?"

Cocking my head at him, for issuing his typical guy remark, I asked, "Do you really want me to answer that?"

"Okay," he sighed. You will have to leave. We don't have any accommodations for pregnancy here."

He picked up the papers he tossed down on his desk and pretended to read as though I was not present. I remained there, frozen, unwilling to move from where I was standing.

He glanced up at me. "What? Are you still here? What are you waiting for?" he snarled.

"Are you *sure*?" I asked. I had nothing left to lose.

He slammed the papers down again, his eyes drilling through mine.

"What did you say?" he demanded.

Few female officers questioned him, and even fewer men did. Reminding myself that I needed to soften up and tone down on my assertiveness, that guys like him did not receive well, I answered, "Are you *sure*? What with this Title VII stuff and the changes about pregnancy? You know, it's not like getting cancer or something."

My heart pounding, I prayed I had not gone too far confronting him with the federal law that offered protections for pregnant women to continue working. Pregnancy was no longer a disability.

Holding my breath, I awaited the Lieutenant's response. Out of desperation, I was taking an enormous risk. The law appeared to be on my side, but the Department may or may not be. It was still very much a man's world where they sometimes made up their own rules. No other choice existed, but to confront it. I needed to keep my job. We had two homes in Wyoming that had not sold and a mortgage payment in California. I was the only one able to work overtime to pay the bills.

If I faced termination, or if they forced me to leave early, it would be difficult for my family. I needed to work through eight and one-half months of my pregnancy since my husband faced difficulty working overtime. If I could endure that long, I could take my sick leave and vacation leave for six weeks before the expected delivery date of my child and six weeks following his birth. It was all that policy and state regulations allowed unless there were complications with the pregnancy.

Fighting the issue in court would be a long, delayed process. The departmental administration manual allowed managers to assign pregnant women to less hazardous positions if it did not require a senior officer to lose his job. Those assignments, in gun towers and gun rails, ordinarily did not exist. They were a kingdom held by older officers until they retired.

Check or checkmate?

He sat back in his armchair, his face expressionless, disallowing me to get a read on him. The first at San Quentin to challenge the department with federal civil rights protections for pregnant women, it was difficult to gauge his response.

"Have it your way," he finally relented, sitting upright, and picking up a paper from his desk. "You can stay, but you *will* do everything the men do."

"Thank you. I can do that," I said confidently.

"And remember this. Because you are here on reinstatement, you are now on probation again," the Lieutenant warned.

Probation again?

I silently groaned. He was going to make it hell and force me to run through the gauntlet of male reprisal. I had won but would dearly pay for it. There was no doubt that he realized the anxiety it created. During the five months since reinstatement, I had not received one probationary report, and there was no notification that I would again be on probation.

For a moment, I stood silently, considering his statement. Finally, I decided it did not mean a thing; it was not worth battling. With the notice of being on probation, issued on the day I reported being pregnant, I would easily win an appeal if anyone tried to force me to leave, especially five months after arrival and not receiving a performance report. Writing anything negative in a report while requiring a pregnant female officer to do everything the men do could be problematic for them. I had gotten my piece of flesh. It was best to be happy with that. A tough road was ahead. I needed to work step by step and get my head wrapped around that reality.

Our eyes locked for a few brief seconds—his reflected anger. Mine spelled out a controlled sense of defiance. He needed to know how serious I was about staying. Still not saying a word about his last comment, he appeared uncomfortable. He realized I knew he had crossed a line.

Breaking the stare-down, the Lieutenant glanced down upon the paper tightly clenched in his hand. We had come to an understanding.

"All right. Now get out of here," he ordered, less sternly.

"Thank you," I offered as I left, carefully closing the door behind me. Racing downstairs, I landed into the arms of some anxious, awaiting women.

"What happened?" "What did he say?" They shot questions at me as we walked toward the snack bar.

"I'm staying, but there is no consideration of any job changes or limited duty," I told them. It was good enough. They were considering starting families, and neither wanted to leave.

It was a start, an advancement for the women at San Quentin. Within the next several years, more than half a dozen more would become pregnant and be able to work wherever they so desired if they had the seniority. I fully supported them.

For the next four months, I remained working on the upper yard. The days became longer, and it wasn't easy. Being pregnant, it was a challenging experience walking the five to ten miles a day. Surprisingly, no one complained about me continuing to work, at least not in my presence. Several of my male counterparts advocated on my behalf, while most of the inmates acted considerately.

One afternoon, a young inmate uncomfortably approached.

Nervously, he asked, "Can I ask you something?"

"Sure," I answered.

"Can a dude get a double-murder beef if he stabs you?"

"What?" My eyes widened with concern while trying to understand the thought process behind the question. It was not what a pregnant correctional officer working on the upper yard at San Quentin wanted to hear from inmates that were most serving life sentences for murder.

"A couple of us were wondering." He gestured toward two others standing near the fence. "I mean, how far along do you got to be to get a murder beef? Would it be a double murder?" he asked.

Not sure how to respond, I decided to pull out my "girl card."

"That's a pretty tough question that would be much better answered by an appellate court which would decide if that were to happen. That is if the person lived long enough to see it that far after killing or harming a pregnant woman," I stated, matter-of-factly.

"That's kind of what I think too," he said, thoughtfully.

Watching as he sauntered away, I understood what he had been asking. Inmates were working out their own sense of justice, much the same as others debated abortion and at what stage they considered a fetus a person. Several intently followed the development of my unborn child.

"Are you taking supplements? It says here you should," an inmate asked.

"You got to eat more, you know," his friend added.

A significant difference in being pregnant while working in the San Quentin yard was the level of violence had decreased. Ordinarily, when the temperatures rose, the numbers of violent incidents rose with it. Different was the level of violence, which fell once the word got out of my pregnancy.

The only thing about me and my job that did not change was the length of my pat-down search line. Our job was to pat-search to find weapons the hundreds of inmates, leaving the lower yard to come to the upper yard, may carry upon them. Most inmates preferred a woman to examine them for contraband. While my male counterparts had two or three inmates in their lines, pregnant or not, mine was always about forty feet long and sometimes extended halfway to the lower yard. Most inmates were quiet and respectful while waiting.

But every circus has its clown, and that summer, I met him. He approached, standing before me, and glaring into my eyes. Then, he turned his back and dramatically readied himself for the search.

"Oh baby," he groaned, performing a cheap Elvis act, gyrating his pelvic area. "You want some of this? Rub those soft, lily-white hands all over me."

"Not at all," I answered, glancing toward a partner, J.J. Hellman, and emitting a sigh of disgust. At six months of pregnancy, and nearing the end of my workday, I was not in the mood to deal with the inmate. My mornings still filled with morning sickness and my afternoons with incredible weariness, continuing to work was becoming more difficult. J.J. offered a sympathetic smile and winked as he stepped behind me.

As I began my search, my face cringed as the inmate wiggled and groaned with exaggerated pleasure. J.J. gently pushed me to the side and took over. Standing behind him, all of us laughed while watching as the inmate continued to rejoice in how good J.J.'s hands felt upon his body.

"You can do this anytime you want, baby," he said, moaning and closing his eyes.

A large crowd of inmates congregated, laughing with us, as I stood, shaking my head in amusement. Done, the inmate turned to leave. His face transformed into one of horror when he saw a male officer standing in front of him, smiling.

"You like that, huh?" J.J. asked, winking at me.

Spouting out a few expletives, the inmate stormed off. We laughed even harder. For a while, my line was shorter.

The day finally arrived when Captain Calderon stopped me outside the institution. "Uh, you can wear a maternity smock now," he offered while looking down at my swollen belly. I was more than ready for it. Over the past months, my body had swelled, more than enough to justify wearing a smock. I was looking like a female Humpty Dumpty with my egg-shaped stomach.

The next morning, when I strode onto the upper yard wearing a green maternity smock over my uniform shirt, all eyes were upon me. It was a relief. A big problem the Department and I faced with accommodating pregnant officers was there were no departmentally approved maternity uniforms. Nor did any written standards exist for the assigning of positions for pregnant officers exist. There was merely one paragraph reading that women should be placed in a lessor hazardous duty position if one were available, and it didn't displace a senior officer from his regular job position. No one had even thought to design a uniform for those of us working full duty when pregnant.

I spent a few evenings designing it and had it tailored at the uniform shop, working off a design I had seen the first pregnant woman officer wore at Soledad. Fashioned from the same material as our uniform pants, I sewed, I sewed a pregnancy panel in the front to replace the zipper.

Tweaking the pregnancy smock into something that resembled a conservative uniform, I added tabs on both sides to accommodate expansion and a tab to affix my badge.

For the first time, I was wearing it on the yard. Many of the inmates were stepping away from me as I passed them. It was comforting to realize they wanted to be as far from me, as possible, to protect both of us. Rather than inviting problems, in the general population of a level five institution, I found my pregnancy was an added layer of insulation from potential harm.

Most inmates aren't any different from anyone on the streets. They have all had a mother figure or a grandmother at some time in their lives. The one respected, consistent person in most everyone's life is his or her mother. Inmates are no different. Like most, they, too, respond to that which is familiar. Besides the relationship with a spouse, the one between a mother and her son is one of the longest, withstanding relationships most men experience.

The women in their lives are their lifelines to the outside world. It is ordinarily the mothers and the grandmothers that write them letters and visit. And it is often the presence of women officers that brings an aura of maternal familiarity and calm into institutions. At San Quentin, women officers fill that void by offering a sense of normalcy to an abnormal living environment.

That summer, at about six months of pregnancy, I raced to an alarm with my partners while a new sergeant was supervising the yard. It had been standard practice. The lieutenant had instructed me to do it when I advised I was pregnant. So, I did. As I passed him, his eyes widened. He ran to catch up with me and grabbed my arm, spinning me around, begging me not to run. He was so concerned with the situation that he and my partners addressed their concerns to his supervisors.

While the assignment lieutenant and others were sequestered in their offices scheduling over a thousand custodial officers in their positions, they had forgotten that I was still out on the upper yard, working. The next morning, I received an immediate job change to the West Block gun rail.

Adapting quickly to my new assignment, I found the only initial difficulties I faced included gaining immediate access to a bathroom and carrying the heavy weight because of considerable armament.

Already carrying over twenty-five pounds of the baby upon my middle, the heavy leather belt holding a .38 caliber revolver, a few dozen rounds of ammunition, a couple of banana clips filled with .223 caliber rounds, and a shotgun slung over one shoulder, with an occasional Mini-14 semiautomatic rifle slung over the other.

Adding a bandoleer across my chest, loaded with shotgun rounds, and weighing one hundred and twenty lbs., in total, every day, I was bearing forty percent of my total body weight. On some days, it was difficult, especially those when I was assigned to work twelve-hour shifts and required to walk an average of ten miles during each.

I learned at Soledad, when one is a sheep, living with a pack of wolves, you do what you must to blend in and become part of the pack, or you will be eaten alive. It was a good training ground. Assigned to one of the two most dangerous institutions in the state alongside some of the toughest guys, I was carrying an equally heavy load as them, along with being pregnant. Continuing to assure myself I could do it, allowed me to get through each day, no matter how difficult, at times, it seemed.

A few years before, I had confided in one of my sergeants that I was concerned I did not have what it takes to do the job, that I was not big enough, or as strong as the men.

He inspired me by stating, "You have to think big. If you think big, you are big. You can do anything you want. It just takes time to develop your own style. Be patient; it will come."

On that gun rail, I made myself think big. Though it helped with the attitude, it provided little resolution about the amount of weight I had to carry that rested upon the swollen breasts and the waistline that I no longer had. Those utility belts the department offered were huge, intended to hold a lot of heavy added equipment. I wore mine upon my lower hips, instead of my "no- longer existing waistline." My service weapon dangled against the edge of my right knee.

That, with the bandoleer worn across my chest, filled with shotgun rounds, created the disturbing appearance of the wife of an 1800s Mexican bandit, rather than a peace officer. While my male peers stood in my corner, asking that I receive limited duty, the inmates approached the administration, complaining that it just wasn't right to have armed, pregnant women carrying weapons on the gun rail.

Trying not to laugh, the administrators debated, "Just don't do anything to upset her, and you won't have a problem."

"But pregnant women? You can't reason with them," they argued.

It was worthy of a chuckle. Only a few had genuine issues. One threw a brick at me and suffered the wrath of Sergeant Read's fury. I had never seen him run as fast as he did up those stairs to confront that inmate.

The gun rail extended the length and the width of the outer perimeter of the cellblock. It was a small walkway attached to the exterior walls, bordered with a protective railing that looked out upon a long row of fifty cells constructed five stories high, and situated in the middle of the cellblock. Back and forth, we patrolled past the inmate's cells. Walking was a good thing. It kept me active and healthy.

Accessing the top rail to cover the fourth and fifth tiers was a nightmare. It required "spider climbing" up a heavy metal ladder affixed flush to a concrete wall. Twenty to thirty feet in height, it had no safety cage surrounding it. Fortunately, I was good at keeping my balance and possessed a fair amount of upper-body strength. Even eight months into my pregnancy, I was still able to do it until June 1982, when all hell broke loose. Boom, boom, boom! I startled at the sound of the rapid gunfire that pierced through the unit.

"My God," my partner said, as he quickly approached. "It sounds like World War III is going on out there. Get ready for overtime tonight."

Twenty-one, twenty-two, twenty-three shots, and still counting, the gunshots continued, and the worry for our fellow staff members consumed us. Neither of us could imagine what was happening out there. That day, officers fired off forty-two rounds, while 1,500 inmates battled one another. Thirty-nine inmates and four correctional officers sustained injuries. Officers were finally able to separate the fighting forces and escort the inmates from the yard. They locked everyone inside their cells.

We were all ordered to work twelve-hour shifts, with no exceptions. Spending the first eight hours on the West Block gun rail, the following four hours were on the gun rail of the institutional dining hall. Perpetually exhausted, I kept myself distracted by quietly singing. Sometimes, I was so tired. I simply wanted to sit down and cry. It was not until driving home after my shift that I allowed myself to release emotion.

- 161 -

After about four weeks of lockdown, and during the final two months of my pregnancy, Connie Chung of NBC television, and other journalists visited West Block to view the institution, while on lock-down. However, most were not paying attention to the public information officer hosting them. They were watching the enormously pregnant officer carrying a shotgun while following them to the top tier of the unit by spider climbing up a concrete wall on a ladder.

Again, I received an immediate, unexpected job change. This time, the personnel lieutenant had safely hidden me away; in the basement of the administration building, where they tasked me with aiding the background investigator. Now, off the gun rail, I had finally worked the required time I needed to work to qualify for pregnancy leave and limited duty. I decided to keep working a bit longer, without opting for either. I had something to prove to others and myself. I needed to be able to qualify to complete in promotability examinations coming up that spring. With my husband unable to work overtime, we needed the money.

During those challenging times, I had filled my mind with the images of our Native American ancestral grandmothers, having heard the stories from our Grandmother of how they often delivered their children alone in the wilderness. Then, childbirth was another part of living. While away from their homes, it was not unusual for the women to leave whatever they were doing, to go behind a log, and often alone, with another, to deliver their baby. After a time of rest, they returned to what they were doing. If they demonstrated that immense amount of strength and courage while delivering their children during far more difficult times, and under the strain of *their* natural progression and routines during life, so could I.

Though I believed it wholeheartedly, my body disagreed. It rebelled. I went into early labor. Prescribed six weeks of bed rest to avoid premature delivery; after a few weeks, my physician expressed concern about the risk to my child's health. His heart rate was stressed. He decided to induce labor early. Twelve hours later, I gave birth to a beautiful son.

Reflecting upon my experiences and that of other women faced with the devastating conflict between choosing between their career or the birth of their child, it is my firm belief no woman should have to risk the wellbeing of herself and her unborn child to keep a job; especially if state and federal governments refuse to remove women from hazardous duty situations into one that is less hazardous when pregnant.

Chapter Sixteen

DAYS OF VIOLENCE

"Man is the only predator who hunts his own." ~Kenneth Eade

A traditional phrase in the (CDC) is "One year of working at San Quentin is the equivalent of five years of experience elsewhere." I can testify to its truthfulness. A little over a week after the birth of my son, I received a telephone call from the new Personnel Lieutenant. "Would you be willing to come back to work early and manage a special assignment for us?" he asked.

It came at just the right time. I agreed to return. My husband and I had separated following the birth of our son. He continued to live in our home while the kids and I moved into our own place. It was a peaceful time, with just me and my children.

My kids were my stability. It was them and my work that kept me going, feeding into my sense of self-esteem, and supplying with an enormous feeling of accomplishment. There was little time to think or even feel sorry for myself while working at San Quentin fulltime, caring for my kids, and attending college classes at night.

The assignment involved overseeing two clerical staff members and an inmate clerk in the writing and processing of "incident reports." The institution was over a year behind in preparing reports for the District Attorney to decide whether to file criminal charges against the suspects.

Our team completed over a year's worth of work within two months, with little difficulty. Following, they assigned me to various temporary supervisory positions, a few projects in the state headquarters in Sacramento, and training San Quentin correctional officers in report writing. Able to prove my capabilities to departmental administrators, it enabled me to stop "dummying up." Staying genuine, I tried to keep as low of a profile as possible. It was essential for career survival.

Rumors ran rampant about the women working in the institutions, especially those women who worked closely with men. Learning early that a few of the staff members could be every bit as brutal as some inmates, not as much of abuse existed at San Quentin as it did at Soledad.

The spirit of esprit décor at San Quentin differed from other institutions. Anyone focused upon petty gossip, or the exclusion of others seldom lasted, unless it was a guy talking about a woman, with another guy. There was only one officer who continually hurled attacks my way. Ignoring him, eventually, karma intervened. He ended up losing his job.

That spring, while feeling the warmth of Indian summer sun that was raining down upon the upper yard, the temperatures were warm enough not to don a jacket. I was disturbed to note a lot of the Hispanic inmates were wearing them. Adding to my concern was that fewer than usual engaged in eye contact as they passed me. My intuition was screaming, "Something was not right."

Acute hypervigilance often develops in an environment where a personal threat exists, whether it be contracting cancer, living alone as a single mom in an urban area, operating in a battlefield, or working in one of the most dangerous prisons in the world. Tension is energy. In institutional settings, before an incident, staff often "feel that energy" just before something occurs, just as those who know "something isn't right," when struck by cancer or other serious illness.

That same hypervigilance learned as a child, had become a lifesaving skill when working at San Quentin. It not only assisted in recognizing changes in inmate behavior at San Quentin but in identifying the changes in me when I contracted cancer.

Fear is a powerful survival tool. When felt, I confronted whatever created it, if possible, to make sure it resolved. If it could not, I made attempts to minimize it with distraction, in the same way as concentrating upon the pain from one area can work to numb the feeling of pain elsewhere. Distraction is a powerful tool to work with during situations over which we have little or no control. I learned it from my father, who spent years using it to help him get past challenging times.

Hypervigilance, that time when the subconscious awakens, and an understanding of impending danger occurs, is a useful survival tool if channeled in the right manner. Learning to recognize even the slightest changes of behavior in others, allowed me to anticipate problems in advance, by trusting in what I felt during those times.

Sergeant Pool crossed the yard and leaned up against the wall, joining me as I carefully watched the activity of the inmates.

"Something's wrong. Feel it?" I stated quietly.

"Yeah," he answered. After a few more moments, he walked over to the phone to speak with Jim DeManche, the gun rail officer patrolling overhead. As they talked, Jim glanced down and nodded. He felt it too.

A small Hispanic inmate suddenly rushed by, hissing, "Got to talk to you. Over here."

Tailing him through the yard, he disappeared into the sea of inmates, rounding into the concealed "slot area," a patio of sorts leading toward a block of housing units to the north and one to the south. No one was there, nor was there any sign of movement anywhere near the South Block rotunda and the West Block yard. The sense of something wrong intensified.

Stopping to listen, I heard nothing but a deafening silence. My heart dropped. *That* was what was wrong. There should have been the lively bantering of inmates on the yard.

Cautiously, I stepped back onto the asphalt of the upper yard and viewed a sea of faces blankly milling around, instead of cloistered together. As I approached, inmates stepped back., revealing a young Hispanic inmate sprawled upon the asphalt, a knife protruding from his neck.

Grabbing for my whistle and blowing it, I noted the high pitched, trilling sound that followed sounded muted, along with the racking of the shotgun overhead and the subsequent thunder of its blast. Everything moved in slow motion. I found myself in a foggy tunnel, feeling like a robot, as I assessed the situation. Slowly stepping forward, the inmates I passed edged back into the crowd. Noting details to write in a report later, I kneeled on one knee next to the victim.

Blood oozed from his neck upon the asphalt, and his eyes were glassy. Turning my head and glancing upward, toward the fence, I locked eyes with a gang leader. Tenths of seconds of contact seemed like minutes. I noted every detail. He grimaced and diverted his eyes to the ground to distance himself from me. His feet and body were half-facing the housing unit. He wanted out of there, badly. Instantly, I knew he was involved.

The gurgling continued as bloody matter spilled from the inmate's mouth as he tried to speak. Calling for a gurney, I noted some of the dozens of officers responding raced off to get one, while more flew toward us, running from nowhere, somewhere, everywhere, pushing the inmates back, away from us.

"Hang on, guy," I whispered as I bent close and grasped his hand. "Who did this to you?"

He looked up at me for a brief second and turned his head sideways.

"Them," he uttered, his one-word sentence vibrating.

"Who?" I asked.

"Them," he repeated determinedly, his eyes lowering toward his right arm. Mine followed, noting the boldly emblazed tattoo, reading SUR 13, upon it.

Glancing up at the men by the fence, I noted they wore the same. Again, following the inmate's gaze, which led to what appeared to be the gang leader, he appeared to be anxious. His right foot was now anxiously tapping upon the asphalt.

What's his name? Alejandro? No. Lugo... that's it. Lugo, the shot caller.

Wearing an expression of desperation, the inmate dropped his head. Jack Read, the security squad sergeant, bent over me. "I caught it," he whispered.

"Lugo?" Read asked the inmate.

The inmate struggled a nod. Read confirmed it. "It's him."

"You five, over there," Read called out to a group of officers. "Secure the yard. Get IDs, shake them down, look for cuts, blood, and weapons." As an afterthought, he added, "and toss their cells."

To the men he supervised, he merely said, "Lugo and the homeboys... over on the fence."

"Gotcha, Sarge." They knew what to do. Instantly, they surrounded the group. Herding them into a cluster, they began shaking them down. Now, standing on the edge of the crowd, I heard the loud bubbling of finality sounding at my feet. Silence followed.

"Oh no," I uttered, looking away.

"I think we lost him," Poole announced, rising, and moving out of the way of officers carrying a stretcher. "Why don't you go into the bathroom and clean up?" he said to me. "I'll wait here."

Standing in the restroom on the upper yard, my hands were shaking. Rinsing the blood off them and dabbing my shirt with icy water, I tried to remove the small spots of blood splatter. Silently, I chastised myself for not keeping gloves on me.

Eyes lit upon some plastic bottles of bleach and industrial floor cleaner set under the sink. Opening them, I poured a large amount into the sink. Dipping my hands into it, I splashed the disinfectant on my face and scrubbed my exposed skin with it. Finally, I felt clean. The tunnel vision subsiding, I could see my image in the mirror more clearly

Wearing the fragrance of a military bathroom, we walked to the captain's porch, where we sat in an empty office and drafted our reports to the rhythm of the soft tapping of my right foot upon the floor. My reaction to the threat of fear was disquieting. The sensation that overcame me had evolved since it first occurred at Soledad. This time it resulted in the newly developed additions of uncontrollable foot-tapping, a slow-motion feeling, and tunnel vision. Looking down at my hands, I again hadn't noticed they were trembling.

Aware Pool was watching, I said, offering a weak laugh, "Bad time to quit smoking, huh?"

In silence, he slid his chair out and walked into the other room, returning with a cup of coffee in his hand.

"Here," he said, "Drink this. First time?"

Nodding my head, "Uh-huh," and offering a weak smile, my hands tightly cupped the mug; and I took a sip. Years ago, having worked in an emergency room while attending community college to be a nurse, I had seen people die on occasion, but I had never seen anyone killed.

"I don't know why I can't stop shaking," I said.

"Happens to most of us, at first."

"Good to know," I answered quietly.

"If you didn't feel it the first time you saw someone killed, something would be wrong with you," he added.

We continued to write. After a few moments, the sergeant set his pen down. "There isn't much anyone can do when they want to get someone here," he said, reading my mind as guilt seethed through me because I couldn't find the inmate. "You know?"

"Yeah," Focusing back upon my report, I added the inmate made a dying declaration, naming Lugo, as a participant.

That day I realized that life is not fair. Monsters are everywhere, existing amongst us. They're not just in prisons; many don't even end up there. And, not all are big, ugly, and scary looking. They can and often do look like everyday people, ministers, teachers, and neighbors. Some may look like police officers, doctors, elected officials, or others holding a position of trust. Most are not identifiable. But if we pay attention to the clues they leave, we can discern between those who are different from us and those who are not.

I learned a lot about survival during that experience. Those of us with hereditary cancer defects continuously consider ways to prevent cancer. We must trust our intuition, recognize the changes in our bodies when develops, and get those regular screenings from experts. By trusting our instincts and knowing the symptoms of its existence, we can also prevent its development; and protect our families and ourselves.

During the late spring of 1982, I pulled out a piece of paper from my shirt pocket and looked at it for the third time since I had gotten off shift. It read, 4:50 p.m. The clock read 3:25 p.m. Sighing, I folded it back up and slid it back inside.

Hanging around in the unit and completing paperwork, I was waiting to take part in an oral interview for consideration of a promotion to the position of sergeant. I didn't want to take the chance of leaving for a short while and coming back. I couldn't afford to be late. With one disabled vehicle on the roadway and traffic blocked off, I could blow a big opportunity and be forced to wait until they again offered the test a few years later.

On that day, and during the last year, I had worked in temporary supervisory and specialized assignments while studying for the exam. Arriving at work at 5:00 A.M., each day for six months, I would go into the Captain's Porch, where I read every single policy manual I could find.

Done with that, I reviewed the state laws governing the operations of state agencies, state and federal case law involving incarcerated persons. I studied the California Penal Code to review regulations regarding incarcerated individuals, the California Civil Code as it related to human resource management, and the regular bulletins that were disseminated by the Department of Justice dealing with federal civil rights violations. I did a lot of reading in preparation for that test.

I had to know all there was to know about every aspect of the institution. Any time there was a question on policy, they would say, "Go ask Linda. She's read the entire library."

The Class A blazer, a clean uniform, and brightly shined shoes were in the car. All I needed to do was clean-up and dress in the In-Service Training Building. With ample time between the end of my shift and the interview, I was playing "catch-up" with completing paperwork.

Violence had been rocking at San Quentin. Someone had murdered an inmate in the gymnasium that morning. While bench pressing weights, someone dropped one upon his head. The victim's only offense was that of being of a different race at the wrong place and at the wrong time. Though on lockdown, the word had gotten out quickly. A war was on, and tensions were high. Retaliation was inevitable.

Our unit was on lockdown. All inmates confined to their cells; we only allowed essential workers onto the tiers. Two tiers of inmates were in the dining hall, and we expected them to return shortly. Those staying inside were anxious. None were looking forward to another night of locking up inside their cells. Leaving the office door open, I kept one eye upon cellblock activities through the window while filling out required state forms for the monthly supplies needed to accommodate the over four-hundred and fifty inmates in the block. Being there enabled my relief to take advantage of the opportunity to deal with matters outside the unit.

Tearing off my copy of the form, and tossing it into a file folder, I slid my pen into my shirt pocket, and sat back in my chair, watching as the first group of inmates entered the unit. They were unusually quiet. Understandable, I thought. A peer had died. But the number of woolen jackets worn by the black inmates were not. It was a direct message. Something was about to come down.

The heavy woolen jackets layered on top of layers of shirts offered padding to soften stab wounds. As I watched them climb the stairs to the second tier, my stomach began its predictable churning. Suddenly, an inmate janitor's enormous body appeared, blocking the doorway. He, too, was wearing a jacket and seemed to be agitated.

"What are you doing here? You're supposed to be gone," he demanded. Managing a smile, I said, "Paperwork."

"Well, I'm closing this door. I don't want none of these guys bothering you when they come in," he said protectively.

"Thank you," I responded, bothered by his strange behavior. As he left, the familiar sick feeling intensified. By now, I was sure something was about to erupt.

Concerned, I rose from my chair and stepped out of the office. Glancing up at the gun rail, I noted the gunman was alert, patrolling back and forth as usual. Looking upward, toward the second tier, I didn't see anything out of order. Nonetheless, I still felt an intense sense of tension and smelled the fear as inmates quickly raced toward the stairs and their cells.

Following, I climbed the stairs. Touching down upon the second-tier landing, I noticed considerable activity was occurring. Inmates were racing back and forth from cell to cell, exchanging items before the heavy bar would grate across their doors. Expecting to be locked down for days on end, they were borrowing and lending items, preparing to tuck in.

Suddenly, a chilling scream echoed through the unit, followed by a flash of black that rapidly raced out of a cell and down the crowded tier, disappearing into the open door of another cell. More war-cries sounded.

Boom! Boom! The sounds of gunshots, war cries, high toned screams for help, and whistles echoing through the concrete hall, from somewhere and everywhere, suddenly filled the unit. Iron doors slammed shut as inmates frantically locked themselves inside their cells. All hell was breaking loose.

Then, as quickly as it occurred, it was over. The unit fell into an eerie silence. Everything happened in less than ninety seconds, and the inmates who were not injured were back in their cells. The only sounds were the occasional ring of metal as the knives they had fashioned from whatever, dropped upon the concrete on the first tier.

"Pull the bar as soon as I get these closed," I yelled to an officer who had reached the second tier. Running as fast as I could, down the concrete tier, stepping over injured inmates, and slamming the opened cell doors as rapidly as possible, I stopped for a second to glance upon the first tier. An enormous surge of relief filled through me as I viewed dozens of responding officers spilling into the unit.

"Look for blood and bruises," I called in a reminder to the troops who worked with me.

"Gotcha, Sarge."

"Where are all the gurneys?" I then yelled down to the officers below.

"They just went out," someone yelled back.

"Get on the phone and call around for more. We need those gurneys *now*!"

"Will do," I heard someone call from the first tier. A couple of officers ran outside to gather gurneys from other units.

I turned around and saw our unit clerk, Yancey, lifting a small inmate from the tier. "He is hurt bad, Sarge. I am taking downstairs so they can get him out."

I nodded as I recognized Bridger. Every officer has their "favorite inmate." The goofy little Bridger was mine. My heart fell as Yancey quickly walked down the tier, carefully carrying him toward the stairwell.

The downstairs door again flew open. Officers from the security squad moved inside. I quickly waved to them. They nodded and headed up to where I was, readied to take over the crime scene.

"Gurneys are on their way," I told the sergeant after debriefing him and before heading downstairs to get out of their way. It was a relief to turn the command of the incident over to him. It was one less cause of worry.

"I'll get you my report tomorrow," I offered.

With others at the scene and the second watch sergeant and lieutenant now in the unit, prepared to leave. Running past me were officers, their gurneys loaded with injured inmates. My face fell as I saw Yancey, standing there at the door, his eyes tearing and wearing a look of helplessness as he still held Bridger in his arms.

I yelled out, "I need a gurney here now!"

"More are coming from other units," someone yelled back.

"Lieutenant, this guy can't wait. I'm sending him out," I insisted, calling to him across the room.

Nodding in agreement, he instructed Sergeant Collins, my relief, "Call Wall Post One and tell him to alert all the gunmen and wall posts we're gonna have an officer and inmate running across the yard carrying one wounded to the hospital."

"Gotcha, Lieu," he responded as he ducked into the office. Yancey's attempts at compressing Bridger's vein were not working. The bleeding from his neck was uncontrollable. The situation was becoming dire.

"Bridger, it will be okay," I assured him. "Just stay calm."

His eyes were glassy. Yancey continued to rock him in his arms, as he anxiously stood by the door, waiting for a gurney.

"Rogers, here, take over what I'm doing, and give me your keys. Please go with Yancey to the infirmary," I instructed the older officer.

"Who says?" Rogers confronted me.

"Me," I answered firmly.

He glared at me for an instant, not moving. None of us had time for his reluctance to follow my order. Especially Bridger.

"Hand over the damned keys now!" Again, no response. Standing silent in defiance, he remained silent, his glare and tightened jaw expressing his hostility.

"That's a direct order, Rogers," I demanded firmly, ticked off by a hostile mentality the older correctional officer was displaying. "Do it, or I'll write paper."

His mouth dropped, realizing my seriousness. He handed them over as Collins came toward us.

"Do what she says, Rogers, or I'll flipping do it," he instructed as he approached. "All clear, Linda," he called out to me.

Keying open the door, I instructed, "Run like hell," I told Rogers and Yancey. "And be very careful with him."

Closing and locking the door, I turned the keys over to Sergeant Collins, and stepping outside, I paused for a moment to take a deep breath. The freedom of getting out of the unit and into the open where I could breathe fresh, clean air. I needed it badly to begin the process of decompressing.

Ten minutes later, as the tunnel vision dissipated, I realized how crazy I appeared, standing in the bathroom of the training department, singing. Looking upon my reflection in the mirror, I was still wearing my concern about Bridger. Glancing down toward my reddened hands, I noted I had unknowingly scrubbed them raw. At least, the inmate's blood was no longer on them. All I could think about was the unthinkable, inexcusable violence. This time I knew the inmate as a person.

Bridger was just another young kid committed from some rural county who, like others, dumped their inmates who should have gotten county jail time, into CDC prison sentences to save money. An enormous disparity in sentencing existed between the number of inmates committed from the smaller counties compared to those in the urban areas.

Every morning the kid skipped down the stairs with his "road dog." Greeting me in a silly, chipmunk type voice, he would say, "Good morning, groundhog." His cellmate and I would laugh. He was a quirky kid who belonged in a youth conservation camp, not in San Quentin.

The duo was *my* project. Keeping an eye on him and his cellmate, who was also small, they were vulnerable as they wandered amongst a sea of larger, more sophisticated, and violent predators.

I shook my head. It was time to stop thinking about it. Trying to rationalize the violence and loss of life was "crazy-making." Picking up my uniform shirt from the floor and rinsing it off in the sink, even scrubbing it hard, I couldn't get it clean. Frustrated, I pulled the plastic bag out of the garbage can and tossed my shirt in it. It did not even phase me. Losing a forty-dollar shirt was nothing compared to the loss of life.

While my mind was still whirling with thoughts, the tense muscles in my body were relaxing; the stress was dissipating. Studying my reflection in the mirror, I appeared worn. My eyes were dull, and I looked as ragged as I felt. Tugging off my t-shirt and replacing it with a clean one, all that crossed my mind was how badly I just wanted to go home. My heart was not in the interview.

Finally, deciding to do the right thing and be a good soldier, knowing I would regret it later, I affixed my tie, washed my face, applied a little eye makeup and some blush, and swept my hair up. Too many people helped prepare me for this day. I could not let them, or me, down.

"It's been a pretty challenging day," I explained to the interview panel of five correctional supervisors, managers, and administrators. "About an hour and a half ago, we experienced a major incident in the unit I supervised. Please accept my apology if I seem a bit distracted. The adrenaline still hasn't worn off. Anyway, most of you know how that is, I'll bet." Managing a smile, I continued, "I'm sure you've all been there."

"We heard it was bad," a panelist finally said, breaking the silence. "Ordinarily, we have some standard questions about commanding incidents. Let's start there. You tell us what you did in commanding it, and we'll ask questions?" a panelist suggested.

"All right." I agreed, taken by surprise. "Today had been uneventful. Our inmates weren't in the gym during the earlier incident, as our unit has been on lockdown, but somehow they got word of what happened…"

Speaking quietly, I detailed what occurred, what I did right, what I should have done and did not, and what I would have done differently. I exercised brutal honesty with my self-assessment of how I managed it. At that point, I didn't care. The only emotion I felt inside was an intense desire to be home.

Time elapsed, and everything quieted down. Weeks later, as I walked through the gate to report for work, I noted an unusual number of officers standing next to a wall filled with papers taped upon its exterior.

Someone called out, "Congratulations, Linda!"

Another approached and shook my hand. "Good job," he said.

"For what?" I asked.

"The list, it's out!" the woman officer with him announced.

"Really? How did you do?"

"Come on! You have to see this!" Taking my hand, she led me over to the wall. Attached to it were dozens of pages of paper, filled with over 2,400 names of all, statewide, who competed for a limited number of positions, as a sergeant. Searching for mine took only a few seconds. My mouth dropped, and my knees went weak.

My name reflected upon the first page, near the top. My heart stopped as my eyes fixed upon the number "six" that stood out in bold print, next to it. I had come in within the top ten in the state. I was number three at San Quentin. Looking again, I wanted to make sure I was reading it correctly.

There were many that I worked with whose names were on that same page. A sizable number of my peers came in within the top fifty. Several of us promoted into existing openings the same day.

Assigned to the third watch, Sunday through Thursday, from three o'clock p.m. to eleven p.m., my position as the watch sergeant meant I oversaw most of the administrative duties and commanded over incidents during the evening watch at the main institution of San Quentin.

Besides checking in the watch and monitoring the work schedules and absences of four hundred and thirty-two officers, along with assigning dozens of overtime positions each day, I was to hold responsibility for overseeing the mass movement of thousands of inmates and commanding incidents in the communal areas of the institution.

"This baby is all yours," the lieutenant laughed when I reported for my first shift. You know the watch commander is God, right?"

Laughing, I said, "Someone has a good sense of humor."

Arriving home, I was excited. Having worked hard for that promotion, I was unable to hold back my excitement.

"We got the results of the sergeant's test today. I came in number six in the state!" I excitedly told my husband, who was watching television. His response was emotionless as it was when I had moved out. All he said before getting up and leaving the room was, "I'll never promote."

I should have felt disappointed, but I did not. I didn't expect much from him. We were nothing more than roommates and real estate partners caring for the kids. We were not a couple. He was married to his job as a narcotics officer, and later as a homicide investigator for a suburban San Francisco community. Seldom home, his household responsibilities were in the mornings, preparing the kids for school and dropping them off at their respective schools and daycare centers. Mine was to race home each day after work to pick them up at their daycare center or school since we could not rely upon his work schedule to be able to do it.

There were some men with whom I worked who were resentful that so many women had promoted. Most were respectful, but one or two disseminated rumors that the women who promoted were having affairs with administrators to get to where they were.

I laughed, I wished. I wished so very hard that my life would one day become carefree again. I hardly had time to style my hair, let alone socialize with anyone, or even get home from work within the forty-five minutes I had to pick up the kids. They could talk all they wanted. During the four years that I worked there, only on five occasions did I ever meet with friends after work. Whatever that person thought was happening, it had to be a pitifully, depressing affair that I couldn't recall.

My life was not unlike that of the women there. They were enthusiastic, caring, educated, and motivated to move forward, and as busy in their home lives as me. Few of us had time to socialize with one another outside work. They, too, lived two entirely different existences. Many of us pursued educational opportunities, attending college when not at work.

Just as we were a different kind of peace officer because we were women, we were also a different kind of woman because we were peace officers. We were mothers, homemakers, cooks, shoppers, laundresses, housekeepers, gardeners, and chauffeurs who were always seeking a balance, and who never had enough time or sleep. Though vastly differing from one another, we were very much alike, with the same pressures, the same hopes, the same fears, and the same stresses of balancing our lives at home with those at work.

Arriving at the Department of Corrections with our applications in hand, our experiences were in education, business administration, human resource management, sociology, clinical casework, and criminal justice. That of our male peers mostly involved engaging in battle in Vietnam and obtaining a two-year administration of justice degree at a community college. Some were also working towards more. Many had a few "lost years" in their resumes.

Former teachers, nurses, administrators of agencies, and women from all occupations sought the opportunities offered. Black, brown, yellow, red, and white women, married and single, urban, suburban, and rural, flocked to the institutions to work in the non-traditional field of corrections.

Many of the first women with whom I worked with at San Quentin became captains, administrators, Board of Prison Terms commissioners, wardens, parole agents, and superintendents of prisons.

Jeanne Woodford served as the Director of the California Department of Corrections and Rehabilitation. She commanded twenty-eight thousand peace officers at the third-largest law enforcement agency in the United States, only behind the United States Department of Immigration and Customs Enforcement and the New York Police Department, housing over a quarter million inmates and parolees.

Chapter Seventeen

ON THE STREETS

When the prison doors are opened,
the real dragon will fly out. — Ho Chi Minh

Bailing out of the correctional institutions in the summer of 1985, I accepted a position as a parole agent. Assigned to work on the streets of Alameda County, and the surrounding area, I was excited about the challenge.

That first morning, as my vehicle crept through Oakland, the city streets were quiet while everyone was deep in slumber. I found myself captivated by the sultry aura of its neighborhoods, with the streets filled with hookers slouched against lampposts, waiting for the final trick of the night. Winos curled up in the nooks and doorways of decaying buildings. Driving through the city, I noticed the colorful shards of glass glittering upon the sidewalks as litter danced in the early morning breeze.

As the sun rose in the eastern sky, the city slowly awakened. Drifting outside, people stepped from their homes, and the city suddenly came to life. Laughter filled the neighborhoods as children skipped on their way to school, and people unfolded card tables and set them up on the sidewalks. Instantly, I found myself captured by the seduction of the Oakland streets.

Oakland was happening. Between 1986 and 1990, the city, with a population of 390,000 people, was entangled within a web of violence, averaging one-hundred and twenty homicides per year. Everything going down on the streets evolved around illicit drug dealing. While dealers gunned down young, parolees were smack-dab in the middle of the mix.

Pulling into the upper parking area of a rundown Oakland mall, I entered the offices of the parole division, noting the grimy smudges, and impressions of handprints covering the glass door reflected by early morning sunlight.

Aging lime-colored walls rose behind a line of cheap, worn orange vinyl chairs where parolees slouched, their legs stretched out across old, stained carpeting. It was early, but the room appeared crowded with heavily tattooed men. Carefully, I stepped over their feet and headed toward the counter.

Walking toward it, I noted a flicker of recognition in the eyes of some and the tightening of the faces in others. Catching the quick movement of elbows jabbing one another, I suppressed a grin. Though I did not recognize any, they knew me, apparently having been some of the thousands I had supervised over the years.

"How nice it is to be remembered," I thought with a restrained grin.

Approaching the bulletproof window, I waited for the clerk to acknowledge me. Sitting at her desk, she glanced upward. Our eyes met. I smiled. She ignored me. My face fell. Continuing to stand at the counter and wait; finally, she hollered across the room, "Sign in and take a seat."

Uncomfortable and noting nowhere to sit, I again signaled to her. Haughtily, she approached.

"I said, sign in there," she snapped at me, pointing at a clipboard.

"But—" I said.

"Do as I say," she ordered as she turned and walked away.

Behind me, I heard snickering. "I sure wouldn't want to be her," the voice of a parolee quietly said, laughing. Spinning around, I caught his head dropping as he covered his mouth, to veil his grin.

Next to him, a scruffy biker type guy was glancing upon his shoes with a half-grin covering his face. I couldn't help it; I caved in and laughed with them. It *was* funny, at least from their perspective.

Shrugging my shoulders, I signed my name and the time of arrival in the assigned places on the parolee log, adding my badge number in the area asking for the "CDC Number" assigned to all felons upon entering prison. Under the final column, with its heading reading "Your Parole Agent," I simply wrote, "Yes."

"Give her your seat, dude," a parolee quietly instructed the young parolee sitting beside me as I stood in the corner. "Let her sit down," he said.

"Why?" the inmate asked. "Who do you think *you* are?" he growled at me. Grimacing in pain, I waited for him to find out while the rest took care of it.

"You don't want to know," another parolee said, looking up at me for approval. I smiled, acknowledging his remark.

"Just do it, man," the older parolee sitting next to him, reinforced.

"Why?" the youngster asked angrily.

The last to speak was his savior, sitting across the way. Rising, he said, "Here, Sarge, sit here."

"Why, thank you," I said.

Across the room, a voice piped up from one of the dozens of males watching the action, "Isn't it lieutenant now?"

"It's parole agent now," I offered, with a smile. "The equivalent of lieutenant."

"Oh," he said. "I remember you being the Watch Lieutenant at San Quentin."

"Occasionally," I clarified, offering a smile of gratitude for his support.

The face of the young parolee fell. Immediately, he stood. Like most men, the one thing inmates did understand and respect, was rank, especially those who held a position of authority over them.

"Sorry, ma'am. I didn't know," he offered contritely.

Thanking him, I patiently sat and waited, while amicably engaged in a chat about the "good ole days" at San Quentin and Soledad. Some may have felt uncomfortable, but not me. I was comfortable speaking with everyone, regardless of race, age, economic status, or otherwise.

As a tri-racial woman who spent years working in traditional and non-traditional professions, growing up in a rural community, going to school in a small midwestern town, and living in an urban city, I had not only worked for America's top entrepreneurs but also worked in some pretty humble positions on my way up.

A single, now married mom, I had traveled extensively when younger, had previously worked in a prestigious Wall Street brokerage house in Boston, the advertising department of a major newspaper in Miami, in a hospital emergency room in Gresham, Oregon, and had picked up college credits in the west, the Pacific Northwest, the Midwest, the East, the South, and the Southwest.

Having worked for top executives in major companies, as their right hand for several years, my experiences offered an intense exposure to diverse cultures. From those experiences, I learned no matter what side of a fence we stand on, if people have a good understanding of boundaries and are open and sensitive to the needs of all and bridging similarities, rather than focusing on differences, encounters are more comfortable and more productive. There was always some commonality I could share with others.

Through the window, I glimpsed a familiar face leaning against the counter, as a man pulled on a string and reeled in the clipboard. It was John, another supervisor I had worked with at San Quentin.

Looking up, he did a double-take, his mouth gaping. I smiled at him and winked. Opening the door, he stepped into the lobby, laughing as he read what I wrote on the parolee check-in list.

"Lindy, what are you doing out there? Get in here!" he said, hugging me. As I entered, I could hear the animated conversation of the parolees as I passed through the door.

"Man, who was that?" one asked.

"You don't want to know," added another.

"At Q, they said if she had balls, she would have been a general," a third said, laughing. "Now, you know why." Walking into the office area, I smiled. His comment made my day.

The lobby incident was not the only thing making my day great. I was pleasantly surprised by the professionalism I initially experienced with the Region II Parole Division. At once, I realized the elevated level of esprit de corps that existed because of an administration with outstanding leadership.

Ed Veit was the Chief, while Ron Chun managed the San Francisco region. Our district manager, Bob Roenicke, was outstanding, overseeing all the planning and operations from San Francisco Bay to Sacramento and managed the supervision of over a hundred agents. The first to supervise our office, Mike Trott, was a parole agent's dream with the exceptional support and the good-natured supervision he offered.

Organized, Roenicke's team was ready for me. Upon arrival, I received a mesh bag holding most of the equipment I needed, including a set of car keys, office keys, a wallet badge, a Kevlar vest, a raid jacket, a duty weapon and holster, and other items. Knowing how to use them all, I attached a kubotan to my key chain, and I was ready to roll.

Spending most my day reviewing the backgrounds and status of the one hundred parolees in the casebook, I carefully studied their histories to set my priorities. One stood out, Louie Pinkerton.

A two-time-incarcerated drug dealer, with a few assaults under his belt, and a history of weapons possession, Pinkerton experienced a run-in with the Oakland Police Department (OPD) street team the night before. According to the phone message from the officer, he had seen Pinkerton swallowing a crystalline bag of drugs before rabbiting on them and disappearing into a darkened backyard. They intended to track him down, hopefully with my help.

Checking the book and jotting down Pinkerton's newly updated contact number, I called it. A recording answered, out of order.

Strike One.

It was clear I needed to dig a little deeper. More was going on that met the eye. Next, I dialed the telephone number for the International House of Pancakes, where he claimed to work. The manager told me no one by the name of Louie Pinkerton had ever worked there, Nobody by that name had ever worked there.

Strike Two.

He told his former agent he was good friends to the Mayor. I called the Mayor's office and spoke with someone I knew from my earlier job. A message was quickly returned to my voicemail stating nobody knew him.

Strike Three.

It was time to visit. Handwritten notes scribbled in the case book reflected Pinkerton recently moved.

With the statement from the police explaining that Pinkerton had run from them after swallowing what they thought to be drugs, coupled with his lies to his former parole agent about having a job, established reasonable suspicion to justify a parole search.

The next morning, I grabbed another agent to get it done. We parked a few houses away from his place in West Oakland and called for police backup from a payphone. It took only a few minutes for an older, weary-looking beat officer to arrive. Taking one look at me, he did not seem too wild about having to contact us.

A second patrol vehicle suddenly showed up, quickly sliding to a stop. The officer hopped out and introduced himself as Paul Musch, the officer who had left the voicemail on my office phone.

"Hey, thanks for calling back," he said. "Sorry I didn't get back to you sooner; I had court this morning."

"No problem," I said.

"Mind if I join you?" he asked. "He has been a problem."

"Please do," I replied.

"I am sure glad you are doing this. We know he's one of the biggest drug dealers in this area, but we haven't been able to determine where he lived." Musch said.

"He reported it to his agent a few days ago," I said. "Seems to move around a lot."

"That's what they do," he agreed.

My partner, the OPD beat officer, and I took the front of the house, while Musch took the back. Climbing the worn stairs to the door, I paused for a second, then knocked loudly on the decaying wood. No answer. I knocked again and waited. Hissing sounded from the side of the house.

"They're running around, getting ready to bail," the task force officer whispered from around the corner. "What do you want to do?"

My search, my call. I had all of five seconds to produce a sound decision. The refusal to answer the door and the running inside the residence served as reasonable suspicion to justify forced entry. They could be destroying evidence.

"Kick the door," I decided, intent on preserving evidence.

"On whose authority?" the older cop asked, looking at me with skepticism, as I stood in my baby-blue business suit, wearing my and sapphire earrings, and sweet pink lipstick. I had accessorized my waistline with a revolver on my right hip and a belt badge attached to a designer belt.

"Mine. I can do that," I said politely.

"*You* can do that?" the officer asked in disbelief.

"Yes! I can," I answered, louder, in a San Quentin tone.

He stepped back, looking at me with widened eyes. I don't think he expected my response in the manner I spent years perfecting it.

"Damn it. Of course, she can!" Musch reinforced in frustration, racing to the top of the stairs. "Step back!" he ordered as he slammed his foot next to the doorknob, yelling, "Police, Parole Search!"

As the door ripped open, splinters of wood flew everywhere. Our entry was far from smooth. Someone had knocked over a table which set in front of the door. Used to weigh drugs, it was topped with large quantities of white powder and a much lesser amount of thick brownish dust. The and brown powders drifted through the air, resembling a Rocky Mountain snowstorm, salt and peppering my hair, and my clothing. I brushed myself off and assessed the scales, little plastic bags, balloons, and other items of drug dealing paraphernalia strewn across the floor. Pinkerton had a nice sized drug operation in his house. It amazed me. For a second, I wondered why these guys did not put as much effort into honest employment as they did into their drug enterprises.

While my partner and I cleared a few rooms, the cops headed straight for the kitchen and returned to the living room, escorting Pinkerton, and his wife into it, wearing handcuffs.

"They were trying to bail out the back," Musch advised.

Cuffed, strip-searched, and questioned, an officer escorted Pinkerton to the backseat of a patrol car that would transport him to the Oakland Police Department jail, where he would be held on a no-bail parole hold. There was no way he would get released from county jail without the permission of the Parole Division and the Board of Prison Terms.

Sitting for a few minutes, I took a "time out." Everything had happened so quickly; I was a bit overwhelmed. Having just finished strip-searching Pinkerton's wife, an officer was now escorting her outside and into the back seat of another squad car.

Through the front window, I could see the squad car carrying Pinkerton pulling away from the curb and heading for the city jail. Sprinkled with white powder, the living-room where I was standing looked like a cyclone hit it.

In the distance, sirens screamed their high-pitched wail, sounding louder as they approached. Squad car after squad car, filled with excited officers and evidence techs, skidded to a stop outside. Laughter erupted as they viewed the room, with the dust of heroin and cocaine sprinkled everywhere. Unbeknownst to me, they wanted to get Pinkerton for a long time. Frustration had festered with failed attempts.

Officer Ignatius Chinn made a beeline straight to Pinkerton's jacket, which was hanging on the wall. He pulled a firearm from it."

"Here it is. I found it. Guys, you got this?" he called out as he dangled the gun from a pencil he was holding.

"Got it," Musch called back to him.

Chinn placed it back. His find offered the prosecution a plethora of options in deciding how to charge Pinkerton, adding a boatload of sentencing enhancements for the weapon and the amount of drugs seized.

I felt good. I wasn't sure if it was because of the natural high from a great bust or because of the drugs sprinkled all over me. My only experience with drugs was confiscating them from inmates after they returned from the visiting room or during cell searches.

The only thing I knew about was the effects the prescription drugs imposed upon my mother and the thousands of addicts in the prison system. My education came about drugs came from that and reading from the textbooks on drug identification and use.

Musch, his partner, Ian Haney, and I went outside for some fresh air. We remained there for a while, about a few hours. Dining on hamburgers, french fries, and coffee, we sat on the patio, taking in the fresh air, and infusing ourselves with liquids. The officers were not comfortable driving me back to the office right away.

"We want them to let you keep working with us," Musch said, laughing.

"You're having a lot of fun, aren't you?" Bob Roenicke also laughed when I got there, just in time for a debriefing later that afternoon. More than ready to head home, with traces of white powder still in my hair and wearing rumpled clothing with white stripes running up my nylons, my day was great.

"I'm having the time of my life!" I confessed.

"You should prepare a ready bag," he said, assessing my appearance and trying to hold in laughter.

"I'll do that," I said, heading for the door.

"Hey, hold up, there," Roenicke called out. "I've got another question for you."

"Yeah?"

"Where did you get those survival skills?"

"I don't know," I answered. Pausing to think of an easy answer, I said. "Maybe growing up in a small town?"

Driving home, I could not stop smiling. It was a beginning to a great career. I had found my niche. Not once did I feel fear. I entered a door, not knowing what was behind it, and I could not wait to get back to work the next day. I often thought of this experience when undergoing treatments for cancer. It served as a reminder that I had been in demanding situations before and lived through it. Challenges offer empowerment.

Each day presented a flurry of activity, starting from the first. On the third day of work, I had barely finished sipping the last of the morning coffee when the phone rang. It was a detective from the Emeryville Police Department.

"We have some useful information from a confidential source that one of your parolees is cooking crank in his house."

"Is your source reliable?"

"Yep. Tried and tested. There's a distinct odor of methamphetamines emanating from somewhere in the neighborhood, but with this danged breeze blowing in from the bay, I don't know where it's coming from." Pausing for a moment, he added: "But, if I were a betting man, I'd place money it's from his house."

"Planning to write a warrant?"

"I don't have enough evidence for the one judge available to sign it. He doesn't like signing search warrants." His voice dropped with disappointment.

"Okay." I thought about it and said, "I'm new to this. Can you give me a second? I'm going to look at his file and check him out." The first few paragraphs revealed all I needed to know. The parolee had priors for cooking methamphetamines, and he hadn't reported in for over forty-five days. Everything was there to justify a parole search.

"Interested in doing a parole search?"

"Thank you, Lord. I was praying you'd ask that."

"When's good for you?"

"Is an hour enough time for you all?" he said.

"You're on. I'll grab an agent to come with me."

Within three minutes, John and I were racing out the door, beating feet to the car. Suddenly he stopped and looked at me. "I don't believe this. You're not going like that, are you?"

"Yeah? What's wrong with me?" I asked in dismay, stopping to look down at myself, then looking back up at him.

"If there is a lab, there's going to be chemicals. Your legs are bare."

Looking down at myself again, I sighed.

"I brought an extra pair of shoes," I responded contritely.

"A lot of good they'll do you. All right. Take the back, and I'll go in," John grumbled. "But you're writing the report. And, tonight, get a ready bag together."

"Fair enough," I said.

Reluctantly, I handed him the diagram of the interior of the house. "Here. Bea had this in the file."

I inherited my caseload from Bea Chavez. An excellent agent, she was thorough with her documentation. It allowed a safer entry. I was grateful to her.

John and I met with the police officers at the station house. With positions for entry and coverage of the windows and exits of the house assigned, we were ready to go. My post was to cover the back of the home, with a rookie. Hopping into his car, we awaited the signal.

"Let's roll," echoed across the radio.

Engines revved. Half a dozen cars raced the short distance to the location, their light bars swirling red. Vehicles skidded to a stop, and doors flew open. Officers bailed and ran toward the porch. The sounds of yelling and banging upon the wooden door were powerful.

"Open up. Police! Parole search! Open up!"

Meanwhile, my face fell as I checked out the side of the house. I had not asked if there would be a fence to scale. There was. It was six feet high. Not happy, my eyes met those of the officer partnering with me.

"Need help?" he asked with a half-grin, bending down, cupping his hand.

"Thanks." Having gained about fifteen pounds during the eight years since I had last scaled a fence, if I had faced difficulty with "the force" not being with me, then, I had no doubt it had abandoned me by now.

"Would you mind turning your head, please?" I asked as I hefted the material of my skirt to my thigh.

Offering a foot up, I pulled myself up and hurled the rest of my body over the top. As I slid down the old splintered wood on the other side, my skirt caught upon it and ripped. An expletive flew from my mouth. The officer chuckled as he quickly hopped the fence. Quietly, we crept forward, passing a partially opened window, emitting a strong odor of rotten eggs.

"Bingo!" he whispered, "Crank."

Peeking around the corner, I saw the enormous black eyes of the biggest dog I had ever seen. Crouched, six feet away, and readied in a pouncing position, it was baring its teeth, growling.

I let out an enormous groan—mistake number two. I did not think about checking the book to see if the parolee had a dog. He did. I waved my hand to the police officer, signaling retreat while wishing I had called Bea to get her read of the parolee and his residence.

Quietly, I spoke to the dog, who was cocking his head back and forth, carefully listening as the officer, and I slowly continued to step backward. Upon reaching the fence line, the officer turned and hopped the fence. The dog bounded toward us.

A second was spent in horror, watching the dog come at us. Leaping upward, my hands tightly clutching the rough boards, I kicked as hard as I could to get my body over the top. One foot lodged between two boards, while I kicked the other at the growling animal to keep it at bay. The officer yanked my foot loose and dragged it over, but not before the heel of my foot slid out of the other shoe. I watched in despair as it fell to the ground. Toppling into the bushes on the exterior of the fence line, I sat for a minute, contemplating how much easier it was to scale a fence, with a dog chasing me.

Finally, rolling off the bush and onto the ground, with one shoe on, one-off, a torn skirt, and abrasions on my arms and legs, I heard a voice announce over the officer's radio, "Scene's secure. Two in custody."

Our eyes met, and the officer and I broke into laughter. Peering over the fence at the dog, he offered me a hand up, laughing, "That's one happy dog laying there, chewing on your shoe. I am not even going to try to get it for you."

This experience taught me that before approaching any situation and making a serious decision, I needed to be ready for whoever or whatever may be present, and for any backfire which might occur. I swore to myself I would never again be fearful of asking for an outside opinion to obtain more information, as I could have done, had I called Bea.

Second opinions are invaluable, especially when dealing with critical issues and life-threatening situations, not just in working on the streets tethering parolees, but in the everyday matters of life, including medical and surgical procedures.

That day, I realized we are all capable of doing incredible things when the need to survive arises, as I found when hopping over the fence. We must believe in ourselves and to have confidence in those around us. Filling our minds with positive thoughts and memories are defense mechanisms that can help us.

The main rules of survival are being attentive, being prepared, identifying threatening situations and behavior, and expecting anything to happen. I learned the hard way it is essential to be ready for the backfire. In my case, it always seemed to occur, no matter the situation. Murphy's Law had a stronghold upon me.

It had not been my finest hour. That evening I packed a ready bag, not only full of what I was sure I would need but with *everything I may need.* There was nothing like the feeling of being overwhelmed. I had not felt it since I had been in the academy. I had a lot to do to adapt and needed to work on finding my comfort zone, so I could put all I learned into practice.

In 1986, the Richmond, California parole office officially opened at the Hilltop Mall, off Interstate 80. A community that experienced strong economic setbacks was experiencing a high rate of homicide, which remained consistent with twenty homicides per year, before 1987. Richmond faced immense challenges. With a population base of 75,000 people, it equated to one in every 3,500 people murdered annually. The numbers remained consistent, though murder statistics cited Richmond as the second most violent city in the country.

My job was to manage the repeat, violent recidivists, notorious parolees, and those posing a severe threat to the public. I worked hard at keeping a handle on it. Four years later, in 1991, the year after I left the Parole Division, the murder rate had exploded, escalating to sixty-one homicides per year or one in every 1,140 people killed.

As the law enforcement liaison for the unit, my job involved performing law enforcement functions, as well as performing casework on my caseload of high-level violent offenders. Endeavoring to keep the recidivism rate of my caseload low, it took a lot of effort to stay on top of their activities.

Working with local, state, and federal task forces, I met with the management and supervisors of the approximate twenty law enforcement agencies within the area. We developed an effective means of resolving the escalating crime problems by ensuring the doors of communication between our agency and theirs remained open. At a minimum of once a week, there were one or more significant operations that went down. It became a pattern. Fortunately, we identified problems before anyone was seriously injured.

Richmond was a tough town to work. Criminals were blatant. One morning, my partner, Al Bousquet, and I were cruising down a city street when a speeding car, filled with young male passengers, donned in ski masks, pulled alongside us. Our hearts were pounding as we tightly gripped our weapons, ready to fire if needed. Watching as they sped off, an immense feeling of relief flooded through me.

"What's wrong with this picture?" I asked.

"Only in Richmond," Al laughed.

Nervously, I joined in as I jotted down vehicle, driver, and passenger descriptions, and we set out to find a rare working payphone. Without radios, and before cell phones, we worked in the blind.

Our lifeline rested in our pockets, the rolls of quarters and dimes to make phone calls at street-corner payphones. Our pagers did little but supply numbers to call back. It was quarters and dimes, laughter, and convenience store hot dogs that got us through the days when our tensions were high.

I seldom feared to work alone on the Richmond streets. I grew up with fear and thrived on avoiding situations that created it. When that wasn't possible, I learned to confront it. After working in the Parole Division for a few months, when the elite undercover Special Services Unit of the Department of Corrections that handled its sensitive and critical investigations nicknamed me the "Dragon Lady," I felt honored. There was some truth to it.

As Ho Chi Minh said, "When the prison doors are opened, the real dragon will fly out." I was once a lamb who learned patience and perseverance at Soledad and San Quentin. Still disarming, when I entered, after what I survived in the institutions, once I was gone, I found myself breathing and exhaling fire.

Though my supervisors filled my caseload with parolees predicted to recidivate violently, my most significant accomplishment was the blessing of only one of the hundreds released, during my seven years with the Parole Division, committed a murder. The fear any would harm someone weighed heavily upon me, resulting in many sleepless nights.

Hassan had broken the tradition. Having known the intense, angry, thirty-something man from Soledad, where I first supervised him in the late 1970s, I found out the hard way that he was passionate about the more radical tenets of Islam.

Refusing to follow my instructions, he held a strong belief that men were not to be subservient to women. Most of the young, inmates that converted into the Muslim religion while incarcerated were polite and cooperative, not as angry, and hostile as was Hassan. Frustrated, I approached the Muslim clergy, asking how I could acknowledge the religious beliefs of the inmates while still ensuring the security of the institution.

"I am sorry this is happening," the clergyman apologized. "While women hold a lower status than men, we teach them to accept authority."

He instructed the entire congregation that they were to treat women peace officers as authority figures. Though Hassan still refused to speak in my presence, continuing to display a hostile attitude, he followed my instructions. I wanted compliance, not adoration.

Now, on parole, the rules he set for himself had changed. Upon release, he reported to my office as instructed. Slouching in a chair, he experienced no difficulty speaking with me.

Smirking, he advised, "I'll be living at Your Muslim Bakery in Berkeley. Heard of it?"

"Got the address?" I asked, dummying up.

"No," he lied, clearly not wanting to help me out.

"No big deal. I can find it," I advised, to rub more salt into Hassan's wound. I knew it well. Your Muslim Bakery was developing a reputation in the community. Yusuf Bey had founded it as a halfway house for young Muslim men with troubled backgrounds. The ex-felons, parolees, drug addicts, and individuals who experienced earlier difficulties with the justice system were baking goods that met dietary regulations of the Muslim religion.

In the latter part of the 1980s, when I visited the bakery to verify a parolee's work or living situation, employees typically ignored me; I was a woman.

Later, when walking to my vehicle, they became bolder. A few followed when I left. Then, in a more explicit attempt at intimidation, upon leaving, someone tailed me to the office. Pulling into the parking lot, I waved to him as he sped off.

As a woman, they expected me to be submissive. It was their belief I should not assume authority over a man. I understood them more than they realized, having an Arab uncle who immigrated to the United States from Lebanon. Recognized as one of the top educators in the country, he was a Shia Muslim. He and my Aunt Marcella partially raised us after our parents divorced. We adored him. One of our top mentors, he faced no difficulty viewing women as equals.

In the first few weeks following Hassan's release from prison, he committed a homicide, proudly confessing his actions to me as he sat on his bunk in his Oakland Police Department jail cell. He was ready to head back to where he belonged, at San Quentin.

While radicalism brewed upon the streets in western Alameda County, West Contra Costa County was rocking with the manufacture of methamphetamines, some of which were reported to be "cooked" by some of my parolees. Members of various outlaw biker gangs and every loser on the street who had a few bucks to "score a bag," or a bathtub to mix a concoction to sell, trafficked it. My job was to keep my parolees tethered, maintain a close eye on their activities, and help them successfully reintegrate into society. That's a pretty lofty goal when dealing with paranoid tweakers who lived in a culture referred by the police as "crystals and pistols," and high-level drug traffickers who dominated the streets, selling cocaine and heroin.

It was about ten o'clock in the morning when I decided to stop by the home of one of my youngsters, a budding, young crank dealer who cooked crank. Matt missed his appointment the day prior. He did not return my calls to his pager and didn't expect me to drop by his new abode so soon after providing me with his address a few days earlier. Ducking me, I figured I would make my bi-monthly field visit a surprise. I climbed the rickety stairs of the graffiti-clad apartment building.

As he opened the door, his face fell. Not wild about seeing me, I had to invite myself inside, to discuss his failed appointment. After meeting his roommate and noting where he slept, we were conversing amicably when the front door flew open, and the silhouettes of three men appeared in the doorway. My heart began pounding wildly as my eyes focused upon the one who was wearing the colors of the Hells Angels inside the front doorway, while I was on the other side of the room. My mind raced, contemplating how I was going to get past them and through that door, unscathed, especially with two violent ex-felons who manufactured crank standing on one side and a Hell's Angels member and two associates parking themselves on the other.

The lyrics of a Stealer's Wheelers' song scrolled in my mind. "Clowns to the left of me, jokers to the right, here I am, stuck in the middle with you," the lyrics went while I was desperately developing exit strategies, to get to my car, unscathed.

Suddenly, I realized why Matt was not pleased to see me. He was expecting them. There was only one reason for the five to be there, at the same place, at the same time. Methamphetamines. Either Matt had a large quantity of the product, or he was ready to make a deal with them to manufacture it. The odds were high; it was the latter.

The chatty cocktail waitress persona came to life. Talking nonstop, I introduced myself and made small talk, as I edged to the door. Keeping their attention upon my face, I did not want them to notice my left-hand tugging on the bulky sweater concealing the one side where I wore a belt badge and the other where I carried my firearm. Subtly herding them inside, they complied nicely. Finally, an opening presented itself, and I slid past them, skipping out the door and racing down the stairs, waving farewell as I backed out of the driveway.

They never realized I had just enough time to memorize the license numbers of their Harleys. Driving a few blocks, I pulled over and jotted the information in my notebook to pass along with their identities to the agents assigned to the ATF and the FBI Hells Angels Federal Task Force.

Chapter Eighteen

MOTHERS AND GRANDMOTHERS

We love our mother unknowingly and only realize how deep rooted that love is at the ultimate separation. — Guy de Maupassant

The incredible capacity of a mother's or grandmother's ability to love is one of the most powerful, passionate dynamics I experienced as I worked in the inner cities of the San Francisco Bay Area.

The elevated levels of death and devastation from the violence of street drug wars left a profound mark upon me. I met mothers who buried child after child due to street violence. It was heartbreaking.

Usually, when a positive change occurred with one of my parolees, it was with the help of their mother or wife. Often it happened when a child was born to them in their mid-thirties. The youngsters drove me crazy.

The firearm homicide rate for fifteen to twenty-year-old youths had increased one hundred and fifty-eight percent in the violent drug neighborhoods of California, where I worked. Mothers lived with an ever-constant fear that their child would be killed by someone with a gun or die of a drug overdose.

My children were safe and well, tucked away in a community that was hardly affordable but offered safety from exposure from the criminal element. Living the idyllic life of innocence, every child should experience, I thanked God I had not lost either of mine, as my father had, and these women, and others that I knew. Many of the parents of the victims were good, hardworking people who were just trying to get by. Most were single moms as I once was.

Early one morning, I maneuvered my car around a city bus and parked in front of a freshly painted house. Meticulously trimmed flowering shrubs, the neatly trimmed lawn, and the raked gravel driveway made it clear the owner held considerable pride in his or her home. A drug-addicted mother with three kids claimed she lived there with her mother. I skipped up the sidewalk to see if what she said was true.

The older woman answering the door wore a worn cotton dress, faded from years of laundering. It hung from her thin frame. Appearing weary, she leaned against the iron gate, asking, "Can I help you?"

"Hi, is Gloria around?" I asked.

"Now, how would I know that?" she asked back, wiping her hands upon a dishtowel wrapped around her waist, and resting them upon her hips.

Taken aback, I apologized and introduced myself. "I'm sorry. I didn't tell you. I'm Gloria's parole agent. She told me she lived here."

"So, she's out again, huh?" the woman asked.

"You haven't seen her?" I responded. "She was in the office a few days ago."

"Lady, I haven't seen that girl in three years," the woman said.

"Three years?"

"Yeah. Most likely, it's those drugs that have got her again."

I didn't believe her. Her eyes darted down as she spoke. She knew Gloria was out, and where she was. But I *did* believe her when she said Gloria was again experiencing an issue with drugs. Establishing a good rapport with Mom was paramount to Gloria's successful completion of parole. It was essential to keep every door open to her so we could work together to encourage Gloria to conquer her addiction successfully.

Tears welled in the mother's eyes. A strong emotion churned within my stomach as I saw the pain of abandonment imposed by the apathy of a daughter whose priorities were getting instant self-gratification from drugs. She needed to talk. I leaned against the porch post.

"So, how are the kids doing?"

She paused for a moment, deciding whether she should speak with me, then finally said, "All right. Most are in school. They get by." Standing aside, she dusted off her apron and offered, "Why don't you come inside for a minute? There's something you need to see."

Stepping through the door, I entered the small, immaculate kitchen, its floor filled with tables, each with three or four chairs. Some were little, and some were big. As we slid past them, I noted two handbags on a chair. One was identical to that Gloria carried into my office when she reported.

Just as I thought.

"I'm sorry there's no place to sit," the woman apologized as she weaved around the furniture. "We're kind of crowded here."

She led me into the next room. Stopping, in amazement, I saw rows of bunk beds lining the walls. In the corner, sleeping children filled a crib.

"Is this a daycare center?"

"No," she uttered. "These are my grandchildren that my children left behind for those drugs."

"You care for these many children?" I asked in amazement while silently counting the number of beds. There were thirteen in total.

"Yes, and now you've seen there is no place for her to live if she's not clean.

"But how do you manage all this?"

"I don't know. Sometimes I don't. Sometimes I dream about running away, just getting up and leaving. But what would happen to the children? There's no one else."

We stepped outside. Mary sank upon the top step of the front porch, appearing exhausted. I sat beside her. It felt good to get away from the enforcement end of my job and relax for a few moments.

"Want a cup of coffee?" Standing up, brushing the dust from my backside, I readied to go to my car.

"I'd die for one, but I can't go anywhere, not with those little ones asleep in there."

"I have a thermos in my car. I'll get it. Get yourself a cup, okay?"

Pulling the thermos off the seat of the floor and bringing it back to the porch, she sat waiting, wearing a broad smile as she extended her chipped mug toward me

"It's got that flavored stuff in it. Is that all right?" I warned, ready to pour.

"My favorite. Oh, yeah," Mary sighed, after taking a sip and sitting back. "I haven't had anything like this in a long time." Laughing uncomfortably, she added, "I can't afford to buy it. It is too expensive."

For an hour, we were merely two women drinking coffee and talking, Mary and me. Her grandmother lived in the same home forty years ago. Times were different. She missed those days, but she has changed, people have changed, and life has changed. She spoke of her five children, recounting memories of when they were younger. Now, as drug addicts, they are strangers to her.

Toothpaste and toilet paper are expensive, as is clothing, but she makes do. She is grateful. She is tearful. Despite Mary's shattered heart, she keeps moving forward, working around the intense emotional pain of loss festering deep inside. She dearly misses the loving people her children had once been. Mary finally stood and stretched her arms upward, toward the warm morning sun. "They will be waking up soon," she lamented.

Picking up the thermos, and glancing around the decaying neighborhood, I said, "Yeah, and I better get back to work."

"It's a beautiful, sunny day," she said. "Good things always happen on sunny days. Thank you. There's been no one to talk to about all this." She reached out her arms to hug me.

"Well, now you do," I said as we embraced. Over Mary's shoulder, I saw a flash of movement with the curtains in the front window. Scrounging in my purse, I pulled out a business card. Handing it to her, I said, "Call me if you need anything."

She held it to her chest, smiled, and opened the screen door. Before disappearing inside, I stopped, deliberated for a second, and then turned to her. I asked in a tone of voice intended for anyone who may be inside to hear, "Mary, if you happen to see Gloria, would you please tell her I'm putting a warrant out for her arrest if she doesn't get into rehab by Friday?"

Mary looked upon me, smiling sheepishly. "I figured you probably knew she comes by occasionally. You saw her purse, huh?"

I returned her smile as I pulled out another business card. "This is a program on San Pablo at the Berkeley, Emeryville border. Tell her to call here, talk to Jim, and tell him I instructed her to call. It is far enough away so she won't be in the mix and close enough where you can go see her."

"I can't afford rehab. I have all these kids," she quietly stated, her arm sweeping toward the house.

"Don't worry about that. We'll take care of it. If Gloria is sincere about rehab, there will be a bed ready. If not, tell her I can guarantee her a cell with a metal bunk."

Tears filled her eyes. "Thank you, Linda. You bet I will. That's the best thing you could ever do for her, and these kids and me. I cannot afford to lose another child, and I don't want to lose her again. This time, it could be forever."

I sang while driving to the office, my mind thinking of the poor grandmother who raised eight kids in the belly of the inner city, three of whom had died and five who abandoned their children to get high.

More than likely, Mary wouldn't realize her dreams. Her hope that her grandchildren will be healthy and do well may not be possible. The odds of it occurring were not good in Richmond, though I wished for her it would happen.

My job served as a buffer between "yesterday" and "someday." It balanced everything. There was no time for reflection, for worry, or fear of the arrival of cancer. But after meeting Mary, I found myself thinking of my mom.

I found myself wondering how and where Mom was living. I had not heard her voice in fifteen years. All I had was a memory, not even a photograph. Did she contract another cancer? Was her hair still long, thick, and jet black, and did she always give thanks for the morning? I wondered if she sang when she was troubled. Was she happy?

Donna said she had been living in Texas. Their oldest daughter had visited her for the summer. While at Donna's home, she revealed our stepfather had sexually assaulted her. Donna immediately notified the police. Knowing she was safe, my goal was to make sure the other children were protected. Mom and Chuck had disappeared again. It was time to track them down again. Fleeing Texas, they were finally found in Maine.

We contacted the social services agency that was investigating the matter there. Speaking with a social worker assigned to handle it, she remained in close touch with us, advising she had done a home visit, and the children were well.

Authorities were monitoring the home to ensure the children would be protected. I offered to take the children into my home. They agreed it was best for the children to remain in the house, with the parents, while pending a court decision to determine suitability.

Then, she shared with me that both Mom and Chuck had been psychologically tested. Their psychologist diagnosed Mom as being paranoid and psychotic, which was thought to be drug-induced. The psychologists diagnosed Chuck with the same. The children were interviewed and denied that abuse occurred.

Through the years, I watched Mom's life from a distance. I had always hoped that Mom would manage to get clean and was living her dreams. I wondered if, during some part of her journey, she had ever taken a moment to think about my siblings and me. Yet, in my heart, I knew she hadn't; we hadn't heard from her in years. A few weeks later, I called to find out the court's determination. They advised that the family had fled from Maine. Nobody knew where they were.

Sighing, then quietly singing to nobody but myself, while heading home that day after visiting Mary, I made myself stop thinking about them and urged myself to divorce my personal feelings from their situation. Today, many families live with the devastation of having a "drug-addicted Gloria" as one of their loved ones. It is far from unusual. Mom was ours. She, like the others of Mary's children, distanced herself from her children and disappeared from our lives because drugs were more important to her.

My mother and her husband were initially my sole inspiration in pursuing work in the justice system. For years, my dream was to one day enter law enforcement and annihilate drug dealing, drug dealers, and those hawking prescription drugs. For years, I longed to bust my stepfather, "someday." I knew, from first-hand experience, the pain inflicted upon the innocent loved ones of addicts. Addiction affects an entire family. But, like most, I couldn't stop hoping she would change, "someday." I kept looking for her.

A year or two later, we again found them living in Spain. Our sister, who had been extracted from the home, was the most fortunate in the family. She had escaped a terrible situation. Receiving counseling, she was able to reveal her dream of one day having a "real mother."

Speaking with her caseworker, I supported her desire to be with someone she could trust; and instead of planning to care for her, I began focusing my energies upon continuing to hunt for the others.

Several years later, Donna mentioned our youngest brother, David, had moved to Maine. Tracking him down, I found him working in a Burger King. Every day, he was riding a bicycle ten miles, through the snow, into work, and every day, he rode it home.

I was able to convince him to come to California to be with us. He moved in with his sister, Stephanie, who was now married, stable, and with an incredibly supportive husband, owned a home together. The mission again changed to finding the last two. Eventually, Donna found the oldest boy. The three reunited for a short period. After he again disappeared into his prior life, none of us ever hearing from him again.

As a parole agent, I applied much of what I knew by living in a home with an addict. I was familiar with addicts and their habits. I was onto the patterns of those I supervised quickly. I could easily tell when they were lying; when they were high, and when the addiction was so deep, they needed to go away. I realized when they were depressed and when they were desperate. Growing up as the child of an addict, my mother's addiction not only motivated me to make a difference in the lives of others but to be a much better parole agent.

Driving back to the office, my mind whirled with thoughts of my children. Chris was now five and in the first grade, and Judi was twelve, as had been dear, sweet Amy, Judi's best friend. Amy spent weekdays at our house, or at least she had until she went into the seventh grade a few months earlier. Judi spent weekends with Amy and her father. Two families blended with the close friendship between two beautiful little girls.

On a Sunday evening, a few months earlier, the phone rang. It was Amy's father asking if she was with us. Earlier, Judi called to see if Amy wanted to join us in going out for pizza, but Amy was not at home. I thought nothing of it as he did not call back.

The next afternoon, I was at my desk completing the never-ending paperwork. It was a fluke I was even in the office. Ordinarily, I was in the field. The phone rang.

"Amy is missing, Mom. They can't find her," Judi cried.

My heart stopped as I reflected upon the call from her father.

"What?"

"They can't find her, Mom. They say she's dead."

"Where are you?"

"Home."

"Stay there. I am on my way."

"Mom. Please hurry. I need you. I'm scared."

It was the longest night of our lives as we waited for the phone to ring. Every time it did, I startled and felt despair when each call wasn't what we hoped to hear. Finally, the call came from the Napa Police Department. It was short. They found her lying lifeless by the creek near her home. Strangled and sexually assaulted, the perpetrator mutilated her body. A suspect was in custody. The seventeen-year-old was talking to the police.

"May we interview Judi?" the detective asked.

"Of course," I said.

"How about you? Are you okay, Linda?"

"Yeah."

"Linda," he half-whispered, his voice breaking as it softened.

"Yes?" My voice, filled with trepidation, dreaded his response.

"Uh, Linda, you guys don't want to come down here."

"Okay. Thank you. I understand," I said, my voice breaking as I tried hard to keep my composure. It was as I feared. The investigator was warning me the scene was bad.

My husband was standing by, waiting. I passed the receiver to him, nodding and confirming the fears. He let out an involuntary, emotional sigh before speaking. As a homicide investigator, he knew the drill. They would supply him with all the details they were holding back from me. But listening to his side of the conversation, they didn't tell him much, either.

"No, I trust your judgment," he said, looking upward, trying to compose himself.

"Yeah, I can bring her there, or you are welcome here… whenever it is good. Thanks for calling, for everything. Yeah, see you tomorrow."

He hung up the phone and walked outside. Being alone was his way of dealing with things. Composing myself, I prepared to break the news to Judi. It would not be easy.

Quietly, I sat next to her, throwing an arm around her shoulders and pulling her close. She knew what I intended to tell her. Tears rolled down her face as she began to sob. All I could do was rock her in my arms as she grieved the loss of her best friend, her tadpole hunting buddy, her roller-skating partner, the sister she never had, and the one friend who always helped wash the kitchen floor by old, wet, soapy socks and sliding upon it.

Judi was the energy who acted before thinking. Amy had been the stabilizer who always thought everything out. Judi was intense and very much a girly girl; Amy had been easygoing and earthy.

"Why, Mom?" Judi sobbed.

"I don't know. Sometimes things just happen. There is no reason."

"Mom, I can't believe she's gone forever," she sobbed.

"Neither can I, Judi, neither can I." Pulling her close and letting her cry for a few more minutes, I said, "This may be hard to understand now, but her soul is still very much alive. I promise you that. All you need to do is to believe and to keep an eye out for the little messages. Amy will be right here with you, forever." I gently tapped my finger atop her heart.

"Really?"

"Yes, really."

"Will she talk to me?"

"I don't know, maybe. Or maybe Amy will do it in another way."

"But how will I know?"

"I don't know, but when it happens, trust me, you'll know it."

The morning of her memorial service was dismal. It rained that November day. The air was damp, and the trees were mostly bare, bravely standing and shivering in the breeze amid a collage of brightly colored leaves that had fallen upon the ground.

After the service, we went for a drive, just Judi and me. She needed to talk it out before we saw Amy's father and her mother, a deputy sheriff who traveled from the Pacific Northwest to lay her child to rest.

Lost amid nowhere, with our broken hearts and a shattered sense of devastation, we were cruising somewhere deep in the forested hills surrounding Napa, on one of its hundreds of twisting, narrow trails. We were finally in sync with where our hearts existed... nowhere.

Suddenly, a doe ran into the road and skidded to a stop, directly in front of us. I slammed upon the brakes. Our tires slid on the wet road, stopping a few feet from it. The animal appeared composed, and demonstrated more interest in Judi, than fear, as her enormous brown eyes locked with Judi's, for moments. Then, as though she had delivered a message, the doe turned and bounded into the forest.

"Mom, did you see that? It was Amy, Mom," Judi said excitedly. "I know it was."

I glanced toward her and smiled reassuringly. "Thank God," I thought to myself. "She is going to be okay."

She now believed, as I do, that those who die never leave us, not really. As Dad and I discussed, life continues within their souls and within those who love them. They will always be a part of us, just in a different way.

"Mom, do *you* think it was Amy?" Judi asked, seeking my approval.

"What matters most is what you think, what *you* feel." Then, echoing Dad's words, I added, "You don't need my approval, ever, and you are the one who will know if it is."

"It *was* Amy," Judi insisted, sitting back with an attitude of certainty. "She wants me to know she's okay."

"Then, I believe it was," I said, patting her leg while I drove.

That following Monday, at work, I longed to be at home with my children, ensuring they were safe. Reestablishing a balance between my work and my home was difficult, especially with an unavailable spouse. Though, for a long while, nothing seemed right. In times of loss, it takes time to adapt and for comfort to wrap its arms around us.

Judi and her friends had lost a good part of their childhood innocence. They were kids who had never ridden the emotional roller coaster of loss and grief. Tenderhearted and broken-hearted, they grieved heavily.

The loss of Amy was a rite of passage my daughter would face again and again in the future. However painful it was and still is, it served as a heartbreaking, young first view into how families like ours and others live. In one way or another, everyone faces the risks of living in a society filled with uncertainty, of cancer and other diseases, violence, and the senseless loss of life in our society today.

Chapter Nineteen

PASSION AND
NOTORIETY

He had a deeply ingrained hatred and dislike of women.
— Asst. Atty General Scott Browne, Florida

The billows of later afternoon fog drifted through the mid-coastal area of San Luis Obispo, California. Doug Filangeri, the high service agent for our unit and I had pulled into the grounds of the California Men's Colony to manage the release of one of the most notorious parolees in the history of the California Department of Corrections, that of the infamous "ax rapist" Lawrence W. Singleton.

When not at sea, Singleton, a sixty-three-year-old former merchant marine sea captain, was either uncontrollably drunk or angrily sober at one of two homes where he lived. Tara Hills, California, was a quiet Northern San Francisco Bay suburban community where Singleton's fifteen-year-old daughter lived with a neighbor after the death of her mother. His other home in Reno, Nevada, was with his second wife. It didn't matter where he bedded. Nothing about him changed. Different houses, same person.

Hostile toward women, Singleton had developed a long history of inflicting violence upon them. Possessing considerable anger toward wives, girlfriends, dates, and particularly toward prostitutes, he was adept in his attempts to disarm others by playing a convincing role as a "kindly" old Dad while out trolling for victims.

On September 29, 1978, Singleton happened upon a fifteen-year-old Mary Vincent, a run-away from her home in Las Vegas, and two others who were hitchhiking on the corner of Fourth Street and University Avenue, next to Spenger's Restaurant in Berkeley, California.

Despite the fact Mary was not traveling alone, Singleton only offered *her* a ride. No one else. Tired of living on the road and dearly wanting to get to Los Angeles where she intended to stay with relatives, she accepted Singleton's offer to drive her to Southern California. The vulnerable, young teen was about to make the biggest mistake of her life in underestimating Singleton and hopping into his van.

Briefly stopping at his home in Tara Hills, then heading east, it appeared Singleton was keeping his promise. Outside Sacramento, he missed the turnoff toward Los Angeles. She called him on it.

Claiming to be en route to Los Angeles, Singleton drove for a while, then turned off, stopped, and began to beat the frightened teen. She fought to keep him off her. He responded by hitting her on the head with a sledgehammer, removing her clothing, raping her, and driving her to the outskirts of Modesto, California. On a seldom traveled country road, he hacked off her arms with a hatchet when she started fighting again, and then threw her over a thirty-foot cliff, leaving her for dead.

As Mary waved in and out of consciousness, her will to survive kicked into play. A little voice from deep inside guided her. "You can't go to sleep," it insisted. "He's going to do this to somebody else. You can't let that happen."

Staggering down a country road, naked, and crying out for help while using every bit of strength she had to hold her bloody stumps upright, she continued down the road. Thankfully, she had the sense to roll in the dirt to slow down the severe bleeding.

By chance, a young couple drove by and summoned help. The fifteen-year-old survived to testify against Singleton, who adamantly claimed he was *her* victim, saying she had held a stick to his neck, so he had dropped her off. Someone else must have harmed her.

Convicted of committing mayhem, he received a fourteen-year sentence. With good behavior, his release was imminent, following eight years of incarceration. Upon his release from California Men's Colony, on April 25th, 1987, he was to parole.

The responsibility of supervising his release landed squarely upon the Richmond parole office until the courts determined where he should live. Previously, he had lived in Western Contra Costa County. However, the courts disallowed situating him anywhere, permanently, until they resolved where parolees were to be released following their prison sentences. This issue created intense media attention. Singleton was now a public pariah. Understandably, nobody wanted him in their town. The media contacts to our office and the Sacramento headquarters were intense. Emotions peaked. As time elapsed, instead of diminishing, the calls were escalating in number.

Days before Singleton's parole date, Bob Roenicke came to the office, announcing two agents would handle the matter. Doug Filangeri was to manage the high-service psychological, and independent living needs, and I would be responsible for the high-control public safety and law enforcement liaison management of the parolee.

I laughed as Bob made his announcement. The day before, Doug had mentioned they were having difficulty placing Singleton in Antioch, California. He advised he was assigning Singleton to our unit. "Notoriety cases are a pain, Linda. I don't want much to do with this," he stated with a sigh.

If I were to collaborate with another agent on a notoriety case, there was no better choice than Doug Filangeri. Filangeri had previously supervised William Parnell, a notorious pedophile, successfully. Parnell had kidnapped a seven-year-old Stephen Stayner, among other children, keeping them for years until Stayner eventually turned him over to the police. The nationally known case eventually became a feature movie on television, titled "I Know My Name Is Stephen."

Bob was the incident commander directing our every move, with Tom Webb supervising the operation and surveillance agents, with other Region II supervisors. They would pull the weight of managing and supporting us and take the heat from the public. Doug and I would oversee Singleton's movement and his needs while hiding in plain sight with him in the back of our car until the public outcry died down, and judges resolved the many restraining orders and court cases from various counties.

"Linda, are you okay with this?" Bob asked gently. I knew what he meant. It had only been a few months since Amy had died. Assuring him I was, I had a job to do, and I intended to put my personal biases aside and do what I do well, keeping some of the most violent and deviant criminals in California on a close leash. It was a responsibility that I took seriously.

Today was his release date from prison. The public outcry was immense. Our mission was to keep him tethered and to protect the safety of the public until the courts determined the appropriate location for him to live. We didn't know how long that would be. What we did know was the courts never moved as quickly as we did.

Doug and I were heading to the office of Warden Wayne Estelle. He was a Department legend. Believing inmates should perform arduous work, achieve acceptable levels of education, and engage in proper social conduct; he had lofty expectations of those in his institution. His staff revered him and mirrored his ethics. As a result, he ran the least-violent, most-efficient, less costly prison in the entire prison system.

Estelle had only one question. "Are you planning to parole him here?" he asked as we sat in his office. Sounding more like a prayer than a matter of strategy, I felt sorry for him, realizing he was suffering from the burning heat of the backfire from a community fearing that the CDC might place Singleton where he spent his seven years of incarceration.

"We know no intent of that at this time," I said. "What we know is the CDC will parole Singleton in Northern California, somewhere between Fresno and the Oregon border."

Estelle heaved a heavy sigh of relief. "You know this is a small community. Thank you. I spent a lifetime building relationships and proving my credibility here. It would be difficult."

Doug and I understood his sentiment. Community leaders throughout California were echoing the same.

"I don't need to know anything else," he said. "Sorry, I have to get this," he apologized as the intercom announced a phone call. He picked up the phone. From his end, we overheard a one-sided dialogue with what was a member of the media.

"No, I don't know what they consider the boundaries between Southern California and Northern California," he said. "If you would like, I'll ask some of our gang members. When it comes to dividing the state, they have got it down. They're experts at it."

Estelle's eyes twinkled as he grinned at us. We chuckled. Gang members were always engaged in turf wars over California's geographical boundaries.

"Yes, I'll let you know more as soon as I find out," he said.

"It hasn't stopped ringing since this morning," he told us. "I don't envy your job. The media are not going to go away. You know that, don't you?"

"Unfortunately, yes," I said with a sigh.

He stood up and grabbed his jacket. "Come on. Let me show you around this place, and then let's get you some dinner so you can get a good night's sleep. I suspect it will be your last for a long time."

The next morning, Doug and I reached the institution in the early morning hours, navigating amongst the heavy billows of fog and through the back gate leading to the Receiving and Release unit of California Men's Colony.

The Receiving and Release Unit is where all inmates process in and out of the institution. Juggling cups of coffee and paperwork in our hands, we opened the back door and headed toward the office.

"He's over there," the receiving and release officer said, nodding toward a corner of the room where some built-in wooden benches set against a stone wall. We headed toward where an older man sat, with a few cardboard boxes at his feet.

"Boy! Am I glad to see you guys!" he greeted, rising as we approached. Watching as Singleton, and Doug spoke, I noted he stood bent, his shoulders hunched over, he appeared old and fragile.

Do not get caught up in his friendliness.

Doug introduced us. Singleton seemed eager to please. As the two discussed his immediate needs, I focused on him.

At fifty-nine years old, he appeared about seventy though he was attentive, and his mind was clear. As he signed his conditions of parole, his face flashed with a few brief micro-expressions of disapproval; however, he did not object to the stringent requirements. If he did not agree to the terms, he would remain institutionalized for another year. Something with him was off. Wondering if the scared-little old-man gig was an act, I continued to evaluate his behavior.

Dad was fifty-eight years old, one year younger than Singleton. My father was vital at that age, working full time, and supporting a second family of three young children. For a man with few health problems, the worst being out of shape, coupled with a history of severe alcoholism, Singleton appeared fine. It was my belief he was not the muddled, older man as he seemed. Anxious to see the former merchant marine in a situation where *he* felt in control, would be the test of his character.

Singleton loaded his possessions into the car, hopped into the back seat, and we followed Estelle out of the back gate of the institution to the highway. Estelle stopped, came to the car, and bade us farewell.

"Good luck," he said. "Now, get driving and don't stop until you are the hell out of my county."

Laughing, we offered our thanks and headed north. We did not envy his job. He had a lot of phone calls to take with little information to provide, except that two armed parole agents had arrived and retrieved Singleton, intending to place him somewhere in Northern California.

As we drove toward the border of San Luis Obispo County, we passed a sheriff's office squad car. He waved. We waved back. Glancing behind me, I saw him pick up his radio and speak. Then, making a U-turn, he headed back toward San Luis Obispo. It was clear they were covering their bases to make sure we were out of their jurisdiction, with Singleton.

At the next intersection, we changed our travel route so the deputies in the next county would not locate us. Having no instructions, and en route to nowhere, we were killing time, interviewing Singleton, and getting a read on him; his level of risk, his attitude, his cooperation, and his demeanor. We only stopped to get coffee, food, and to call into headquarters at the designated time for instructions of where we were to report at the day's end.

As most parolees, Singleton seemed compliant at first. But it was early in the game. He was on his best behavior and did not know us or the lay of the land. One thing was clear. He knew how to take orders and not to rock the boat. Used to living in close quarters, Doug noted he would be comfortable tucking in and keeping to himself.

Suspecting he was a chameleon, being able to be what he wanted to be, dependent upon whom Singleton was around, I sensed at some unknown later date; that he would become a parole agent's nightmare. His commitment offense, alone, indicated he was control-oriented. Having spent a lifetime being a ship captain, I was confident he would follow his own desires. Right now, he was trying to appease us. After the honeymoon period elapsed, we would know the real Singleton.

As he became more comfortable around parole agents, he would swagger, pretend to be off-balance, and wildly waving his arms. Often Singleton would perform an exaggerated act of being a dry drunk, engaging in barroom type behavior to entertain them.

Constantly flowing from him was an underlying sense of anger toward women and an ongoing inappropriate sexual overtone in everyday casual conversation, which he felt to be normal.

Whenever two or more were present, Singleton physically placed himself in the middle of agents, dominating the conversation and making himself the center of attention. While he regularly played the role of an innocent old man, or that of an endearing father, the aging merchant marine face difficulty not concealing the escalating hostility and anger he projected toward the child he victimized, who he insisted set him up. A couple of weeks following his release, Singleton made a mistake in conversation with me. He referred to his victim as "a two-bit whore."

His eyes widened as I tore into him, flatly instructing him never to address her in that manner again. As quickly as he reacted in anger and made the remark, his mood at once transformed back into the compliant role of the happy dry drunk, saying, "Yes, dear."

That night, we settled Singleton into a cheap, nondescript hotel room, in a rural farm town. Giving him paperwork to fill out, we told him to get some rest. We would see him the next day. Circling the block and pulling into the parking lot of a shopping center, we met with agents of the Special Services Unit.

From the moment we dropped him off at a hotel anywhere, to the moment we were to retrieve him the next morning, several sets of eyes remained upon Singleton always. Unbeknownst to him, he was always under the constant surveillance of the Special Services Unit or of parole agents, when not with us. He believed he was on his own.

After a few weeks, the honeymoon period inmates often experience on parole rapidly faded as Singleton's real character began revealing itself. He was getting testy and was still making inappropriate comments about his crime victim, displaying his unhealthy obsession with her. Doug finally had enough. While pulling the car over, his deep brown eyes glared at Singleton through the rear-view mirror. A good minute of uncomfortable silence prevailed until he firmly confronted him.

"Larry, do you want to ride in the trunk?"

"No, I'm just fine, right here," Singleton answered.

"Do it again, and you'll be walking," Doug threatened.

"Then, you can just let me out here, and I will go sing for my supper at the mission," Singleton bluffed.

Doug played along with him and slowed to pull over, saying, "Just say where."

Singleton remained silent as Doug pulled back onto the highway and continued driving. I noted Singleton accepted criticism and direction better from men than he did from women.

One morning, a few weeks later, when Doug and I were driving into Sonoma County, we heard the radio announcer state Sonoma County supervisors had instructed deputies to keep an eye out and to report our movements.

We glanced at one other with shared concern. The radio announcement did not say what would occur if they found us. We didn't want to know. The rules of the game had changed. Not only did we need to duck the media, but we now had to evade law enforcement officers, with whom we worked with closely and depended upon for backup. The situation was getting serious. Pulling off the main roads, we traveled deep into remote areas.

Stopping for breakfast at a coffee shop in one of the less populated areas, Doug left our table to make the morning phone call into headquarters, while Singleton and I placed our food orders. Noting a group of men glancing toward us as they engaged in lively conversation, I covered my discomfort by fidgeting through my purse, carefully attempting to catch a bit of their discussion. My heart stopped as I realized it was about us.

"Is that him?"

"Sure looks like him."

"Yeah, but she doesn't look armed."

"I'm not so sure of that," one man said.

Damn, he sounds like a cop.

Singleton and I continued our conversation, while I pretended to ignore them, all the while wishing Doug would hurry. In the meantime, no reaction was the best reaction. The more they questioned themselves, the more uncertain they would be. My mind was racing as I developed exit strategies.

Where is Doug?

Standing in front of a row of payphones, Doug noted a big logger kind of guy, with an enormous bruise spanning across a swollen nose, towering over him as *he* spoke on the telephone.

"Yeah, we're going out hunting that Singleton guy today," the man said. Doug's ears perked. He instantly turned his back to him. Though finished with his conversation, Doug continued holding the phone to his ear, pretending to be engaged in his call, while hearing the man speak.

"Did I say Singleton's name?" Doug silently asked himself, running through his memory to determine if he had made any reference to Singleton by name, during the call.

"No, I didn't," he decided.

Doug remained at the payphone as he heard the man boast about what he intended to do when he and his buddies found Singleton. It wasn't pretty.

Anxiety raced as I waited for him. Relieved, I finally saw him walking toward us. As he filled me in on everything happening at the phones, he suddenly groaned.

"Oh, Lord. They just seated the guy from the phones behind Singleton," he whispered.

Glancing up, I was holding back an enormous laugh that was building inside but went with a chuckle instead.

"Yeah, well, check out the guys in the corner," I quietly responded, taking my turn to apprise him of what had been happening at the table during his absence. "One has him made, and the others aren't sure."

"We'd better get out of here. You pay the bill, and I'll get the car. I'll meet you out front."

"Will do. See you in a few," I said.

It was *my* job to protect the public from Singleton. It carried the misfortune of often having to be alone with him, for extended periods, in situations where I might have to act. It was getting old, and I was not sure how long my good luck would hold out. A minute or two after Doug left, I sighed, calmly picking up my handbag.

"Ready to go?" I asked Singleton.

Making no sign of rising, he ignored me. It was clear he intended to take advantage of the situation. Without saying a word, my eyes caught his, firing off a piercing look that had him looking down at his shoes for a second. It gave him the time to think of his next course of action, and hopefully, the ramifications of those actions. Fortunately for him, he decided to slide off his chair and follow me.

We exited the main door of the restaurant just as Doug pulled up. Hopping into our station wagon, loaded with luggage, some drooping tropical plants, and other miscellaneous treasures we found throughout the state, we pulled out of the parking lot and headed down the road. It was doubtful anyone would expect the vehicle to hold two state parole agents and the most notorious, parolee in the country, hunted by vigilantes. We hoped those on the lookout would be searching for black vans with darkened windows. We were working alone in the open and hiding in plain sight.

The day was tense. Singleton bent his head toward the front seat of the vehicle and commented to us that he was sure glad to have a couple of bodyguards there to protect him. We shot back with the same standard curt response that our mission was to protect the public from him. He sat back, silent.

"I don't want to be in a situation where I will have to shoot someone who is coming at us because of this guy," Doug confided to me later, when alone.

"I don't want to see us putting ourselves into the situation where that could happen," I haughtily responded.

Charged with an enormous responsibility to the public, to the department, and ourselves, I often wondered if we were sitting ducks, with a pack of hungry wolves waiting to chase us down if we were not alert. The vigilante Doug met in the restaurant was unnerving. We needed to tighten up the way we worked and not allow ourselves to become too comfortable.

After a few days, a report appeared in a newspaper. Someone had spotted Singleton at that specific restaurant. Countering that information was another reliable source that said we were traveling up Interstate 5, over a hundred miles away. The fact was we were long gone, and far from both the coffee shop and Interstate-5.

As weeks passed, Singleton grew unhappy as his name had all but disappeared from news headlines. We were glad. It had been our goal. But not Singleton's. He was dependent upon reading about himself and was interested in little else for distraction. By then, we had arrived at the point of insisting he dine alone and act independently. It was a welcome break in the routine, yet one to which Singleton did not adapt well. He thrived on receiving attention, good or bad, from anyone.

As the honeymoon period elapsed, he attempted to test us, as I anticipated. On one occasion, as I passed the lunch counter where he sat, and noted he had placed our business cards upon it, in front of his plate. As the server passed, he tapped his index finger upon them. Fortunately, she did not notice.

Discreetly, I stepped forward, retrieved them, and whispered, "Let's go." Caught, he hung his head and could not look at me, like a scolded child as he submissively followed me outside.

In May, the court finally released its decision. Singleton would parole to West Contra Costa County. I felt immense relief to be back home, in familiar territory, at home, with my family.

Our mission was evolving. Doug and I now worked with Bob and Tom, developing a residential plan for Singleton. It was no longer one of playing blind man's tag in avoiding everyone. They tasked us with the difficult mission of seeking a proper site for Singleton to live during his remaining months on parole supervision.

Each community presented legitimate concerns of having him as a resident. Richmond, West Contra Costa County's most populated city, posed a challenge with its empty storefronts, graffiti-covered walls, neglected homes, and glass and litter covering the streets. Vying with Oakland and one or two other towns for the title of murder capital of the United States, we felt concerned for the safety of our twenty-four-hour surveillance teams, who would be keeping surveillance over Singleton's activities. We were also worried about the safety of the police who would need to respond to assist them if called. That particular part of the city was too volatile for him to live.

Carefully, we assessed each of the other communities in western Contra Costa County, starting where Singleton had lived at the time of his commitment offense. Filled with middle-classed families, unsupervised teens roamed the neighborhood. Not fitting our needs for covert surveillance, we determined it was detrimental to the protection of the public.

Of all the other surrounding communities, only one option stood out as an appropriate location. We homed in on a large, rundown apartment building at the end of a road, in an emaciated business area on the far west end of Rodeo, California. There were few homes in that part of town. Once a booming business area, it was mostly deserted, hosting only a couple of thrift shops and secondhand stores, a bar or two, and a convenience store. San Pablo Bay fronted the building; two of the sides of the building bordered vacant lots. Dilapidated buildings existed in the back.

No neighborhood centers or schools existed nearby, and no young women lived in the building. Quiet, with insignificant foot traffic, children did not play outside. Parolees lived there. Developing a plan to place parole agents covertly into a position where they could perform 24-hour surveillance of him worked well.

Before moving in, we transported him to the Contra Costa County Sheriff's Office in Martinez, California to make sure he registered as a sex offender, in compliance with Section 290 of the State of California Penal Code. It imposed a legal requirement that all convicted sex offenders registered, with the agencies revealing their addresses in the communities where they lived. I noted the clerk's eyes widen as we supplied the address to punch into her computer.

Instantly, I realized it would not remain a secret long, not with a couple of hundred deputy sheriffs knowing, all with their contacts with the local and major San Francisco media moguls. Added to a dozen or two more in the Parole Division now having the information of Singleton's location, there was sure to be a leak.

Early the next morning, after placing Singleton into his new home, our planted surveillance team kept their eyes glued upon the building from their concealed location.

I had stopped by Singleton's apartment to do a welfare check and make sure he was adjusting to his new living quarters. Within minutes of returning to my office, I received information from the surveillance team that a journalist, riding a bicycle, had stopped, and peered into my work vehicle while I was performing the welfare check.

I wasn't concerned. Nothing about the vehicle, except it was a standard make and model for the public and government alike, suggested it belonged to a parole agent. It bore undercover plates. Inside, a car seat, some kids' toys, women's magazines, and cosmetics made it appear like any other messy public auction car often seen in those neighborhoods. I hoped it would throw off any counter-surveillance from members of the media and others who were seeking us out.

A nagging concern arose over why a journalist would bicycle to our specific location within twelve hours after the business department of the Sheriff's Office had closed. Throughout the months on the road, we had experienced no leaks. Less than a half-dozen people in the Bay Area knew the details of our operation, and only a few top-level government officials in Sacramento knew of our activities. After only twenty-four hours in Rodeo, we suddenly had a member of the media hanging around, scouting the site. It wasn't a coincidence.

With the media scouring the area, crowds arrived. The communication network in Rodeo was lightning fast. The apartment manager called the Sheriffs' Office and asked for a deputy to confirm the identification of a tenant. He did and called me, asking that I have him removed. I advised him it was a civil matter and an issue for the Sheriff's Office and passed the information to headquarters.

During the day, dozens of people began forming outside the building. A man traveled through town with a loudspeaker, announcing Singleton's presence. Meanwhile, in the front of the building, a woman suggested a lynching party, and demonstrators began throwing rocks at his windows. My telephone was burning with phone calls, from the Sheriff's Office to my supervisors, and from the media, all demanding information. I had none to offer anyone. The Singleton issue was being handled far above that of my supervisors. It had become an issue for the community of which he was a product.

Calls continued to flood my home--from the sheriff's office begging for help, parole administrators working on a plan, members of the press asking for information, and the usual threats of violence from the more radical protestors. Instead of their attempts to intimidate me, they ticked me off.

Nobody could do nothing until the powers to be gave the word. The decisions were rocking at the highest level of state government. There, things never worked as rapidly as we did.

Matters were getting out of hand. After I stepped out for a moment, the phone rang. My twelve-year-old, Judi, picked it up to hear a woman threaten, "We are going to bomb you and your house." At the site, matters were intensifying.

Lea Anne Branch Snowden, a parole agent, was working on the surveillance team that night. Assigned to perform surveillance on Singleton, she watched as the numbers within the crowd swelled.

Protesters lined their vehicles outside the building, using headlights to illuminate the windows of Singleton's apartment. Branch contacted administrators, reporting members of the crowd had made Singleton. Directed to access his apartment, she and other agents noted he was frightened, his hands shaking as he tightly clenched a butter knife, he had pulled from a drawer.

She heard the hundreds standing outside the apartment building, making threats. The surveillance team of peace officers stayed with Singleton in his apartment while vigilantes pounded on the door, threatening them and Singleton. Receiving a call from Ed Veit, the Chief of the CDC Parole Division, instructing them to vacate the apartment, they retreated, leaving Singleton alone. If he feared for his safety, he was to call the Sheriff's Office and report his concerns.

Within minutes of their departure, Singleton made the call. Sheriff's officers responded at once. Placing Singleton into a bullet-proof vest, they extracted him from the building and put him into a transport vehicle. At once, the crowd surrounded it. They rocked the SUV back and forth, trying to turn it over, with Singleton inside.

I watched the demonstrations on television, while the calls continued. Finally, I received instructions to act.

"Linda, can you retrieve Singleton at the Sheriff's Office?" Bob Roenicke asked.

"Will do. I am on my way," I responded. Hanging up the phone, I went to the cabinet, and after unlocking it, grabbed my duty weapon, badge, and cuffs.

"Keep Judi away from the phone, please," I called out to my husband as I headed out the front door.

"What do I do if it rings?" he asked.

"Just don't answer it, please."

"All right."

Shaking my head, I grabbed my handbag, raced out the door, and headed toward the Contra Costa County Jail.

Sheriff Warren Rupf was awaiting my arrival. Pulling me aside, he was apologetic, saying, "Linda, people far higher than us need to talk." I agreed.

The problem was not just one of the Sheriff's Office or the CDC. It was created by the elements of a violent society living in western Contra Costa County; the "other Singletons" who reacted violently against others, and as vigilantes had no problem taking the law into their own hands. Their actions reinforced to never put an older and weaker animal in with a pack of others. The nature of the beast is to work together to stalk and attack the most vulnerable. It was also the nature of the culture demonstrating in Rodeo, California.

Frustrated with the realization of the lost chance to assess Singleton's socialization and his risk to society, by clandestinely surveying his activity after he settled in, I was upset the opportunity to track a potential serial killer and put him away for good was lost. We would never know if he would recidivate when left on his own. I feared the backfire of that created in Rodeo, coupled with Singleton's propensity of violence toward young women, would drastically affect women's lives.

Out of frustration, I suggested to Doug that Singleton live in a small camping trailer set upon San Quentin grounds. It would resolve the problems, save a lot of money, and put the matter to rest. Doug discussed it with Singleton. He agreed. Bob and Tom embraced the idea, and Bob Roenicke, Ron Chun, and Ed Veit got it done. Within days, Governor George Deukmejian ordered just that.

With Singleton under wraps at San Quentin, again under surveillance by parole agents twenty-four hours a day, I could focus on my caseload four days a week. It offered the opportunity to reconnect with the drug dealers, robbers, burglars, gangsters, methamphetamine cookers, murderers, and sexual offenders assigned to my caseload. Returning to the familiar semblance of disorder was a pleasant change.

My week was less stressful. Conducting casework and continuing to supervise the activities of Singleton, every Thursday, we escorted him into the community to buy needed items and engage in some recreation or transport him into San Francisco for psychological assessment and counseling. Sometimes, we took him into San Francisco for medical treatment. It was a welcome change. Little existed for anyone to worry about since he was always under a set of eyes at San Quentin.

Missing from the team was Doug. He received a well-deserved promotion as an investigator with the Board of Prison Terms that he had been wanting. Departmental administrators assigned Cindy Haagenson as the relief agent to Singleton. She had a motherly calming effect upon him. Her presence freed me to track down and tend to the other eighty, some-odd violent and volatile parolees on my caseload.

With Haagenson taking over most of the transport duties, I had a chance to destress, allowing my days to return to normal. It was not long before Tom danced into the office, dropping a folder on my desk, and playfully racing out the door, as was his practice whenever handing off a challenging assignment. My role was to laugh.

Intrigued by new cases, I immediately picked it up. My face tightened as I turned the pages. Booming laughter echoed from the hallway where Tom stood, carefully watching me. Finally, he got the courage to stick his head through the door. Deciding it safe to enter, he stepped inside.

"Boss, can we talk?" I asked.

"Sure, but I don't know if it is going to do you any good," Tom said.

"This guy wants to play Rambo by standing on top of a hill in camouflaged clothing, blackening his face, and arming himself with assault weapons to pick off parole agents, right?"

"Yes, that's what I read."

"Okay," I sighed, turning a page in the file. "And when he becomes upset, he writes federal representatives, the governor, the director of corrections, the director of parole services, the regional manager, the district manager, the president of the United States, and the mother of his parole agent, right?"

Glancing up at him, I returned Tom's big, toothy grin with an uncertain one of my own.

"I think you covered it quite well," he said, "though I didn't read the part about the agent's mother. Good thing it's not a problem for you."

"Yeah, thanks for small favors," I retorted facetiously.

"Linda, I want to assure you that Ron, Bob, and I all hold the utmost confidence in you. We know you'll figure out how to manage him effectively."

"Again, thanks a lot," I growled. "But you *do* remember our office is at the bottom of a hill. And he *is* from the other side of the county? Right?"

"Yes."

"So, why is he on *my* caseload, and why is he here?"

"Linda, because you are good at what you do," Tom said. "Just be sure and wear your vest, and I will be keeping the drapes closed," he said with a wink before walking out the door.

Glancing toward my partner, who was chuckling as he took in the conversation, I asked: "Do you buy the line he gave me, or do you think they're trying to get rid of me?"

"The latter. You can bet on it," my partner said, laughing.

When parolees proved a propensity for threatening the safety of the community or the police, I served them with conditions of parole at the institution ahead of their parole date, and then picked them up personally. It was a strong message I sent. Asking them to sign the papers in my presence implied an understanding between them and me. It decreased the likelihood of recidivism.

If they chose not to sign, I placed a hold to retain them in custody. The parolee remained in custody until the Board of Prison Terms held a hearing. Realizing he no other choice than to return to custody, like all the others, Tim had no problem signing his. En route to Richmond, he talked nonstop. I listened, trying to get a read on him.

Needy and dependent, like Singleton, Tim had an insatiable appetite for attention. Like most of my parolees, his actions reflected poor impulse control. I gauged his emotional age to be about fifteen years old.

"Damn, he needs a mother," I groaned to myself. No wonder Ron and Bob wanted me to deal with him. There was a lot to do if we would get him through parole successfully.

Sitting in the passenger seat of my car, Tim was looking forward to his return to society. I patiently listened as he informed me of the many needs he had. I needed to get him a job, go shopping for new clothing for job hunting, find an apartment where he could live, and provide him with funding for food and job-hunting expenses.

"I don't have a problem with that," I said after he finished with his long list of needs.

His mouth fell open in surprise. "Wow! I'm impressed!"

"Good," I said. "Because I already have a room reserved for you at the Richmond Mission. The rent is low, forty dollars a month, and you are right on the bus route. We'll get you a bus pass to get around, unlimited rides, and you can hop right on board and go wherever you desire without having to pay for parking."

Watching his face drop, I continued, "There's a little place just around the corner from where you live. A terrific little soup kitchen, it serves two home-style meals a day. After we get you settled in, we'll go through your things and see what you need in the way of clothes. There are several reasonably priced thrift stores in town."

"Ooh, you are a cold woman, Linda," he laughed.

"Ooh, *that* hurt." Laughing, I threw a hand up to my chest and feigned pain. "And right after I took care of all your basic needs."

He laughed even harder. "This is going to be a lot more complicated than I thought."

"You think?"

"Yeah."

"So, what are you going to do? Are you going to throw a tantrum and write the president or call my mama?"

"Maybe," he said with a big grin.

He did well. Within forty-eight hours, he had found a job and had a line on a new place to live. Excited, he sat across my desk, handing me paper after paper that outlined his health insurance and job benefits.

I expected that he would test boundaries once the honeymoon period was over. It occurs with most young parolees. One common denominator with all parolees is the absence of a father in their lives. Only on three occasions, of the thousands of parolees on my caseload, did I ever have a parolee that came from an intact family. Most lived in homes where their mothers were too busy trying to feed half a dozen kids and overwhelmed with the responsibility of solely supporting and caring for the children in their young families.

The need for a stable, older role model that they can emulate is essential in the lives of adolescent males. This young man did not have an ongoing relationship with either a father or a mother. It was apparent he was seeking direction and needed someone to help him set boundaries.

In 2012, a clinical researcher, Ronald Rohner at the University of Connecticut and his co-author Abdul Khaleque performed a review involving 10,000 individuals involved in thirty-six different global studies. Their focus was upon the effects of rejection of children by parents of all diverse backgrounds. They found children rejected by parents were more anxious, insecure, hostile, and aggressive toward others. More importantly, they also found if that rejection continued well into adulthood, it made it difficult for rejected children to develop trusting relationships with others.

Their study conducted over fifteen years evidenced that the emotional trauma of rejection affected the same areas of the brain as physical pain. If the psychological distress of rejection repeatedly continues for the child for years afterward, that anxiety, insecurity, and the hostile aggression toward others, as mentioned, often results in children ending up institutionalized at one point or another in their lives.

Typically, the emotional growth of the young becomes stunted by their first institutionalization. Many become dependent, especially if incarcerated in a facility with little responsibilities except for following the institution's program. They are not learning responsibility but only complying with a disciplined pattern of activity. It does not replicate real-life experiences. As a result, many parolees live a life without ever making an adult decision. Court sentences filled my caseload with parolees who functioned at an emotional level of thirteen- and fourteen-year-olds in men's bodies.

Complicating matters were studies evidencing male brains often develop less rapidly than that of the female, frequently not until the age of thirty or even later. This phenomenon is helpful when recruiting the young into the military, with a supervised mission of battle during a time of war. It becomes a threat to public safety when dealing with young men in low-income drug neighborhoods, who are hard-wired into an environment of violence and fighting for survival. Most are simply not capable of making good decisions.

There were some parolees I could work with and get past that so that they could develop positively. Many paroled successfully, and many I sent back to prison. And, then there were those I could do nothing with but lock them up and try again in a month or two upon release.

The day of reckoning finally came when Tom stomped into the office, holding a phone bill, hollering, "What's this? That parolee of yours, I swear... "

"Let me see that," I asked, sighing.

Tom handed me the phone bill, and I carefully reviewed it. Someone had billed over eighty dollars in telephone calls to Saudi Arabia to the office. The debt equaled a week's minimum wage in 1988. Tom had correctly pegged Tim as the person who did it. He was calling his mother, who had moved while he was in prison.

"I'll take care of it," I sighed, as I arose and searched for volunteers to back me up. Nobody wanted to go. They were still not comfortable with Tim, and just now, they were finally getting accustomed to scanning the hill behind the office before going out to their cars. Tom drafted someone to back me up since I would have to play a role tougher than a mafia wise guy to collect the debt.

My recruited partner and I drove to Tim's place, a little hovel in the Rescue Mission, the size of a prison cell, the kind where the locks on the door are a hook and an eye, secured with a single deadbolt. A dangling light bulb completed the scene. Upon arrival, we found him lying in his bed, listening to music on headphones and reading a book. The door was partly open. Walking straight in and holding the bill high for him to see, I asked: "Tim, what is this?"

His eyes grew wide. He laughed, his face reddening in embarrassment.

"I had to call my mom."

"And you billed it to the parole office?"

"Yeah," he said, shrugging his shoulders. "Where else would I bill it? I don't have a phone."

"I want eighty-seven dollars and fifty-six cents, right now. Hand it over, slick," I demanded.

"I don't have it," he said.

He was lying. His eyes diverted downward and to the left as they did every time in the past when he was untruthful. Mine followed as they drifted toward the top of his bed, noting he slightly shifted his weight to obstruct my vision of his pillow.

My eyes rolled. He was too easy. Tim unknowingly revealed where he hid his stash. My kids were even more sophisticated than that.

"Yes, you do," I stated confidently. Tim stared blankly at me, in silence.

"Okay, we have two choices," I announced, deciding not to play with him. "We can do this the hard way or the easy way. I can toss your flipping room and search for it, which is the hard way, or you can dig under your pillow and save me some time. Your call, Slick."

"Oh, my God, how do you know these things?" he muttered in frustration as he reached into his pillowcase and pulled out a wad of cash. Peeling off four twenties and a five, he asked, "Can I pay the rest later?"

Glancing toward my partner, he added, "She's frigging scary, you know?"

"Yep," my partner agreed, with a straight face.

"Don't you have anything to say?"

"I'm sorry," he said contritely.

"Thank you. Don't do it again," I said as I walked out.

Tim's honeymoon was over. He was going to be more difficult than I had thought if this was the beginning. My partner was also unusually quiet until we got to the car. He stood by the passenger door for a minute, just looking at me.

"How *did* you know?" he asked.

Laughing with relief, I thought he had a problem with the way I managed the parolee.

"Tim glanced toward his pillow and positioned himself in front of it."

"Dang! When did that happen?"

"As soon as he got up, while I was confronting him."

"You caught all that?"

"Yeah. Tim is pretty smooth," I laughed.

A big part of what some interpret as intuition is observational skills we develop when young. Our mother taught us to pay attention to details by playing cards and memory games. It helped me to learn to recognize my mother's sharp mood swings and avoid volatile situations.

These skills became even more finely tuned after attending advanced interviewing classes. Silently, I echoed a note of gratitude for Agent J. J. Newberry of the Department of Alcohol, Tobacco, and Firearms for his excellent instruction in analytic interviewing, a class I had taken on a day off. He taught us how to read what people were not saying. It paid off.

Those same skills I learned, I used later, when battling cancer. Feeling changes in my body, I reacted. When I felt the muscles aching and burning, I drank lots of chilly water, took a good, long shower or bath, and relaxed. When I felt an urge to move, I walked. When I was hungry, I ate, and when I felt an unusual gnawing pain, that was different, I saw my doctor. Listening to what my body was telling me, and to my "intuition" that was telegraphing subconscious warnings, I realized physical needs. Paying attention to details, whether it is what happens around us or within us, is essential to survival.

Tim completed parole successfully as was our goal, but he faced difficulty being able to adjust to life without support and attention. He kept reporting in, just to talk. I arranged for community-based psychological services for him. Reporting back to me, the psychologists issued a "duty to warn," and that he presented as a danger to me.

It had been a challenging year and would only be more so until Singleton was back in Florida with his family. A calendar on the wall counted down the days for him to leave. As that date neared, his anger and hostility intensified. One morning, I answered the phone to hear Singleton's voice barking instructions.

"Be ready to take a ride tomorrow and bring a lunch. We're going a long way," Singleton ordered before suddenly hanging up.

Moving the telephone away from my ear, I looked at the receiver in amazement, before hanging up, wondering what prompted his audacious attitude. Singleton felt empowered. He had been acting out for the past several months. Attributing it to the difference in the way I worked and dealt with him and that of the new agent who had a softer approach, I thought that was why he felt empowered. The only problem with that was a disconnect in sharing information. Everything filtered through the unit supervisor. Little information came my way. The consistency of dealing with Singleton was nonexistent. Inmates and parolees need a sense of stability. It helps reduce recidivism. Sighing, I glanced up at the calendar.

Just a few weeks left.

Deciding to call him back, the agent working surveillance at Singleton's site answered just as Tom walked into my office.

"Singleton's planning to take legal action against his victim," Tom whispered into my ear before he plopped into a chair across from my desk.

"No way! I'm calling him now," I informed him.

"Can't wait to hear this," Tom said, his eyes sparkling as I put the phone on the speaker. He knew by the seriousness of my voice that Singleton was in trouble.

The news took me by surprise. No one had told me. There should have been some information passed along from the surveilling agents, my relief, or anyone who knew. Singleton was not quiet about anything he did, especially when it came to his crime victim. There was nothing in the documented notes, and I had heard nothing, yet I was the case agent.

"Hey, is Singleton in there with you?" I asked the agent who answered the phone.

He chuckled. "Wondered how long it would take for you to call. He's outside."

"What's going on with him?"

"Nothing much. Singleton is just making arrangements to file a lawsuit against his victim."

"You're kidding, aren't you?" My stomach fell.

"Unfortunately, no," he said. "Bet it sucks to be *you* right now."

"Don't you know it?"

Damn!

"Would you mind putting him on the phone?"

"Gladly… can't wait to hear this," the agent laughed.

"You're not the only one," I said, glancing toward my supervisor, who was sitting in the chair across from me, laughing.

"It's not going to happen," I firmly told Tom while waiting on hold. I did not know whether to scream or to cry. "That poor girl..."

"You've got that right," Tom's low, raspy voice boomed in support.

Singleton was not a complicated character. He was not mentally ill, nor was he an evil genius as some sociopathic killers. There was nothing brilliant about him. He was demonstrating his sociopathic tendencies, intense anger, and hatred toward women without any impulse control. He was just another good old boy from the South who could not stand women and wanted to control them through violence. It did not matter whether he was drunk, though most of his violent acts toward women took place when he was under the influence of alcohol. He tried to kill women he could not control, and every woman who had been prominent in his life was fearful of him, his former wife, his current wife, his daughter, and his crime victim. That said something about *him*.

A minute or two later, Singleton came on the line, sounding contrite. He was taking his time, and his approach was softer. Given a few moments to consider his prior call, he appeared more self-disciplined and constrained while pouring on a superficial charm.

"Now, dear, I just wanted to let you know we will be taking a long ride tomorrow."

"Singleton," I interrupted, "Let's set something straight before we continue. We need to set some boundaries here."

"I was just telling you—"

I could not allow him to think he could manipulate me or be the domineering influence in the parole agent/parolee relationship. This new behavior that developed in him needed adjustment.

"Well, that's the first boundary, Larry. I am your parole agent, and you do not tell me what to do; I tell you. Got it?"

"Yes, but, dear—"

Singleton's use of the term "dear" was an apparent attempt to demean and to lessen my position with him.

Don't let him get away with it.

"Hold up, there. That's the second boundary, Larry. Don't call me 'dear' again. And there are "no buts" while on parole."

"Yeah, but," he interjected

I didn't give him a chance. "However, what I will do is grant you one minute to think seriously about what you intend to do and how you wish to communicate it."

"I'm going to sue that bitch who ruined my life," he angrily spewed, giving up on the manipulation tactics.

"Really? You are expecting me to drive you to some unknown place so you can do that?"

"I'm expecting you to take me to Auburn to do it."

"Well, Larry, I hate to be the bearer of unwelcome news, but it's not going to happen. If you need to file something, you can do it by mail."

Tom vigorously nodded his head in agreement, giving me a thumb-up.

"But your job is to take me where I want to go and…," Singleton argued.

Oh boy, now he really feels empowered.

"Okay, boundary number three. As I have repeatedly told you, my job is to protect others from you. I am not your chauffeur, your bodyguard, or your mother."

"But..."

"There you go again," I said, cutting him off. "What didn't you understand about using the word, "but? When you can communicate appropriately, shoot me a call. In the meantime, have a lovely day."

Hanging up the phone, I said, "Sorry, boss. I lost it. He's going to sue that poor girl. Can you believe it? What in the hell is empowering him, making him want to do these things?" Banging my head up and down on my desk, I asked, "Why didn't anyone tell *me*?"

"You did great. It was exactly right. That leaves us with how many days left?" Tom asked, deliberately not answering my last question.

"Forty-six," I said, after glancing up at the calendar on the wall. Then looking down at my watch, I added, "Oh, and about twelve hours and… about thirty-three minutes."

Tom laughed as the phone rang.

"You know it's Singleton, right?"

"It might be."

"I don't want to talk to him right now. I'm tired of being a mean Mommy. You want to answer the phone?"

Tom merely shook his head. "Nope."

"Coward," I said, laughing. "Hungry?" I asked.

His eyes lit up. "I'm starved."

"Let's grab lunch and give him some time to think about it. I'll even buy," I offered. Reaching for my jacket and tugging it on, I grabbed for my handbag and followed Tom, making a mad dash out the door, toward fresh air and sweet freedom.

Most days, I would have taken the burn of the heat and exercised patience and self-discipline. This day, Singleton went too far. He had the papers ready to sue his victim. There would be no way to change his mind. I was not going to help him. Why would he think I would?

After ten and a half months of babysitting him and burned out, I was weary of his antics. Today was just one of those days when a girl did not want to sit around and wait for a probable serial murderer to call her back and tell her he would act compassionately with his victim. No longer into dealing with Larry Singleton and his adolescent tantrums, I needed a break, or a drink, or something else to escape from it all. I was quickly putting myself in check by reminding myself that it was my Mom's thing, not mine. My way of managing it was to dial it back and suck it up, staying strong, and doing whatever I had to do to complete the mission.

Later, sliding across the cold vinyl seat in the booth where Tom and I were sitting in the back corner of the restaurant, my stomach was grating, and my heart was pounding, fearful Singleton would stage a scene at the courthouse. That he would call all the media there, and I would be standing somewhere nearby charged with keeping him from harming someone.

Unable to eat, I was silently praying my earlier hardened stance would not backfire. It was consuming me. Backfire was something we had to always expect from our "clientele" to allow ourselves to remain emotionally healthy. Human behavior is difficult to predict. As parole agents and risk-takers, we hoped for the best of those we supervised but readied ourselves for the worst.

"Are you sure I didn't take it too far?" I repeatedly asked Tom, second-guessing myself throughout our lunch.

Returning, I saw a pink message slip lying upon my desk. The name Singleton reflected in large print on the top. My heart raced as I picked it up. The message read that Singleton had taken his legal papers to the San Quentin post office and filed the matter by registered mail.

"Hold up, Tom," I said, excitedly. "Check this out."

I handed him the telephone memo to read. First, his face was serious upon scrutinizing it; then, a smile slowly crossed his face as he set it on the desk and heaved a heavy sigh.

"Phew, that was close," he said.

Laughing, Tom and I slapped each other's hands, with a high five. We had again thwarted a major public relations nightmare.

Being able to clean it up, we made sure there was not a showdown at the courthouse. Neither Singleton's victim, the parole division, or anyone else deserved that. By the time he would get a court date, he would be out of state and wouldn't have the means to appear.

A few weeks before his release from parole, Singleton launched into yet another tirade of anger, this time against Donald Stahl, the elected district attorney of Stanislaus County. Stahl had prosecuted his case, and Singleton held no love for him.

"A desperate man has nothing to lose," he loudly heralded, with bravado. "There's gonna be a showdown at the courthouse."

"You know what to do, Linda," Roenicke sighed after I reported Singleton's intentions.

Once District Attorney Stahl was on the phone, I issued a duty to warn, directly quoting Singleton's threats. The District Attorney did not seem surprised. He expected it.

We spoke for a good while, with him desiring my read-on Singleton. Exercising complete honesty, I advised I felt he was extremely hostile toward women, that he was incapable of exercising impulse control during an episode of anger, and, if able, he would continue to react violently. I stated I wouldn't be surprised if he recidivated in the same manner. He agreed.

As Singleton's release date neared, People Magazine ran an article on him, despite our best attempts to dissuade it. Film crews were in San Francisco, Oakland, and Richmond interviewing employees. It was mostly the male agents filmed, primarily supervisors who had not encountered Singleton. The public never realized the man who hated women, and who had sexually assaulted a young girl, dismembered her body, and left her for dead, had his parole supervised by three agents, one man, and two women, Cindy Haagenson, and me.

On a cold, snowy evening in March 1988, upon the eve of the termination of his parole, a team of agents joined Tom and me in transporting Singleton to Reno, Nevada. We planned to put Singleton on a nonstop flight to Florida. En route, he uttered a statement that brought discomfort, that the best thing about leaving was he would be getting a hug from me.

I watched from a distance as he boarded his flight to Tampa, Florida. He shook hands with the team of all-male agents, who wished him well. Before disappearing down the ramp leading into the plane, he expectantly glanced back toward me. Waving farewell to one another from a distance disallowed him the opportunity to create the scene he fantasized about earlier.

With my major distraction now ended, I began hustling at work to find some clandestine methamphetamine labs. It only helped fill a part of the void. Without the madness that accompanies working notoriety cases, the thoughts about the "family cancer thing" intensified, along with the constant emptiness and loneliness existing in our home.

My empty marriage offered little more than a false sense of security of hedging my risk of "someday," when it was sure that I would become ill. For my husband, our home was merely a stable place with a family waiting for him to arrive so we could sit at the dinner table and eat.

We needed more than merely having a job in common. And, security doesn't equate to happiness, though my mother consistently argued it did. She was a woman of the 1940s, taught to be dependent upon others, and never questioning the poor choices she made in her life. She lived in the moment, seldom thinking about the past and too fearful to contemplate what the future may hold. I was different. A woman of the 1970s, I embraced the opportunities that presented themselves during a time of immense change for us. I welcomed the new status women held and embraced the chance to be more than I had ever dreamed of being. By the end of the decade, I had finally worked my way to a point where I didn't need to depend upon anyone to care for our family and me.

Each year, the reality of our "family circumstances" grew stronger while the lonely nights grew longer. The older I became, the more disillusioned I was with everything around me as I anxiously awaited for what was or was not to be. I was just biding time, waiting for "someday" to come.

Working at the lowest level of the grittiest of life, I learned that being released on parole doesn't guarantee rehabilitation of the parolee any more than being treated for cancer doesn't mean it won't come back. And, like cancer, it does not mean it is no longer a threat. It may only serve as a warning, such as the quiet of the calm before the storm. Bottom line, life is uncertain. I finally gave up thinking about it. I was doing too much of it, and that can drive a person crazy.

In life, there is never a guarantee, just a lot of hedged bets, no matter who or what we are. The one certainty we have is we exist "now," and that is there where I try to stay… in the moment.

Moving on, I continued working. In 1997, nine years after California law resulted in the release of Lawrence Singleton from parole supervision, we finally learned what we needed to know. As I predicted, Singleton returned to his old patterns. He bought a van, trolled the streets for vulnerable women, and murdered one with an everyday kitchen tool, repeatedly hurling a boning knife into her six times. In 2001, he died of cancer while awaiting execution on Florida's death row.

The only question I had was shared by Florida's Attorney General, Scott Brown. How many others had he killed before he was apprehended?

Chapter Twenty

THE FINAL YEAR

"I've learned that making a "living" is not the
same thing as making a life." —Maya Angelou

The remainders of 1989, I spent ripping apart the illicit methamphetamine manufacturing industry in Alameda, Contra Costa,
and Solano Counties. Methamphetamine manufacturing was a
booming business. The product was far less expensive than cocaine, and
the consumer was readily available. Any idiot could make it, and many tried
in Contra Costa County.

With a stable caseload and having developed a rapport with many of the
parolees, they often revealed the criminal activities of others, most of
whom were involved in manufacturing methamphetamine. It was a
popular activity in our part of the county. We took down two or three meth
labs a month. Methamphetamine users, known as cranksters, were tough to
supervise. Living a lifestyle of a primitive culture, most were transient and
uneducated.

When under the effects of methamphetamines, many were prone to
violence. In the advanced stages of addiction, side-effects of paranoia and
extreme aggression often occurred. Dealers carrying substantial amounts
of drugs and cash usually carry guns. Mixing the two often spells out
devastation for anyone involved with a meth addict. Street police officers
and narcotics officers referred to the Contra Costa County culture as being
involved with "crystals and pistols."

In October, Agent Dave Herrington and I spoke at an assembly at a
local high school, discussing our experiences with those affected by drug
use as a program we set up for Red Ribbon Week.

Intended to honor Kiki Camarena, a DEA agent murdered in Mexico
by Mexican cartel members, after finishing our presentation, Carolyn
O'Connor, a reporter with the California Correctional Peace Officers
Association, and I drove to North Richmond, where many of the students
lived. I hoped for her to be able to experience, firsthand, the culture and
environment where the kids came from, so she could write from a unique
perspective of their life experiences, living in a culture of addiction.

Exposed daily to a tough neighborhood, filled with drug trafficking,
most of the kids engaged in one of two activities involving drugs during

their high school years. They either battled against its use or became caught up in dependency and became baptized into the criminal justice system. There was no in-between for them. The pressure to use drugs was powerful.

As we drove down the street, I was comfortable taking her there. It was my turf. Having worked here for a few years, I had even taken the Chief of the Parole Division into that area when he rode with me. The only thing different that day was the streets were eerily quiet for that time of the afternoon.

"Sorry, Carolyn. I guess no one is here today," I apologized as I turned right onto a major thoroughfare where a few of the locals usually congregated. Immediately upon doing so, I regretted it. Ahead, I saw an enormous crowd of seventy people assembled on the corner.

Damn, they turned it into a drug turf!

"Be cool; we're on a drug turf," I said. "An active one."

Glancing into the rear-view mirror, assessing options to turn around and leave, I spotted a vehicle directly behind us.

I can't back up.

I searched for a chance to turn around. A vehicle was coming from the other direction. There was nowhere to go but forward. Ahead, another blocked the street, engaged in a transaction. Trapped between traffic, we slowly crawled forward as we drove past people openly buying drugs.

Suddenly, a young black man dressed in white raced to my side of the car. With his right hand, he raised a .45 caliber revolver and pointed it at my head. Noting his quick movement through my peripheral vision, I instinctively turned to the right, just as he fired.

Instantly, the sensation of slow-motion set into play. The gunshot that drilled through the driver's window, hitting the windshield, and ricocheting down into the dashboard, sounded muffled. Though a slight pain was developing on the left side of my head, I could not feel it. Creating the uncertainty of whether the bullet had hit me, was the feel of a sting, not a penetration by a larger, more solid object. Unable to ascertain my level of injury was difficult. I felt nothing, not even the small amount of blood trickling down my scalp onto my neck and my shoulders.

Carolyn screamed. "Your head! Your head!"

"I'm okay, Carolyn. I'm all right," I reassured her. "It's okay."

Stay calm, stay calm, find help.

As the symptoms of PTSD kicked in, I tried to get in sync with the tunnel vision. After seeing others stabbed and shot at San Quentin, I knew, if I had been hit, I had only a few moments of consciousness left. If I could keep my blood pressure down, as I had seen others do, the odds of survival would be better. I had seen inmates who had done the same and lived after repeatedly being stabbed, even in the heart. It offered hope.

"We're getting out of here," I quietly said to Carolyn. "Keep your eyes out for cops, okay?

"Okay," she sobbed.

Humming a made-up tune that even I didn't recognize, I was trying to keep myself together. My navigational skills eluded me. I searched for the sun. Seeing it setting over the horizon, which was on our right, we turned toward town. My first concern was Carolyn. Terrified, she was sobbing. Quietly speaking nonstop, I attempted to maintain an aura of calm.

"Boy, you sure have a story, now, huh?

"Yes," she sobbed.

"It will be okay, Carolyn. We *are* getting out of here."

The truth was, I had no idea where we were. I realized we were still in North Richmond, but war was raging between my survival instincts and that of reason. I was driving with a complete loss of navigation skills. Desperate, I tried to stay composed in contradiction to the little voice screamed, "Faster, drive faster! Get out, get out now!"

Finally, I recognized the emergency light bars of a law enforcement vehicle rolling toward us. As it approached, my eyes teared, and I sighed in relief.

Thank the Lord, Contra Costa sheriffs.

Their vehicle came to a rapid stop. The two deputies quickly hopped out. One ran toward my door, and the other raced to the passenger side.

Lindy, you okay?" the deputy asked as I sat in stillness, viewing the white knuckles of my hands still tightly gripping onto the steering wheel. Caroline sobbed as the other deputy peeled her from the vehicle.

Placing my left hand upon my head, I gently felt my scalp. I felt a stinging sensation on the upper left side of my head. The warm stickiness of blood melted onto my fingers while shards of glass that had penetrated my scalp and that which had become tangled in my hair fell onto my upper body and lap. Watching sparkling drops of bright red blood dripping onto my arms, my lap, and onto the floor, I answered, "Yeah, I think so."

My scalp burned. Bringing my hand down and studying the blood upon it, I tried to muster the courage to look at the window.

"Someone threw something at the window," I told the deputy, continuing to look forward.

"No, Lindy. Someone shot at you," the deputy gently advised.

Turning slightly to my left, I decided to confront what I knew I would see. My heart stopped. Level with my eyes, was the chilling pattern of a gunshot etched through the glass. Viewing it jogged my memory. I recalled the image of the young man racing to my car door and pointing a gun at me.

Phew, that was close, too close.

Remaining in my seat for a few minutes, until I could compose myself, I whispered a grateful prayer for being alive. The ability to feel came back, the wetness of blood upon my collar, the dripping of it down my scalp, and the burning sensation. Most of it was the result of the shattering of glass fragments puncturing into my scalp and my neck.

As I sat, taking a moment or two to compose myself and to allow time for the sheriffs to photograph the car and my position, my hands trembled, along with my knees. The adrenaline was wearing off. In the distance, I could hear the high-pitched wails of sirens. They were growing louder, piercing through the air from distant Richmond and the communities beyond after the dispatch call went out as an attempted murder upon a parole agent.

Dozens responded to the scene. Everyone available was there, except for my supervisor. He had sent an agent who cared for Carolyn. I felt disappointed. As usual, I dealt with it on my own. It had been a pattern in which I had worked for a few years. Any time I needed direction, my supervisor instructed me to call Roenicke, who, the few times I did call, was always there for me, offering support.

During a time of crisis, peace officers need to have someone of knowledge and authority around to support the troops and voice their concerns for their agents or officers. Failure for the supervisor to come was not a sign of support.

He lived in the same community as he worked. He never came into the field to see any of us. We were left on our own while he remained in the office. I believe his circumstances created discomfort for him to act in his position in the community.

The deputies and I drove to the scene where dozens of police officers were searching for the bullet casing. Dave stayed behind with Carolyn. I could not recall exactly where it happened, but they somehow knew. Someone must have called it in. Everything looked different, with the street empty, than it did when the crowds were present. Now, it was eerily silent and devoid of any signs of life.

Nothing remained but litter floating across the asphalt, shattered glass on the roads and bullet casings scattered everywhere. It reminded me of a shooting range after a week of qualifications. The search to find the casing of the specific round was futile. We returned to where Dave and Carolyn were waiting by the car.

"When you're ready to go out in the field again, be sure to call us. I'll go out with you," one of the deputies offered. "We know it is going to be tough for you to want to get back out here."

My heart warmed with their support. The police officers realized we had a difficult job working out in the field alone, without a means to call for backup in the community that was vying as the murder capital of the nation. It was a kind offer. They entered the same neighborhoods we did in two-person cars. I was incredibly grateful. After, Dave drove us to Kaiser Permanente for examination.

"Looks like a minor graze," the physician said as he sat back upon his stool, after examining me. "You're one lucky girl."

He cleaned my wounds and removed the fragments of glass. Then he handed me a small brown envelope holding a couple of Valium tablets. I tucked it into my purse, figuring I would need them more when I was alone and facing the reality of what occurred, head-on.

The next morning, Tom instructed me to attend a departmental arranged appointment with a shooting psychologist in Berkeley.

"Who brought you here?" the psychologist asked, looking around.

"I did," I answered.

"You drove yourself?"

"Yes."

He groaned. "That's great. Simply great. Are you working today?"

"Yes."

"Well, how do you feel about that?"

"Okay, I guess. I know how to drive," I laughed.

"Do you know what PTSD is?" he asked.

"Yes. Post-traumatic stress disorder."

"Do you understand the symptoms?" he asked.

"Yes."

"Are you experiencing any?"

"Of course. Someone tried to kill me."

Suppressing a chuckle, he laughed.

"Of course," he reiterated, rolling his eyes. "Silly me."

The bit of humor was disarming. I felt comfortable speaking with him. We spent a while discussing the side effects of PTSD, me telling him when I first learned about it and how I managed the effects… the heart palpitations, the hypervigilance, the uncertainty, and the occasional feeling of depression.

After, he said, "I still can't believe they sent you here by yourself."

"I realize it is not the recommended procedure, but it is the nature of the beast, Doc. We work by ourselves. I have been doing it for several years, supervising the most violent in our office. I think they expect more of me. You know?"

Pausing for a second, I continued, "I don't fault anyone. Everyone is swimming in uncharted waters on this. There is no certain procedure for treating field shootings but time. That's it. I'm just grateful I am alive."

"But how do *you* manage it? How do you cope with all this?" He sounded surprised.

"I compartmentalize it until I'm ready to confront it."

"Wow. I'm amazed that you openly admit this."

"Why? I've adapted to it."

"But most cops aren't this open…"

"But I'm not a cop," I laughed. "Maybe that has something to do with it?"

He again laughed. "Touché. Okay, you parole agents *are* a different breed. "So, tell me how about your brothers and sisters? How did they adapt to everything growing up?"

"My brother was defensive and angry. His veneer wasn't as strong as he thought it was. My sister was dependent, like our mother." I answered.

"But what about you?"

"I was defiant as all hell, the mother we didn't have."

"Never a kid, huh?"

"Oh, yeah. I rebelled in high school. I hosted a lot of high school beer parties. Then, again, I've always felt responsible for taking care of everyone and everything."

As he cleared me back to work, he asked one final question. "Where did you get those survival skills?"

My heart stopped as the question floored me.

Why does everyone ask me that?

Sighing, I pondered how to answer it. It was far too complicated to share with one or two sentences, and with those who authored reports and condensed hours of conversation to a paragraph or two that could become public record. Everyone has a history and a closet where we store our most significant memories, especially those which are traumatic and painful. I wasn't ready to get into it with him or anyone. What was, was. I had moved forward long ago and gotten past everything but my sensitization to stress. I simplified my answer.

"Through life experiences, I guess."

It was intentionally vague. The truth was, long ago, when I was a child, I gave up running away from fear. Empowerment comes from confronting it. Viewing how our mother managed difficult circumstances when young, I learned denial does not serve anyone well, not the person unwilling to accept the reality of their situation or those who love them. I confronted her and the fear I felt every chance I had.

I found this to be especially so, knowing how my ancestors survived under far more difficult conditions than I could ever realize. Compared to them, we had it amazingly easy. I subscribed to Dad's philosophy when he stated, "You don't have to look far to find those worse off than you.

The legacies of those who came before us offered strength and inspiration. If they could live despite the incredible odds against them, so could I, even with the unknowns that I was not ready to confront, specifically cancer. Grandma was right. What she revealed *did* help me when "someday" rolled around... when I needed it most.

We all face tough decisions, requiring us to make conscious choices. Accepting reality makes life less complicated. Those of us affected with Lynch syndrome accept our lot, no matter how painful it may be, adapting to the fact little choice exists other than going through uncomfortable screenings and prophylactic surgeries if we want to live.

We can view it as a positive experience that allows us to confront it, or we can live in denial, limiting our experiences. We have choices in how we choose to live, doing it either the "hard way" or the "easy way."

Changes usually occur when we are ready for them, and when we make them happen. Living is difficult; loyalties are often fragile, and nothing is "forever." Our existences upon this earth are temporary, and if we are to survive, we must be able to depend upon ourselves and others. We can ask those who have survived to mentor us or look to the past and learn from those who lived, and consider what our ancestors endured, allowing it to give us strength. Help is available through support groups, nonprofit organizations, and counseling services. And, we can take on the responsibility of how we react to life's more difficult circumstances. Sometimes all we need is to alter our perspective.

Through the years, I learned to become proficient in choosing either to confront or not to face whatever issues that appeared before me. Prioritizing *my* needs in balance with those of my work and my family, I now choose my time to decide when and how I will act because it is best to do so when it is advantageous to me and others when I am ready.

Making sure every major decision I make is on my terms is a crucial element in developing a sense of empowerment and the furtherance of my goal of survival. Along with managing my situation with confidence and feeling in control of myself, I make sure everything has its time and place. Like my father, dozens of little compartments exist within me. It is where fears, thoughts, and everything that needs to be resolved is stored until I am ready to confront them, head-on.

Compartmentalization and disassociation from negative or distracting situations are typical methods of dealing with trauma. It is practiced by many who work extensively in harm's way. Used by soldiers, peace officers, physicians, medical professionals, first responders, crime victims, survivors of life-threatening situations, and others, it is no different for those of us affected by life-threatening health conditions. The fight-or-flight response is not discriminatory in who it affects. It touches all of us in diverse ways.

By minimizing negative thoughts and experiences, we can better focus on immediate priorities. In concealing negativity, we can achieve a balance that allows us to accept responsibility and take control of ourselves and the situations we face. Crucial is we learn to adapt. The longer someone experiences adversity, the more fine-tuned one's survival skills become.

Living with PTSD is tough for any peace officer to manage. Though common, with an estimate of one in every eight peace officers affected, finding others to serve as a support base is difficult. Most keep their PTSD to themselves as I did. I did not discuss it with my supervisors or my peers. There was too much of a stigma of weakness surrounding it. The best support I received came in a telephone call from a sergeant at the Oakland Police Department, a few days after the shooting occurred.

"The guys and I are wondering, how are you doing?" he asked.

We spoke for a while. I relayed what occurred. It was good to speak with someone I could trust with my thoughts and my fears.

"It was eye awakening," I said. "I was so lucky to see him through my peripheral vision and turn my head at just the right time. I swear, there was an angel perched on my shoulder."

"I thank God he wasn't aiming at a vital organ," the sergeant teased.

"Huh?" I asked, initially stunned by his comment, not knowing how to react. He repeated it, this time, laughing. Suddenly, catching on to his teasing, I could not stop laughing. At that time, what I desperately needed most was some of that dark police humor to help get past it all. Releasing an incredible amount of stress and tension. It was the most helpful contact I received.

When a crisis hits, sometimes people disappear from our lives. One or two of those who were close, and who rely upon us, distance themselves as far as possible. And it is incredibly painful.

It does not matter what created the incident and the crisis. When co-workers stop looking you in the eye and are uncomfortable around you, because they know what happened with you could happen to them, it is tough. Even for those viewed as solid, working through a crisis can be lonely. Support can be hard to find, especially from those who have leaned on you for their help in the past.

It is not uncommon for those with hereditary cancer syndromes to experience people they love disappear from their lives. A crisis is a crisis. In our situation, both our parents vanished from our lives. Not only did they detach from us, which was strongly encouraged by their spouses, each disconnected from their parents either by rejection, the death of the parent, or a feeling of being too inadequate to help. That pattern continues with some of our children detaching from my siblings and me. It is heartbreaking.

We need to understand they may fear that which has happened with their parents or siblings, will happen with them. An enormous difference exists between the uncertainty of living with the blindness of fate, living with a life-threatening disease.

Previously diagnosed with PTSD, I then sought support and help from the outside. I had no problem seeing a counselor or spending time with good friends who ensured privacy and confidentiality. Sharing everything with them without fear of judgment and needing to get it all out of my head and out of my heart, was necessary to recover. My counselor supplied the best support and guidance on how to adapt that money could buy. He taught me how to live effectively with my PTSD. There was a lot to manage. Subsequently, it was a good experience while living with a hereditary cancer gene.

Though some friends and family members disappeared when I went through the shooting incident, and while I battled PTSD, those equipped to offer support remained by my side. Those who were invisible are still so to this day.

And, there were a rare few who were unable to adapt to my cancer diagnosis. When a close family member disappeared, it was heartbreaking. Regardless of how she felt, I felt it was essential to continue to stand behind her. Though it stung, I have not been able to get past it. Neither has she. The bottom line is when this happens, which is not unusual; it has little to do with us and everything to do with them. There is nothing like a life-threatening crisis to destroy long-termed relationships.

Having worked alone on dangerous city streets and continue functioning at an elevated level with a keen sense of awareness of my surroundings, one by one, I used my skills to realize the triggers creating the anxiety. Problems occurred when I drove. When I saw someone crossing a freeway pedestrian ramp while holding an umbrella, my heart would stop, then pump furiously. From a distance, my mind interpreted the umbrella as a firearm. Realizing it to be far from probable, I "talked myself down," while approaching the threat.

Stay calm. It's okay. It's just an umbrella.

An immense relief would surge through me when I realized I was right. Though I realized it was just an umbrella, it did not stop the natural survival response of blood from continuing to race through my head or the rapid heartbeat accompanying it. After a while, those incidents became less threatening, the more times I experienced them and minimized the threat. However, it never totally went away.

When a vehicle backfired, or if a gunshot sounded, an instant startle reaction occurred, followed by an instinct to cover my head with my hands. On crowded highways and city streets, this is a severe problem. When driving in inner cities, someone is always firing a gun, and in lower-income areas, inevitably, there will always be older vehicles that backfire. There was no way to avoid it.

Seeking a transfer closer to my home, I found no positions were open. Despite feeling trapped, it was still difficult to ask for help. Bob and Ron were available. But I was not comfortable contacting them. Ingrained in me as a child was to stick it out and find a way to resolve it myself. I could not make the call.

To get past this involved finding out who had tried to kill me. Most people do not become shooting victims when driving on city streets. I needed to know who they were and why.

I had not been in contact with anyone in the Sheriff's Office, and I couldn't call the investigators. My biggest fear was doing so would make me look weak. Asking my husband for help, he refused, saying he could not interfere with another officer's case. The response was one of a police officer, first, and of a husband, second. It stung, though it should not have. Nothing had changed with him. But everything *had* changed with me. I couldn't accept it any longer. We were no longer good partners, nor were we a couple. It was time to prepare to move on. Waiting any longer wasn't good for either of us or our children.

A month later, while working with the Contra Costa County Sheriff's Narcotics Task Force and performing a parole search upon one of my parolees-at-large, the issues of whether I was reliable in "shoot/don't shoot" situations were tested.

Narcotics officers reported Michael, one of my parolees who had absconded parole, was cooking methamphetamines and had weapons. At six o'clock A.M., one autumn morning, we decided to serve the PAL (Parolee At Large) warrant to take him into custody.

A cadre of law enforcement officers and I awakened Michael that morning, surrounding him as he sprawled beneath the covers of his bed. Beside him, upon the floor were dirty bed linens and miscellaneous items of clothing. Suddenly, in the reflection of a mirror set next to his bed, my eyes caught upon his fingers crawling toward what looked like the recoil pad of a shotgun.

"Is it a gun? Does he have a gun?"

I frantically questioned myself as I desperately focused upon his hands. Seconds seemed like minutes as I kept second-guessing myself. Then, I saw it, a quick glimpse of the stock lying beneath the dirty clothing. It allowed me to believe in myself and my perception of the situation.

"He's got a gun," I yelled. Instantly, I drew my weapon and leveled it at his head. Firearms flew out of holsters. Within seconds, the air filled with the distinct odor of Hoppe's firearm lubricant, as Michael found himself with a dozen guns pointed at him. Surrendering, his hand dropped to the side of his bed, dangling where I could see it.

"Don't shoot, don't shoot! I've got him," called an officer as he leaped upon Michael, flipping him over and cuffing him up. Another on the other side of the bed immediately grabbed the shotgun, pulling it from his reach.

After securely tucking Michael into a jail cell, and while driving back to the office, I felt overcome by an incredible sense of anxiety. My heart started racing, and, this time, it would not stop. This event set a pattern that continued for weeks, beginning every time I got into my car. It did not end until I was safely at home. The adrenaline rushes were not dissipating, as usual. My stomach rocked incessantly.

The negative office conflict that was always in existence contributed to the stress. The effective action by the supervisor and my high level of sensitivity, allowed it to escalate. I stayed away as much as I could or kept my office door closed while I worked. Burned out, I found trying to manage the physical effects of the stress, while at the office, did not work. They managed me. My blood pressure continued to race out of control until my vehicle climbed the hill overlooking Napa Valley, where I felt safe.

The MMPI test that assesses, and measures personality and psychological health came out fine. It showed no character defects or other serious problems. Used to determine mental stability in persons in high-risk professions, it is the determining factor for the continuation of employment in law enforcement following a shooting incident.

"It shows you are well-grounded," the psychologist laughed, "especially since someone tried to kill you, and nobody has figured out who did it, or why. I do think your work is creating an intense amount of stress for you. If it becomes too much, you need to leave."

Something changes in people once one experiences a life-threatening situation, whether it be working on the streets or contracting cancer. For each, what we experience is different. Sometimes nothing matters, but those we care about and our ability to continue. Sometimes, everything matters, focusing on anything but the root problem. Some of us tend to take life for granted, and when something occurs, we experience an awakening. The realization that a clock is ticking is powerful. In the months to come, I saw a few more workers' compensation doctors. They asked more questions—different ones.

"How was your childhood?

"Early or late?" I asked.

"Let's try early when the character forms."

"Idyllic. It was stable. I grew up in a small town with an intact family until junior high school."

"And your relationship with your husband?"

"All right, I guess. We share a lot in common with work."

"What if you grow apart if you left your job?

"I don't know. I guess we'll deal with it then. To be honest with you, I am just dealing with today."

The conversation progressed into a discussion about my parents and my relationship with them.

"I don't know much about my Mom. She left the country when I was twenty-one years old, and we didn't hear from her much after that." With my attention focused upon the wall to conceal emotion. I added, "My dad was just diagnosed with cancer."

"I'm sorry."

"No need to be. It's part of life. It runs in the family."

"Leaving your family and moving to Europe?" he asked.

I laughed, concealing a thought that had clicked in my mind. The psychologist had focused on my mother. He was, exploring my past with a woman who not been a part of her children's lives for decades. I had never hidden the fact from anyone that my mother was a prescription drug addict who abandoned her family and moved to another continent.

"No," I laughed. "Cancer."

"Ah, your dad. It must be hard. But how do you feel about your mother?

"I love her, of course. She's my mother," I sighed heavily. "I just hope wherever she is, that she is living the way she always dreamed."

"Don't you miss her?"

"I used to… terribly. You know, it's been a long time.

"Where in the devil did you get those survival skills?" he asked.

Good Lord. Again?

"I don't know. Growing up in the foothills, I guess."

The shooting psychologist was the final one to get down to "brass tacks," zeroing in on the million-dollar question with the answer everyone sought, including me. It was the only one that mattered.

"Okay, my only concern is whether you will shoot too fast or too slow. What do you think?"

"I don't know. Nobody knows until it happens. We have this policy…"

Explaining my dilemma to him and the stress I felt having to write "drawn weapon" reports whenever we pulled our weapons, I admitted to him that I never did it. First, if I did, I would be writing them day in and day out, and I would not get any work done because I was in situations many agents never experienced, with my demanding caseload of repeat violent offenders. Secondly, I knew the extra seconds taken to second guess ourselves, and "think it through," could be life-threatening. Those few extra seconds are precious in "shoot, don't shoot" situations and can make the difference between living and loss of life.

I was performing high-risk arrests once or twice a week. I did not want anyone who hadn't experienced what I had, judging me. I knew what would happen. It would be the same as what was happening since I had gone through the shooting incident. Everyone had been drawing their weapons and not saying anything to anyone. None of us knows what any of us will do until we are in a life-threatening situation, whether it be on city streets or while fighting cancer—none of us. I found myself in a quandary, fearing I was a liability to the department, and that nobody would ever want me in their unit.

"Well, do you want to stay or leave? What do you think?" the doctor asked.

"That is something I am not certain of either. It doesn't appear there are vacancies anywhere else. I have explored that. I would have to see if I can go back and work effectively in the same environment, which is doubtful. I think everyone is trying to figure that one out."

In the days after, two agents speculated what they would do or not do if the same occurred with them. One was the agent who came to the scene. He boldly proclaimed, "I would have gotten out of my car and shot back at them!"

I found myself shaking my head in wonder. With seventy people on a drug corner, his rant was nothing less than reckless. The other agent didn't even want to think about the possibility of such a situation as I had found myself in. He expressed anger that the circumstance I experienced jeopardized *his* safety. His thought was I brought it upon myself. I was too aggressive with my high control caseload. He didn't understand I was committed to doing my job.

Despite being office mates and working as partners, they stood as opposites on two extreme ends of accepting risk, one who seldom ventured outside the office due to fear, and the other who was extremely aggressive and unstable. Yin and Yang. Both managed a caseload of younger, untested parolees than mine. Mine had proven what they were capable of doing. I knew what to expect from them with their level of violence. I made sure to be prepared for violence from them and for anything that could happen. I was working with the most violent in our office.

That morning, after those statements occurred, I placed my files on the boss' desk and said, "I need to leave." My heart was not into it anymore. The support wasn't available in the office. Too much uncertainty existed on behalf of myself and others that fed into being able to move past it. A part of myself was gone, the passion for doing the job. Both Bob Roenicke and Ron Chun encouraged me to remain and offered various forms of accommodation and support, not involving fieldwork.

Our bodies have a natural way of dealing with stress, crisis, trauma, illness, loss, and other often life-changing events. Many intricate internal workings are involved in our responses to them. We all react differently to situations. Much of that reaction depends upon our level of resilience. I had to listen to my body and what my heart was telling me.

It takes time to heal and recover from traumatic situations and from crises, whatever they may be. The interaction between my genetic makeup and my past will decide how much I will need to adapt and how well I would be able to continue to survive in the future.

Chapter Twenty-One

TAKING A BREAK

*Reflect upon your present blessings, of which every man has many,
not on your past misfortunes, of which all men have some.*
— Charles Dickens

No longer working a high-stress, dangerous job, I took life easier without the distractions. Dad and his wife had separated. He was stressed and came to visit more often. We spoke on the phone several times weekly. That first summer he lived alone, we camped with him and his children at the same place we camped with Mom and Dad when younger.

"Someday" had arrived for him. His physicians had diagnosed him with cancer of the renal pelvis, a small round cap atop the ureter, funneling urine into the bladder. Dad underwent resection of his kidney for the same cancer that took the life of his father's brother—facing the possibility of death encouraged Dad to resolve the regrets in his life.

Though there is no evidence that stress can cause cancer, a link to it does exist. Dad still had a family to support while undergoing cancer treatments. Not living in his home, his response to being displaced and alone was to smoke more. Smoking causes cancer, especially in those who possess a high predisposition to contract it.

As Dad learned during the time of his separation in the twenty years leading up to it, chronic stress can accelerate the growth of cancer. When the body becomes exposed, transmitters release and stimulate cancer cells. It makes the disease spread faster.

While Dad dealt with that, we were in the process of selling our Napa home and settling in Vacaville, California, a small agricultural town, east of San Francisco. A better place to raise children, we wanted them to attend school with everyday kids who were doing everyday things while living a less pretentious lifestyle. My hope was for my kids to grow up with an appreciation for life and to recognize the value and beauty of others, not for designer clothing and flashy cars.

Quickly adapting to the move, I headed east toward Sacramento, to seek some type of work that would boost my value and contribute to helping others. Driving in that direction was more comfortable than toward where I previously worked. Volunteering with crime victims' rights organizations, authoring articles for local publications, and working on some political campaigns, including participation in "Three Strikes" legislation, advocating for longer sentences for repeat violent offenders, kept me busy.

My involvement in the review of legislative issues with the California Correctional Peace Officers Association was rewarding. As one of the five members of the legislative committee of the largest law enforcement agency in the United States, I remained busy and felt value in our efforts to ensure public safety legislation.

Continuing to sit upon the State Board of Directors of the California State Parole Agents Association, representing the Bay Area and Silicon Valley parole agents, I testified in legislative hearings on criminal sentencing. Working with another parole agent, we authored a paper on parole for the United States Department of Justice.

Finally, becoming more involved in the community, I hopped into some local political campaigns, which lead to working a gubernatorial race and a few presidential campaigns. Friends and I founded two nonprofit organizations, one for women's rights and one for crime victims' rights. Soon, I was as active as I was before the shooting. Finally, with the help of my vocational rehabilitation counselor, I applied for and received a license to conduct investigations in California.

Working in some way was my lifeline. I needed the distraction. My counselor and I found ways to keep doing what I had done, on a limited, controlled basis, and doing so on my terms in situations that did not trigger the many symptoms of PTSD.

Being in crowds or congested areas drove me crazy. My stomach still churns every time I shop at a Walmart. Aisles are narrow. Items are stacked high, and the shelves are crowded. People violate personal boundaries and bump into one another in lines. My lungs feel heavy—blood pounds through my head. If I avoid overcrowded situations, I am fine.

I haven't been to a movie in thirty-six years, nor do I go to concerts or other large venues. I went to a few professional hockey games, but the crowds set off anxiety. Driving in Europe drove me crazy, as did standing on London's busy street corners and using public transportation.

Accepting a case here and one there, within a period of a few years, I was investigating matters full-time. Besides working with the courts and receiving contracts to perform independent investigations, I worked with former federal law enforcement officers involved in counterterrorism investigations with the US Immigration and Customs Enforcement Division of the Department of Homeland Security.

Following the 9/11 attacks, I performed risk assessments of public venues and of American schools desirous of accepting international students. Verifying the schools' academic programs and assessing the risk of international students wishing to attend United States educational institutions, they kept me busy.

The time had come to make changes in my life and explore the question the psychologist had asked. After I retired, the realization hit both my husband and me that we had little in common but our work. In 1993, with my eleven-year-old son, I left our home with a $10,000 T-Bill, a few rooms of furniture, my vehicle, and a lot of positive thoughts. I walked away from everything from the past, the investments, the savings, and our home. My son and I moved into a small apartment in Sacramento, set next to a human-made lake filled with ducks.

I desperately wanted out, out of the relationship, out of the house, and out of everything from the past. Leaving almost everything I owned behind for my husband and taking enough furniture to fill a two-bedroom apartment, a small t-bill, and leaving our home, the rest of our fourteen years of investments and savings behind, I accepted total financial responsibility for our child. I exited my marriage in the same way I did during the three-month debacle with the first husband, with little. All I desired was peace, comfort, and support, away from conflict and discomfort.

I loved the feeling of freedom and solace that little place offered, with the natural morning alarm clock of the ducks swimming beneath my deck and loudly squawking for bread. That one year, alone, was when I was able to focus upon and resolve issues.

Shortly after moving, I received a call from our younger brother, David. He informed us that Mom had died on the mainland of Spain, neither he or anyone else knew for sure how or when it occurred. David advised he heard she had fallen ill following an allergic reaction from snacking on some appetizers at Christmas. For months after, she did not get better. He later said she eventually died from responses to the medications the physicians prescribed.

Bill, our other brother, relayed that Mom had died after undergoing treatment for breast cancer. He stated she expressed worry that Donna and I might contract it, someday. That sounded more reasonable. At the least, it was comforting that she was concerned about us if it was what occurred. And, in all fairness, we could not discount the possibility she could have overdosed on her prescribed amphetamines and Dilaudid.

Donna reiterated statements from embassy officials that revealed an emergency airlift transported Mom to Barcelona from the Mediterranean island where she lived. She, too, had no idea where, when, or how Mom eventually died.

Over the years, we have been able to find little documentation on the date of her death or its cause. Hospital records from the small island where she lived reflected one medical visit years earlier. She had to receive care elsewhere or didn't make it to the hospital.

Burial records of the isle were nonexistent. Graves were reused. No death certificate was ever received upon request from Spanish authorities.

Police officials were only able to very that she had died. Hopefully, Mom finally found peace.

Decades later, we found Chuck had returned to the United States and first changed his name to "Chris," and later, to "Austin Heelee," moving around the country and eventually settling in Washington State with their youngest adopted daughter, whom he had married.

Relinquishing what little hope we had held that we would see her again, we finally accepted the fact she would never return. The endless search for a glimpse of her unexpectedly appearing at family events and the ever-constant anticipation it may be Mom at the door when the doorbell rang, ceased. Our mother was gone forever.

At forty- two years old, I was now the second oldest woman alive in our family. Our seventy-one-year-old aunt was dancing her nights away on a Hawaiian beach and living her life with gusto after surviving one bout of uterine cancer and two rounds of colorectal cancer. Everyone except for Grandpa and Dad were gone.

That summer, a letter arrived from Grandpa's wife telling us he, too, had died. He had outlived his two children and left this world peacefully at eighty-four years old. Grandpa's tired, and old heart could not take his vicarious lifestyle any longer.

For the next two years of my life, I began slowly but surely unpeeling the layers of sensitivity and vulnerability, trying to resolve that which could never be fixed. I had to learn to accept everything that happened and clear my head. It was over. There was nothing I could do anymore. My mother no longer existed.

Overwhelmed, I found everything was happening too fast. The only control I had, in my own life, was to invest time in making some meaningful changes, by focusing on recovering from the challenging few years of loss of two of our uncles, our mother, and our grandfather, while attempting to navigate a route forward following the end of my career. It was difficult, especially since it's journey ended at the same place of fear where it all started, learning to face the same cancer and heart disease affecting me that had taken and was taking the lives of our loved ones.

Feeling trapped by everything happening around me, I realized I needed to do something about it as soon as possible. Once my feet had been planted firmly on the ground. Now, while confronting it all, I was precariously dangling in mid-air. Now planted on the ground, I felt off-balance. Those years spent "being strong" had caught up with me. I had lost my emotional footing. Again, I sought counseling to get through it.

With no one in our natural family left but my brother, his children, a sister, and her child, a dying father, my aunt, and my two children, I decided to take a year's break from all distractions and begin viewing life in a more deliberate manner. Loss encourages us to rethink our purpose and to reset priorities.

Considering moving to Costa Rica with my son, Chris, to pursue work opportunities in Central and South America, I felt a strong urge to live my life as vicariously as possible, if I could. The same thirstiness for living as I did when younger had again returned. The compulsion to pick up and leave was building while a clock was ticking loudly. I was unable to stop my compulsive need to keep moving. Then, as always happens, fate intervened. While readying ourselves for the big move, I accepted an assignment to interview a witness to a legal matter.

That day, I met Steve. He was a solid guy who reflected the values of his industrious Italian father. Immediately, I felt a familiar sense of comfort around him. Kind, responsible, and soft-spoken, it was clear he loved sports. Stepping into his home, I looked around.

The family room was filled with his sports trophies, and with plaques setting upon shelves, a large, elaborate stereo system set in his family room, resting across from a big-screen television that was flashing a football game. His home screamed bachelor. It was clear he loved sports.

Interviewing him at his kitchen table, I found his answers to my questions reflected a refreshing sense of honesty. Appearing kind and sensitive, when he spoke, his eyes revealed his sincerity.

When he asked if I would join him for dinner, I felt terrible about declining. Apologizing, I tried to be as gentle as possible when I explained it would be a conflict of interest. My heart winced as I handed him a subpoena, instructing him that he was to appear in court, or the attorney may ask for a warrant for his arrest.

Weeks later, the phone rang. I was elated to hear Steve's soft, easygoing voice on the other end. "Now that the case is over, do you *still* have a conflict of interest with having dinner with me?"

After agreeing to his condition that I would not have a subpoena with his name upon it, either on my person or in my handbag, that one evening of conversation evolved in getting to know one another better.

During that first dinner, I asked, "Why haven't you ever been married?"

"Every woman I have met has some kind of problem," he stated sadly.

I just stared at him for a moment, my eyes widened with fear, before banging my head on the table. Then, looking up at him, I said: "Well, there are some things that I need to tell you…"

Holding nothing back, I revealed every aspect of my life, describing every bit of the emotional baggage I had hauled around with me. I didn't want to take a chance upon getting involved in a relationship that may end later. I was at a point in my life where I was willing to accept "forever," no matter how it was to be. So, guided by a blind trust, I put it all out there for him to chew on.

Unlike most guys, he didn't care. It prompted me to wonder why I let it bother me. At that moment, I fell in love with him, for that, and because he was easygoing, fun, and possessed a joyous laugh. My relationships in the past had been like hit and runs, intense and severe, with me driving guys off with my honesty and settling for those who were not worth caring if they left or not. Those relationships were far less painful when they ended. I knew what to expect, a quick encounter, and a "goodbye."

We married five weeks after Dad died. Most everyone I cared about was there. It was a wonderful time, a large Italian wedding in a public hall, with a gazebo in the corner where a Catholic bishop performed the service.

The only thing missing was my father. I missed him terribly. Dad couldn't hold out long enough to attend. At least, when he died, he knew he no longer had to worry about me.

This year, Steve and I are celebrating our twenty-third wedding anniversary, and there is no end in sight. Finally, blessed with a strong foundation of stability, we have been married longer than anyone in the last several generations of my family.

Chapter Twenty-Two

THE INEVITABLE

We spend precious hours fearing the inevitable. It would be wise to use that time adoring our families, cherishing our friends, and living our lives. — Maya Angelou

I t was in 2001, when Jim and his daughter, Jill, joined us in Lake Tahoe to spend the Fourth of July holiday, that cancer again began to rear its ugly head. Having turned fifty, two months before, Jim was far too young and fit to appear as tired and rundown as he seemed. But something was wrong. My suspicion was confirmed when he awakened us in the middle of the night.

"Lindy, I'm bleeding," he whispered, his eyes filled with terror.

Jim's voice was heavy, holding back his constrained fear as he revealed a significant amount of blood was spilling from his rectum. I had no doubt he had contracted cancer. He was at the right age as all the rest, in his early fifties. His symptoms of colorectal cancer were loudly screaming an alarm.

Since the death of our father over a decade earlier, I had researched every article on hereditary cancer I could find. Day after day, I was on the internet seeking the root of the genetic disease that plagued our family. Then, late one night, my fingers tapped out a search, "hereditary cancer, colon, uterine, kidney, skin, bladder."

My eyes widened as pages upon thousands of pages of research papers referencing hereditary cancer flashed on my computer screen. Stumbling upon over eighty-five thousand citations of research papers involving hereditary colorectal cancer (CRC) and other cancers, I noted research had been occurring for years. Some of the studies were the same as those with the long name that I had discounted years earlier. Immediately, I realized those studies was what Dad's physician had found when my father cautioned me to tell everyone to "get checked."

Many were accolades announcing a genetic test had been developed in 1993 to detect hereditary cancer, four years before the death of my father. To qualify to take that genetic test, one had to have three individuals in a family, one of which was directly related to the other two, to have been affected by colorectal or endometrial cancer. Because we didn't meet that criterion, I discounted it.

Dad had died from what he called kidney cancer, also known as renal pelvis cancer and cancer of the ureter, at the time. The renal pelvis is a bowl-shaped cap sitting atop the ureter that filters urine from the kidney into the bladder. The cancer had metastasized into Dad's kidney, bladder, stomach, esophagus, and, finally, to his bones.

In layman language, he was affected by a "kidney cancer" or "bladder cancer" because the standard treatment that Dad underwent was a resection of one kidney and the cancerous parts of the urothelial system. The esoteric medical terms used by experts in diagnosing hereditary cancer threw us off when seeking the root of our family cancers.

A myriad of cancers, stomach cancer, skin cancer, uterine cancer, breast cancer, kidney cancer, esophageal cancer, bladder cancer, and ureter cancers existed in our family. Still, until our generation, only one incidence of colon cancer and one of endometrial cancer occurred. Not recognized as part of Lynch syndrome, physicians and genetic counselors discounted most of the cancers found within our family.

With Jim and Aunt Marcella now having contracted colorectal cancer, we realized we would have to wait until a third person from our generation would become a sacrificial lamb and contract one of the more common Lynch syndrome cancers. In the interim, we worked hard to keep cancer at bay and work with diet, exercise, and to reduce stress as much as possible to remain cancer-free.

In 2001, Jim became diagnosed with colorectal cancer. Fortunately, Jim's physician detected it at an early stage. My mission was to search for its cause. At night, and into the early morning hours, I worked at it, looking for something, anything that matched the cancers in our family. Every night, I curled up with a medical dictionary to consult, as my eyes scanned every significant research paper on hereditary cancer, that I could find.

In late 1998, a year after Dad died, the criteria for Lynch syndrome had again changed. It required a family history of colorectal cancer or a cancer of the endometrium. However, the study wasn't well-publicized. The articles that addressed the changes were published in medical journals, which was only made available at a high and often prohibitive cost for physicians and the public, alike, to review. Therefore, physicians only subscribed to those publications that directly affected their specialties. Gateway physicians exercised a tendency to ignore the hype about hereditary cancer and continued to focus on the usual and most common ailments and injuries of the public.

We didn't find those 1998 changed guidelines until around 2001, after my father had died and my brother contracted cancer. Within them was mention of other cancers of hereditary nonpolyposis colorectal cancer, including the small intestine, skin cancer, and cancer of the ureter and the renal pelvis.

Patients are not medical professionals trained in the correct medical terminology for the intricate parts of human anatomy. We do not speak in an esoteric medical language when discussing parts of the body. We speak in common everyday language. Thankfully, today, the standards of care address bladder and kidney cancers without the use of esoterical terms making Lynch syndrome more easily identifiable.

Through the years, I continued researching. My medical dictionary was tattered and full of notes, its page corners becoming dog-eared. If researchers had published research studies in a layman's language, and if research papers involving publicly funded studies had been made available to the public, the opportunity to review more studies may have occurred. We might have found our cancer syndrome sooner before loved ones died.

But, the silos in existence, at that time, disallowed for that. Little information was provided to those who were outside the medical field. Overworked physicians didn't have time to read the large numbers of studies relaying advancements in cancer diagnoses. And poor communication skills in releasing the findings of the research communities didn't make it out to practicing physicians.

Merely publishing a paper and distributing a single press release about a medical condition isn't adequate to inform physicians of new syndromes, due to the immense number of trade journals in existence to which they subscribe. Had the information been issued on a more frequent basis to gateway physicians, cancers could have been deterred with cancer screenings, and the thousands who died may have lived.

I didn't read those studies hidden by publishers, which were only available to those with subscriptions. I couldn't afford the hundreds of dollars to subscribe to each, or the $35 to read the article. Then, research institutions were profiting from the results of publicly funded research. Mostly, the profit came from those of us with Lynch syndrome and other hereditary or rare diseases who were desperately scouring the internet for information that would lead to us being able to protect ourselves and our loved ones.

Eventually, the situation improved a bit. Publishers allowed patients free access to their publications, with "conditions." Often, so much was required in procedures to gain access, it deterred efforts, rather than providing what was needed. Today, taxpayer-funded research papers are still published for profit, disallowing patient access, and the ability for us to protect ourselves, despite recent legislation, gaining access remains difficult.

Jim left early that next morning to undergo a colonoscopy that his physician immediately scheduled. The gastroenterologist detected an anomaly upon the lower left side of his rectum. Once removed, they shipped it out for a biopsy. Upon its return, Jim found he had contracted an early-stage colorectal cancer. His surgeon recommended that he have a colectomy (the resection of the colon) based upon our family history of cancer. Unfortunately, the physician did not refer Jim for genetic testing.

Jim refused the surgery. A single parent, he had a mortgage to pay and five kids to support. Jim was frightened. By changing his lifestyle and exercising incredible willpower, he focused on eating a healthy diet filled with fresh vegetables and healthy teas. He cut sweets and processed foods from his diet.

Getting more exercise, reducing stressors, not drinking alcohol, and keeping a cheerful outlook, he did well. Fortunately, his cancer did not metastasize. They caught it at an early stage. After the removal of the tumor, the margins were clean. Jim was lucky. In the nineteen years since, he has not contracted a second cancer.

Steve and I worried. We discussed the cancer history of my family with our physician. We shared with him the cancers that struck my father, my aunt, my grandfather, our grandfather's siblings, and now my brother. All the cancers affecting our family were those that appeared below the belt, gastric cancer, bladder cancer, renal pelvis cancer, colon cancer, and endometrial cancer, as well as skin cancer, and esophageal cancer.

We informed him of the family history of cancer that existed on my mother's side with my mother, her mother, and her mother, all contracting breast cancer and how it met the criteria for the testing of BRCA1 and BRCA2.

"Don't worry. I will monitor you," the internist promised after listening to my concerns. I wondered how he intended to do it. Every physician I had seen, said the same, "I will monitor you." None did. Not one knew of hereditary nonpolyposis colorectal cancer (HNPCC) or Lynch syndrome. None bothered to search for it.

There were no laboratory tests, colonoscopies, or other radiological treatments, MRIs, or screenings ordered for us. They gave us nothing except empty words intended to provide comfort. It was clear everyone in our family was contracting cancer between the ages of fifty to fifty-six years old. That was a fact. Many had died, and what we found was there was nothing anyone could or would do to protect us.

I visited my gynecologist. Refusing to take hormone replacement therapies, fearing they may cause cancer, he, too, promised to watch me. Again, neither he nor I knew how he intended to do it. He scheduled no tests, nor did he refer me for genetic testing. He was one of the many who didn't know of it. He did nothing to find out. My gynecologist was the chief of his division. Despite Lynch syndrome as the cause of some women's cancers, he did nothing to protect me from contracting cancer.

Desperate to find the reason, I located a study that might help us. My aunt, brother, sister, and I took part in a clinical study through Case Western University who was researching the prevalence of hereditary colorectal cancers within siblings. I asked my gynecologist to prescribe a blood draw and send it to them. He did, which should have turned on a light in his head, encouraging him to investigate sibling hereditary cancers.

In 2002, I underwent a colonoscopy after light rectal bleeding. The gastroenterologist assessed my family history, and after not finding cancer, he diagnosed me with a familial cancer syndrome, prescribing colonoscopy screenings every five years, instead of every two to three years as prescribed as the standard of care for us with Lynch syndrome. He joined the others in not referring me for genetic counseling, despite now meeting the Amsterdam II, and the Bethesda criterion for HNPCC/Lynch syndrome.

All three physicians I saw were specialists. One was chief of gynecology, the second, a gastroenterologist, and the third, an internist. We provided each one of them with a regular family history of cancer. For over twenty years, it had been documented and updated in my medical records for more than two decades. Not one of those physicians referred me for genetic testing, despite the test for Lynch syndrome becoming available in 1993, fourteen years earlier.

By then, the standards of care had changed. To qualify for a referral for a genetic test, one had to meet the criteria set by the Amsterdam criteria, set up by physicians and researchers, with knowledge of Lynch syndrome.

Also known as the three-two-one rule, it required a minimum of three relatives with a Lynch syndrome cancer (cancer of the colon, the uterus, the ovaries, the small bowel, or the renal pelvis.) One of the three persons must be a first-degree relative to the other two, with at least two successive generations affected, and at least one family member had to be diagnosed with cancer before the age of fifty. It also required they exclude familial adenomatous polyposis (FAP), another hereditary cancer syndrome, and a pathological examination is conducted to verify if the resected tumors possessed microsatellite (MSI-h) activity. The presence of microsatellite instability suggests the mismatch repair process of correcting errors in cell reproduction is working incorrectly.

Later, this criterion again significantly changed immediately following the launch of the 2019 New Year. These revisions developed by the National Comprehensive Cancer Network "standards of care" team have resolved many of the problems with the Amsterdam criteria.

The difficulty with using family history to qualify for genetic counseling was that they were applying the most stringent requirements that proved inadequate to be a national standard. The rigorous qualifying criterium presented itself as a barrier for families to become genetically tested and diagnosed with hereditary cancers. The researchers and experts who developed that criteria are brilliant, oncological, and genetics scientists, but they were not social scientists nor historians.

Recent studies show a generational interval of today to be thirty-four years for a man and twenty-nine years for a woman. A three-person survey could span one hundred and two years. For those born in 2019, the three-generations would date back to around 1917, during the heyday of the eugenics movement. It didn't end until the mid-1960s.

From the 1800s until then, many physicians rarely documented cancer as a primary cause of death in "cancer families." Instead, they wrote other associated health issues such as heart attacks, nephritis, and tuberculosis on death certificates, as a primary cause of death. Physicians listed the more socially acceptable causes of death to protect surviving members of the family from mandatory sterilization.

Today, most single-family histories of hereditary cancer of persons with an American ancestry that dated back to 1850, may have had at least one person threatened with eugenic actions, or had a family member who faced mandatory or coerced sterilization as an "undesirable person." Without the existence of medical records, the diagnoses of family members became lost to history and replaced with family lore.

A long-standing tradition was not to discuss cancer outside the family. To protect loved ones, people preferred to die rather than seek treatment. Causes of deaths often listed anything but cancer, diabetes, and other diseases listed by eugenicists as causing a deterioration "in the quality of breeding" of people.

Further complicating and diluting the three-generational histories were the mass numbers of deaths of men and women during the Depression, when health care was unavailable and unaffordable; and with young men who fought and died during our wars. World War I, Korea, and Vietnam. All these events imposed a negative influence upon being able to obtain a definitive three-generation history of hereditary cancer today.

Many Americans died young before they reached the age in their families when hereditary cancers were ordinarily contracted, as what occurred with the tens of thousands of immigrants who could not survive the rugged pioneer lifestyle. Without physicians in the rural towns and villages, there were no medical diagnoses or documentation of death as required by geneticists today.

The experts did not consider the life-threatening epidemics that created mass deaths and left orphaned children behind who knew little about their parents, or their family histories. Families such as those in my mother's family, who still live in Appalachia, do not have any historical documentation of causes of death. Neither do those adopted immigrants in our families or those with a Native American history. In black communities, there was little health care provided, and physicians were few and far between. Minority and rural families were not considered in the guidelines.

Some policies involving requirements for genetic testing are not consistent with federal and state laws. One is the practice of requiring medical records of other family members being submitted to genetic counselors to prove they contracted cancer. This requirement is a barrier to genetic testing as many families cannot supply the medical records of others, especially those who died.

Most medical professionals and institutions archive records for only ten years, and the federal regulations of HIPPA require that only the executor of an estate can release medical records of the deceased. Some physicians have been able to get them, but by law, they are not allowed to be accessed unless in compliance with HIPPA.

Many were denied genetic testing because of the above. Today, barriers involved in obtaining traditional genetic testing from healthcare providers, insurance companies, genetic counselors, and medical providers, based upon the standards of care guidelines, are many. These conventional processes of germ-line testing are burdensome and costly for the patient and insurance companies.

In our family, the eugenics movement, which existed from the 1880s to the early 1960s, was a frighteningly negative influence in the lives of our parents and grandparents. Those practices resulted in the mandatory sterilization of over sixty thousand people in the United States, and tens of thousands more were sterilized upon the recommendation of their physician.

One-third, over twenty thousand of those sixty-thousand sterilized, were from California, as was our family. This occurrence created a tendency for families to choose not to discuss the existence of hereditary cancer. A culture of family silence developed due to them. As a result, many deaths from cancer were documented as heart failure, tuberculosis, and other associated diseases of cancer.

Genetic counselors often ask why patients refuse to submit to genetic testing. In the past, when I attempted to explain what some of our families had been through, some did not understand their level of fear and the reasons why patients needed to develop a relationship of trust in their genetic counselors and medical professionals to maintain confidentiality. Several argued with me about my family's response to genetic testing and refused to listen. One supervisor of my network's genetic counseling program hung up on me. It was then that I realized another serious barrier existed. Raised in a foreign country, she didn't understand the past of our history as experienced by the Americans who lived it.

Several years ago, genetic counselors developed the Lynch Syndrome Screening Network (LSSN). Its purpose was to collect medical records on those diagnosed with LS, to provide for the genetic counselors' research purposes. Some genetic counselors typed on the pages of their website that they were currently copying all the medical records of those in their institutions who had received a diagnosis with Lynch syndrome. Some were doing so without the knowledge or permission of patients, stating it was permissible by HIPPA.

LSSN had been advocating for these records to be placed in a public governmental database hosted by the Michigan Department of Public Health. Their online conversations were held on an open website hosted by that regulatory agency. Disturbingly, every major cancer institution in the United States supported this effort, except for mine.

When questioned, they claimed they did not need the permission of patients to harvest the confidential medical records of others that would be publicly available to other genetic counselors and health professionals. They were using it for "research purposes."

These actions are precisely the reasons some patients are concerned about the confidentiality of genetic testing, primarily when non-medical professionals like genetic counselors are gleaning entire medical histories of patients without their permission and retaining them in public databases, "for research purposes," and "to better their educations."

I held several discussions with members of the LSSN, and when that wasn't effective, with the management at HIPPA. I also spoke with several research professionals at major cancer institutions.

The decision by the federal government was that they could not legally collect confidential patient records. Further, their intent to educate themselves did not present a valid reason to access and distribute patient records without patient permission. It is my understanding medical records are no longer being collected by them. None had been kept in that specific database, though there was no formal confirmation. I do not know what happened to the records of those counselors who wrote they had copied the medical records of others, though I was unable to confirm it with the State of Michigan. They have not returned telephone calls.

After receiving that information, it was written upon their website, that a patient advocacy group at San Francisco State University Medical Center, Kinfolk, which is managed by genetic counselors and a gastroenterologist, was considering the same.

California has some of the most stringent confidentiality laws in the nation regarding genetic privacy. Over the years, we have spoken with legislators and health care administrators across the United States, but specifically, we worked with those in California, where our advocacy organization was registered. It was there that we received baptism into legislating genetic privacy. The rule is to get permission from the individual. Pure and simple.

Other states have or are intending to introduce state legislation for the privacy of genetic information. There are robust laws on patient confidentiality of medical records, both state and federal. These need to be realized and adhered to during this heyday of rapid genetic technology. It appears those in the genetics communities are not up to date with the laws. This deficiency in providing patient assistance presents a substantial void in the two-year advanced degree in genetics.

Today in their desire to bank patient medical histories in databases are genetic counselors and employees of commercial pharmaceutical companies who are sitting upon the seats of the Board of Directors of patient advocacy organizations. There they are properly recruiting volunteers with Lynch syndrome for their research studies. The genetic backgrounds patients provide are like gold for commercial and medical research companies and benefit everyone.

It is essential to realize that when we provide our genetic information to anyone, that we must make sure we receive assurances of exactly who receives it, what identifying information is used, how and where it will be stored, what security will be utilized for its storage, who will have access to it, who it will ultimately be distributed to, what will occur to our information after it is used, why it is being used, and that you obtain written guarantees that it will not be provided to anyone else except for those persons specified in the patient consent document.

Make sure information about third parties and family members are redacted, so it will not contain the names and other personally identifying information about other persons in the family or be distributed to others. The release of such personal data, without permission or knowledge, or the public dissemination of their medical information can be devastating for family members, especially those who participate in conversations on behalf of those family members, or others, as we experienced in our own family. Be sure you receive copies of the detailed policies and your consent of patient information that is distributed to third parties *every time* you authorize the distribution of your medical information.

In the spring of 2004, I felt a time bomb getting ready to explode. I was extremely ill. Nobody knew what was wrong with me, except for me. I had no doubt it was cancer; I was certain I was next.

A war was raging through my body. Suffering from severe reflux, nausea boiled inside. Often, I was light-headed. My muscles were on fire. Everything I attempted seemed to be an effort. Eventually, my bowel habits changed, alternating between constipation and thin, loose stools. A gnawing feeling pressed upon the top right side of my abdomen, under my rib, along with a tenderness found on the bottom right-hand side. Meeting with my doctor, I discussed my symptoms and fears.

He claimed it was merely a flare-up of the fibromyalgia that he had diagnosed me with a few years earlier when the signs of colorectal cancer began appearing. Prescribing guaifenesin, a decongestant that clears up mucus and congestion, the internist again promised to watch over me, assuring it was not cancer. His focus was more on my psychological distress and my fear of getting cancer instead of performing diagnostic testing to detect or rule out disease.

Growing up during an era when people implicitly trusted their physicians, I believed in mine. Our medical providers are our lifelines, an extension of us. They hold the same position of trust, as did our parents, our priests, our pastors, our police officers, and our teachers.

When my care providers said, "Everything is fine," I believed them. And, when my doctors promised, "I will monitor you," I trusted them— that is until a telephone call came from a clinical researcher at Case Western University.

The day she called asking for information for a diet study she was conducting of those with family cancers, she requested if changes in information about my family history occurred. Nothing significant had changed since we joined their research sibling study several years earlier.

"Have you experienced cancer yet?" the researcher asked.

Yet? What does she mean "yet?"

"No," I said, "The colonoscopy I had in 2002 was clear."

"Well, what happened with the one since?" she asked.

"There has only been one," I answered, anxiously. "Every five years, the doctor said."

"What? You haven't had one since?" She sounded upset.

Oh, my gosh, I've only had one!

Anxiety built while I explained to her the gastroenterologist had prescribed colonoscopy screening every five years in 2002 following prior guidelines, which had since changed. He prescribed preventative methods for familial cancer syndrome, not for those with HNPCC (Lynch syndrome.) Adamant I was to undergo a colonoscopy every two to three years, she insisted I speak with my doctor.

Steve and I scheduled physicals. While waiting for our appointment dates, we obtained full-body CAT scans from a commercial testing center, concerned our doctor would again not order diagnostic tests for cancer.

Little did we realize CAT scans could not see inside of the colon to detect colorectal cancer. We were naïve in thinking they might help our physician, especially since he was reluctant to order testing to diagnose disease.

Steve's results turned out great. He had the best arteries the examiner had ever seen. It was no surprise considering his strong Italian background. Mine was not as good as the CT scan reflected an anomaly in my right lung. We took the results with us to our shared appointment. Upset we had obtained them, the internist said, "Why did you do this?"

"Because I do not want to get cancer," I said. "I need testing."

"I wish you hadn't done this. All it does is present bad things."

"That is what we should look for, right?" I asked. He ignored my comment.

"Could you please refer me for a colonoscopy?" I pleaded.

"You don't need one," he insisted. "It takes ten years for cancer to develop."

My mind kept reflecting on my conversation with the expert from Case Western. "Hereditary cancers can develop in one to three years."

"I need a colonoscopy. Our cancers may be aggressive. The clinical researcher said every three to five years."

He claimed she was wrong. Researchers only wanted money. He was adamant I wasn't in any jeopardy.

"I will monitor you," he reluctantly grumbled after I advised him of it.

"With what?" I angrily muttered to Steve as we briskly walked toward the Jeep, and after hopping inside, slammed the door shut.

"I don't know, Lindy," Steve said. "It probably wasn't wise to ask him if he intended to use X-ray vision and Kryptonian superpowers."

I left his office with two referrals that day. One was for a chest x-ray to see if the anomaly still existed, and the second was a referral for anger management counseling.

As the months elapsed, and the seasons changed, I didn't get better. More symptoms of cancer developed. I had little stamina. Walking more than a block was exhausting. Pain radiated down my back and my right shoulder. I couldn't sit at the computer for prolonged periods. Unable to work much, I gained weight.

Summer came and went. I spent it at home, sleeping. Keeping up with full-time work and investigating major cases had become impossible. I cut down on my work and turned down assignments. Losing energy, I found short distances to be challenging to walk. My muscles were still burning; I felt my body was engaged in battle with something unknown. Bowel functions were irregular, and I was weak. My strength was no longer readily available. My body had ballooned from a size eight to a size eighteen. My cat was distressed. She would not leave me alone. Meowing loudly, she frantically pressed her paws up and down on the right side of my abdomen, where the gnawing pain radiated.

Overcome by a need to prepare for the future, I didn't know for what. Suddenly, I found myself flooded with a sense of urgency that I could not shake. It continued for over two years. I had to get things done, "just in case..."

Compulsive, I began preparing for Christmas during July and organizing everything in our home. I tagged sentimental items with the names of my children and grandchildren to pass down to them. I insisted on teaching the kids the family recipes and telling them stories of our ancestral grandparents. I was working hard on finishing our family history to leave to family members while cleaning up loose ends as Dad had done when he lived by himself while battling cancer. Like him, I was seeking redemption and preparing to die.

Steve and I searched for property to build a retirement home, far from everything and everybody. We hoped it would resolve my health. I craved comfort and held an ardent desire for a peaceful place to live. We found it in the remote foothills of Northeastern California.

Spending a day trekking through the tall grasses and wading in the water of a river that ran through the eighty acres, surrounded on three sides with U.S. Forests and BLM lands, we were considering purchasing it; finally, we rested upon its banks. There, we sat for what seemed like hours, not saying a word. Fish jumped, creating beautiful rings in the water, while the flapping of the wings of soaring eagles gliding overhead sounded in rhythm as the water trickled through rocks on its journey downstream.

Steve stood and brushed himself off. Helping me up, he asked, "So what do you think?"

"It's perfect," I answered.

"For our retirement home?"

"For our final home," I said.

"So, you think you could live here?"

"I could die here. I think we've found the place," I answered.

We were grasping at hope. A sanctuary and a quiet end to whatever was ahead. Never mind the fact I had now grown to a size 2W, and I desperately ate everything in sight to relieve the reflux and to alleviate the pain in my abdomen. Never mind that my hair was thin and stringy, my eyes reddened, and my pallor was pale. I could barely walk, while my physician thought my fear of hereditary cancer resulted from some form of hysteria.

Though I did not have the strength to work a ranch or develop eighty acres of land, I was reaching for anything that could provide me with as much denial of having cancer as I could muster. Reluctant to admit that I was extremely sick, I subconsciously readied myself to die. I resigned myself to the fact I was no different from anyone else in my family.

Without physicians taking me seriously, for a while, I bought into their dialogue that something else had to be wrong with me. That it was not all that serious as I thought it to be, but it was more psychologically-based due to my fear of cancer following the death of our father.

Consulting a new physician three months later, she didn't do any of that. She took a family history and at once made a referral for me to obtain a colonoscopy. "You should receive a telephone call with an appointment date in a week or two," she reassured.

The months came and went without hearing from the schedulers, and I consistently called, asking when it would occur. They instructed me that it would be a while before I could get in. They had a lengthy waiting list.

In the meantime, my father's sister, Marcella, had telephoned during the late summer of 2006. She reported contracting another colorectal cancer. It had metastasized and "spilled into her gut." Participating in chemotherapy treatment, she was taking "Xeloda" (capecitabine). Though tolerating treatment, she was still worried, feeling it may be best for us to come and celebrate her eightieth birthday party earlier than later, just in case she didn't make it, this time.

At seventy-nine years old, Aunt Marcella was the poster girl of strength. She had faced cancer three times before and was hopeful she would not have to do it again. Not wanting to die the same devastatingly painful death as her father, her aunts, and uncles, her grandparents, and my father, Dad's only sibling, Marcella, lived her life with urgency. She hiked and danced several times a week. Our aunt kept moving and embracing as much of life as possible. She said the moment she stopped was when she would be "ready to go." I wanted to be like her.

We were frightened for our aunt as she spoke with a sense of finality. None of us knew what we were facing. Without knowing what was causing the cancers responsible for killing our family members, we had no way to protect ourselves. All we could do was wait.

Finally, I decided to act. I called the gastroenterology clinic every single morning, insisting on being able to get a canceled appointment. The clerks laughed, thinking it was funny. I was the "crazy lady" calling all the time and begging for a colonoscopy.

The clerks told me: "You need a referral from a physician." I told them I had one.

"Colonoscopies are for people over the age of sixty," they then said.

"But I have a lot of cancer in my family," I argued.

"No, you don't," they said. "And, you're too young to get colon cancer."

They, too, thought it was merely patient hysteria. Getting scheduled for a colonoscopy proved itself to be as tricky as later trying to get genetic testing. The level of frustration I felt fed into a sense of hopelessness, and eventually, depression.

Steve kept a firm grip on me after that occurred. Not having the strength to keep bucking an unrelenting system, I wanted to quit trying; to spend the rest of my days in my home, preparing to die. To do it the way my father had done during his last year of life. But, giving up wasn't in my nature. Caught in a Catch-22, I found myself trapped in a senseless situation where one resolution was confronted by another that worked against it.

Every morning, I made myself dial that number, no matter how difficult it seemed. Not getting anywhere, I began to make calls to others in the same health system begging for someone to help me. I could not let my kids down and leave them alone. No matter how old we are, there is a considerable comfort knowing Mom and Dad are around when things go wrong. Our children will always be our kids, and they will never stop needing their parents. I wasn't going to let them down or anyone else.

Finally, I attempted to find an appointment outside of the system, where I faced the same problem. I needed a referral from a doctor. That required seeing another general physician and paying the $350 out-of-pocket cost. It was worth it. I tried. The appointments in our area to see a physician without having insurance coverage to cover it was two to six months out.

Upon attempting to set up an appointment, they told me that without being sixty years old, when colonoscopies were offered to patients, I would need screening tests for cancer first. Without that testing to provide evidence of the need and the expense of a colonoscopy, obtaining an appointment would be difficult. Then, few physicians knew or understood hereditary diseases. Many still didn't believe it existed. Most felt I was buying into the research hype.

Therefore, I continued calling those in my health system. While reviewing studies, I found the name of a physician who was involved in Lynch syndrome clinical research. When I asked his clerk if he worked with those with hereditary cancers, she advised, "No, he just works with regular cancer," whatever that was. I told her I wished to speak with him, anyway.

The physician called back. He compassionately listened but did not schedule me for an appointment. Instead, acting as my savior, he used his ability to pass my information through to my facility. Then, someone patiently listened to me, and his actions fired up a series of events that saved my life.

"I have a family history of cancer," I revealed to Dr. Ralston Martin of Kaiser Permanente, Vallejo, California, during that telephone call, after finally being put through to him.

"Tell me about it," he quietly asked.

Finally, I had gotten through to a specialist, and he was compassionately asking the right questions. Quickly explaining my symptoms and telling him of our family history of the kidney, bladder and esophageal cancers that took my father's life; the colorectal cancers and endometrial cancer my aunt contracted; the stomach cancer that took their father's life, the malignancies of all of grandfather's brothers and sisters; and the colorectal cancer my brother had been diagnosed with a few years earlier; I confided I knew I was next. I feared it might be my birthright. I was the next in age, and it was when most contracted cancer. I was also extremely sick.

"You *do* need a colonoscopy," he said. "Someone *will* contact you with an appointment date."

The amount of relief that a ten-minute telephone call brought when ill was immense. Upon receiving an appointment notice in the mail with a confirmed date for a colonoscopy, an enormous weight lifted from my shoulders. I felt like dancing.

Scheduled following Thanksgiving, it was not soon enough but, fortunately, time flew. Before I knew it, in the third week of November 2007, I awakened in the gastroenterology clinic, on a gurney, feeling groggy. Someone had covered me with warmed sheets. The stress I once felt had dissipated, knowing the procedure was over, and someone was finally looking after me.

As I laid there, I watched as Dr. Martin stood at the end of the bed, his back facing me. He was intently focusing on the images upon the large screen in front of him. I strained to see what he was studying. My vision, still foggy from anesthesia, could not make out the details. I watched as he sank his head into his hand, and took a deep breath, before slamming his fist onto the stainless-steel counter in front of him.

This cannot be good.

I quietly asked, "Didn't turn out so good, huh?"

Startled, he spun around and managed a reassuring smile.

"You rest for a few minutes and let the anesthesia wear off. Okay? We'll talk then," Dr. Martin suggested.

I nodded. Rolling over and closing my eyes, I tried to calm myself down. I knew "someday" *had* come. It was no longer a figment of my imagination or a creation of my mind. Though I had expected a diagnosis of cancer, and I was trained to appear collected on the exterior, my mind was racing. I was able to slow it down, but I could not stop the silent screaming.

Oh, my God! My kids, my grandkids, my kitchen drawers are so messy!

In retrospect, when I realized I was facing a life-threatening condition, my first concern involved my intense need for approval. I was worried about what others would think when they rummaged through the contents of the drawers in my cabinets after my existence was no more.

The thought of anyone combing through the personal remnants of my life was devastating. No one could ever realize the sentiment contained in them. To the average person, it was junk. The stretched and faded fifteen-year-old Oakland Police Officers Association T-shirt; the seventeen-year-old parole agent hat; the now misshapen Notre Dame T-shirt won in a poker game twenty-three years earlier, and the little, silver cross, without a chain, that had been blessed by the "Brown Pope." The beautiful, porcupine-quilled barrette handmade by an old Choctaw woman was my most cherished possession.

Mixed with torn ticket stubs from events, were photos with friends, a lot of pens, and business cards with little notes written upon them. A lifetime of birthday cards and Christmas cards mingled with the dozens of "get well soon" cards. Short notes from my children, wrist bands from their birth, and the dozens of other little items were reminders of the most memorable moments of the special people in my life.

When setting out to remove complications in my life, I would open those drawers with an intent to discard everything. But I could never do it. Everything in them represented people who had once been or were a significant part of me.

Suddenly, I realized my thoughts were of one who was preparing to die. It was not what I wanted. I wanted to live. Then, predictably, it happened again. Slipping into the slow-motion foggy tunnel vision of

PTSD, I felt trapped within that protective, familiar tight scope that enveloped me. I could hear that reassuring little voice inside quietly reminding me to remain calm. My training instantly kicked in.

Look around you. Assess your surroundings.

My eyes searched through the room. Nothing threatening existed.

Slow down and think. Step-by-step.

My first thoughts were about Steve and my kids. My life still held value. I was not going to leave my family alone, not now, to experience the same that we faced as children. I wanted to grow old gracefully, travel with my grandchildren, and die peacefully in old age. Dying of cancer wasn't part of my life plan. As the anesthesia wore off, my mind continued to race. I had to alter the course of fate, somehow.

Images of the past flashed. My almost-two-year-old granddaughter, Sonny, racing around the house with excitement as she experienced her first memorable Christmas morning; my three-year-old grandson Scott only wanting wings for his birthday, so he could fly up to the roof and retrieve his beloved ball, and the numerous occasions we apprehended our toddling, youngest granddaughter, Jaycie, who had escaped into the front yard, and was joyously sloshing barefoot through mud puddles during the midst of a winter storm.

I thought of my two kids who were just beginning to learn the intricacies of surviving everyday life with a young family of their own while putting themselves through school and working.

"I am not done yet. I need to teach my kids how to protect themselves," resounded determinedly in my mind. With everything happening, I realized what I needed to do was to sing. Bursting into song had always gotten me through everything in the past. But I couldn't think of any songs for days like today, so I hummed. It didn't help. Nothing did, not while the devastation was building.

Slow down. We do not know how bad it is.

Working my way into a quasi-calm as they wheeled me into the recovery area, I was more alert. By the time I arrived, I could think clearly.

"I don't think things went so well," I whispered to Steve.

"Okay," he replied softly.

"If it is not good news, just nod your head at what he says. We'll talk about it on the way home. All right?" I asked.

Steve's eyes were enormous, expressing sheer fear. He had seen enough during the past few years to realize the situation was severe. He had stood beside me when my father had summoned his sister and his children to be with him one last time before climbing the stairs to his room to await death. And he was always there, with me, standing with my brother and my aunt when they both contracted colorectal cancers.

Steve felt the fear as much as we all did, if not more. I passionately believe those who love us face more difficulty adapting to our cancer than we do. Most of us possess instinctive, natural defenses that help guide us to survive. Not so for our loved ones, our friends, our co-workers, and those who care for us. What we share are fear and hope.

Fear is a natural survival tool. It keeps us alert and prepares us to protect ourselves. What is unnatural is when no one resolves the root of that fear, and the information to fix it exists somewhere but is only known by a privileged few. I had spent my entire life in denial of fear of hereditary cancer, just waiting for it to come, when the uncertainty would be justified. "Someday," was bittersweet, a combination of fear, devastation, and relief. Steve deserved time to adapt to what was sure to be.

"All right," he said. "But, are you okay?"

"I don't really know," I admitted. "But we're gonna find out in a few minutes."

As we waited, I reflected upon his family and how differently they live. They are first to third-generation Italian Americans. His Aunt Ange turned one-hundred and two years old this summer. Mowing her lawn and doing the gardening herself, she finally stopped at age ninety-five when her strength waned, and her eyesight failed. Her voice sounds young, and her thoughts are always positive. At ninety-seven years old, Steve's father's mind is clear, and his hair is still dark. The two of them and their two remaining brothers and sisters are all in their nineties, except for Ange.

"Why complain? What good is it going to do?" Aunt Ange says.

Steve's father consistently echoes the same. They focus on the everyday beauty of living, not the complaints, or the aches and the pain of arthritic hips and knees, and their failing eyesight, and stiff joints. Much like Vito Corleone, in the movie The Godfather, Steve's Dad's only desire is to sit on a chair, soaking in the sun for a few hours each day. His greatest joy is being amid everyday life, watching birds fly overhead, and the squirrels play on the fence line. All he desires from life is in his backyard and his monthly dinner at the local Italian Club.

Steve's grandparents, their children, and their grandchildren worked on the family farm that set on the banks of San Pablo Bay until it was sold as part of the estate of the elders, following their deaths. Eating pasta, the vegetables they grew, and the soups they made, in which they dipped focaccia bread, drank red wine and raised children who grew old while our family worked and waited for "someday," when they would face a devastating death.

Dr. Martin quietly slid through the worn, faded curtains, and stood at the side of my bed. An epitome of strength, he offered us a reassuring smile, aiming to appear rock solid. I knew it was difficult for him, having to tell me what I needed to know. Not only did I hear what he was saying, but my training allowed me to listen carefully to what he was not saying.

I believe that our cancers are more difficult for those who care for us than they are for us. An instinct blesses us with the ability to roll with what our body is telling us. We intuitively know what is occurring in our bodies. Neither our loved ones nor our physicians can feel the changes we feel in ourselves. All they can do is sit back and comfort us while we wait to see if treatments will work.

Wishing to be anywhere other than standing at my bedside, Dr. Martin's foot pointed toward the curtain. As he spoke, he rubbed his hands. My heart was breaking for him. Along with being my savior, he was charged with the misfortune of being our harbinger. Nobody wants to tell someone he or she has cancer. No doubt, it was a daunting task.

Detecting a slight break in his voice, he said, "We found three tumors, two in the lower right colon and one on the transverse colon. It may be a hereditary condition called hereditary nonpolyposis colorectal cancer, or HNPCC, also called Lynch syndrome. I scheduled an appointment for you the first thing on Monday with the surgeon. If you can, try to relax over the weekend. Let's see what he has to say then. Okay?"

My ears perked. A sense of positive anticipation stirred inside, despite the devastating news Dr. Martin had to present. He offered me a tremendous sense of relief and hope... for my children, siblings, and me, at a time when it was dearly needed. If true, he knew about our hereditary cancer syndrome that my father could not recall the name of thirty-six hours before he died, ten years earlier.

A name may mean a treatment.

Doctor Martin's sense of compassion touched my heart. It was more difficult for him to tell me I had cancer than it was for me to accept. I spent a lifetime preparing for this moment, hoping it would not be my fate, but if it were, I would be readied, at least psychologically, to battle it. I no longer had to wonder, wait, or deal with the uncertainty of "someday." It happened just the way it had for Mom, Dad, and all the others.

All I wished for was to go home and get to work on it. I so very much desired to be somewhere else, dealing with something else, with anyone else, as I always had. I desperately needed a distraction to avoid all of this, and there was none. Wanting to be normal again, I dearly wanted to be anyone but me. The last place I desired to be was there, though little did I know it was the best place for me because I am who I have always been, predisposed to cancer, and what I am now, a cancer patient. I needed to learn to adapt to it because that is how we survive.

Finally released, Steve and I stepped outside. Fresh, cool air swept across our faces. Looking toward the sky, I saw beauty evolving in the ominous, darkened clouds gathering overhead, their ragged edges protecting the silver lining that I held no doubt was hiding somewhere inside. The thoughts filling my mind were changing from that of pure devastation to that of empowerment. I was committing to a continuation of life if it could be possible. We had a lot to do in a short amount of time. A storm was coming.

Chapter Twenty-Three

DEALING WITH CRISIS

*Courage is being scared to death
and saddling up anyway.* — John Wayne

The kitchen of our home reflects the heartbeat of our family. Like others, this is where we spend most of our time. There is something about holding a cup of hot, steaming coffee in our hands, and feeling the warmth and the comfort it brings to a distressed soul while sitting at a table with those we love.

It is where we first sat to eat and learned to read from milk cartons and cereal boxes. Here is where we hung out with our young friends after school and where everyone in our family gathers to discuss our day. It was where honest and sensitive discussions happen. It is where we decide everything of importance. Here, we await births, plan weddings, and grieve over those we have lost. It is here where comfort always exists. In our kitchen. Where we know another pot of coffee is brewing and available when we need that extra bit of warmth.

Naturally, this is where we parked ourselves after arriving home. With the laptop, paper, and pens at the ready, and our heavy hearts dragging, we set about untangling the complicated processes of dealing with a cancer diagnosis within a family plagued by an unknown hereditary cancer syndrome. We had much to do in a brief period. Deciding where to start is always tough. Receiving a cancer diagnosis in real life is nothing like what they depict in the movies.

Hollywood's version of cancer diagnosis and treatment is a team of doctors and nurses racing into a room, zapping the patient's heart with electricity, and pushing a stretcher down a long hall. At the same time, family members run alongside, holding the patient's hand. Slamming through double doors into a sterile room where machines beep endlessly, physicians perform a quick surgery, and nurses wrap a rag around an instantly balding head. The patient is dead or cured in hours, and everyone lives happily ever after.

In the real world, following a diagnosis of cancer, we go back to our homes, and we grieve. Most of us experience incredible devastation, and we cry. Initially, we are in shock, not knowing how to react. As reality sets in, so does the will to survive. We begin to prepare for the journey ahead.

Many of us leap through hoops in our attempts to ready ourselves for surgeries. We put our homes, employment, and financial affairs in order. We focus on our families, making sure they are cared for and supported to ease the crisis that follows. Nothing pulls a family together or tears one apart than a life-threatening illness or the loss of a family member.

We ready ourselves for surgeries, make plans for treatment, and worry whether we can afford a prolonged period of recovery. Revising budgets repeatedly, we pray we can pay the bills, and that our employers will hold our jobs until we get better. In dealing with insurance agents, attorneys, priests, rabbis, imams, ministers, and with creditors and employers, our underlying concern is if we will survive.

During those long waits of listening to elevator music on the telephone, while attempting to make appointments or resolve issues, fleeting images, and thoughts flash through our minds of the concerns we had kept to ourselves, not wanting to upset those we love.

Silently, we hope we will endure, and we worry. Some of us wonder if our bodies will still function after surgery, as they had before. We hope we can get back to normal, not realizing there is no return to normal after recovering from major surgeries for cancer. Our bodies and our lives change. The future depends upon how well we adapt to a "new normal."

Most of us focus on the immediate, getting through the surgery. Seldom do we realize recovery is not always smooth. Regaining strength takes time and patience. Few are prepared to endure the length of time it takes to heal. Many are not able to accept the temporary and permanent changes that occur in us, for good or for bad. Nor are we prepared for those that may arise later down the road, and to those close to us.

Some research the "what ifs" that may or may not occur. Most discuss them. What if I become disabled and can't work again? How are my children going to get to college if I am ill? Can we afford the medical bills, the co-pays, and the deductibles? If I die, who will take care of my kids? What is the cost of burial? How will my family care for themselves? Do I have enough insurance? Will we have to sell our home? What if I can't continue working? And all the other uncertainties to living with a cancer diagnosis.

Those and hundreds of other questions emerge out of nowhere when one receives a cancer diagnosis. Few of us are ever really prepared for the answers we receive. All these thoughts and more are typical for those battling cancer. It is a rational response to a challenging circumstance.

When one has something medically wrong that is unknown, life becomes even more complicated. What if my kids get this? Can I afford the cancer screenings for my family? Where am I going to get the $4000 for the genetic test and the $500 for the genetic counselor and still be able to pay the co-pays for the doctor? How am I going to pay for genetic testing and annual cancer screenings for an entire family, especially when it is more than the equity I hold in my home?

If I see a genetic counselor, are they going to report my condition to an insurance company or put my medical records into a database that is open to others, without telling me? Will my insurance company list us at an elevated risk in their national database and jeopardize health care for my loved ones? Can we afford the cost to travel to get an appointment, the test, and the appointment with the genetic counselor?

Steve and I were fortunate. We had excellent insurance through an HMO that supplied exceptional care and didn't report to insurance companies. Our priority was to find the best physicians who would serve as members of our medical team. Every critical condition needs an experienced team. Establishing one should be the priority of any cancer patient. Fortunately, Kaiser Permanente allows patients to choose their own. There are thousands of great physicians on staff.

Spending years as an investigator, I am an expert at researching people and unraveling the issues involving difficult circumstances in their lives. Proficient at seeking out the best expert witnesses for court cases and other matters, I never thought I would be doing it for myself. I had always held a blind trust and confidence in my doctors. But after a late diagnosis of cancer, I realized it was a naïve luxury I could no longer afford.

Then, I felt a doctor was simply a doctor. I ignored the red flags in favor of the removal of inconvenience. The late diagnosis was devastating, and I was heartbroken over the betrayal of trust I felt due to the lack of care provided by three of my former physicians.

The first medical professional we homed in on was Dr. George Berndt, a surgeon specializing in colorectal surgery. Scheduled to see him on Monday, I needed to learn everything I could about the man to whom I would entrust with my life.

Not only did I want to learn about his abilities in performing colorectal surgeries, but I also wanted to know his character, and who and what he is as a person. Driven by an insatiable desire to learn as much as possible, I swore I was never going to make the same mistake I made in getting myself into something so profoundly serious, which should have been preventable.

"Steve, listen to this. He grew up in New Mexico, worked his way through med school, and is a military reserve officer in the army, a colonel.

And he is regularly deployed to Iraq, where his son is in the Special Forces," I added.

Emotion flooded as I considered the steadfast love and commitment between a father and a son and what parents will do for their children. It placed him at the top of my list.

"No kidding?" Steve said, bending over my shoulder.

"Yes. Cancer patients are not the only ones undergoing colectomies; our soldiers are too. It says the trajectory of IED injuries arise upward, damaging the gastric system. Of the two hundred surgical procedures he performed, he has lost less than five." I glanced up at Steve.

"Incredible," Steve uttered.

Reflecting upon the thousands of young people living with colectomies today, I wondered how I would have managed it at a younger age. Their resilience and courage inspired me. If they could do it, there was no reason I could not.

The reports flowing back from those familiar with Dr. Berndt revealed he was stable, focused, enthusiastic, and committed. We decided he was the perfect surgeon to oversee my independent nature.

Arriving early, we checked in and sat in an empty waiting room. A nurse at once ushered us into an examination room. Uncertainty struck as my feet dangled from the table. I was again that three-year-old girl I once was, waiting for the doctor to make her better. Just as she realized the doctor was going to make her feel better, I realized how much I needed this doctor's help to live.

Dr. Berndt's tall frame bent as he cleared through the doorway. Like my father, he was not a man of many words, but one of action. His eyes expressed what his face did not. As Dr. Martin, he had trouble keeping eye contact as he confirmed the diagnosis. It offered the reassurance of his compassion, dedication, and competence.

We spoke matter-of-factly. It was how I best communicated with others after spending decades working in nontraditional justice system occupations, with men. His mission was as an expert in the surgical removal of cancer, not in comforting the soul or in trying to untangle the labyrinth of emotional upheaval. Healing the soul was for later. Therefore, the discussion focused upon the first step, the medical aspects of the removal of aggressively growing cancers. I had done the research.

"We won't know how cancer will stage out until we explore and see what's occurring," Dr. Berndt said. "We need to receive the results of molecular testing. Until then, we won't be able to determine its extent," he explained.

"Are we going to do a hemi?" I asked, wondering how much of the colon needed removal.

His eyes narrowed. "No, that's a partial removal. We are going to do a subtotal colectomy. An almost-total removal, it leaves a little of the colon. Considering your family history of cancer, it is best. We'll also do molecular testing to see if it is hereditary," he said. "The risks…"

"Please. I don't want to hear the risks." I put my hand up to stop him. The thought frightened me. I was not ready for it. I had to prepare myself psychologically for living, not for anything else. Informed consent was irrelevant at my stage of illness.

"I'm well-grounded in the reality of my situation. I know the only chance I must survive is to do this. Either way, there are risks; and they are irrelevant."

"Yes, but bleeding—"

"But I'm not worried about that. You *are* a trauma surgeon."

"Yes, I am." He looked at me, his eyes squinting quizzically.

"And Dr. Berndt, it makes my odds much better. I spent years working in the justice system, and I have some experience with being in the military."

"Yes, but…"

"Please… I'm a strong woman who has lived a high-risk life. I can manage most anything. But, right now, I want to trust *you* to make the important decisions. You do what *you* think is best. You are the expert in this. What I am good at is being a good soldier and following instructions."

"That's how it is supposed to be," he said.

"So, do we have a deal?" I asked, my voice breaking.

"We do," he said. "How about we all enjoy Christmas and do this the first of the year? It won't make much of a difference."

"Sounds good," I agreed. "It will give me time to adapt."

I left his office feeling much better, knowing the beginning of the first step was covered and considerable relief that I didn't have to deal with the "what if's" of the surgery. We had an outstanding surgeon on our team.

Chapter Twenty-Four

PREPARING FOR THE HOLIDAYS

Our hearts grow tender with childhood memories and love of kindred, and we are better thought the year for having, in spirit, become a child again at Christmastime.
— Laura Ingalls Wilder

December was an excellent time to prepare for surgery. Ordinarily, I would be engaging in holiday revelry, but I did not have the energy. The shopping and planning for Christmas had occurred months before when I was cleaning up loose ends.

When diagnosed with cancer, not only are people sick, but they and their loved ones are adapting to a change in life circumstances. It requires developing new priorities, and sometimes new traditions for themselves and their loved ones.

The holidays can be tough, especially if entrenched in a crisis, as what occurs when diagnosed with cancer. With any diagnosis of severe disease, feeling overwhelmed is not unusual. Besides dealing with emotional upheaval, a whirlwind of preparation for the upcoming surgeries and treatments is not only needed to treat cancer, but we also need to prepare for a major holiday. If one is seeking a distraction from the uncertainty of an impending surgery, it is a perfect time. My thought was we should continue as many traditions as possible to keep consistency in our family. It was emotional and challenging.

The processes involved in preparation for the removal and treatment of cancer are complicated. Thrust into an entirely different culture; patients often feel they have little control. Learning the ins-and-outs of battling cancer is a challenging situation, emotionally and physically.

As an investigator, I had kept a busy lifestyle, working, traveling, spending time with my grandchildren, and often visiting with our elderly in-laws, in addition to working on the city streets, and always functioning in a survival mode.

Staying positive and active kept me alive. Now, I was gearing up into an entirely different type of survival mode, battling cancer. I held a cavalier attitude with my certainty I would beat it if it ever occurred. Initially, certain I would triumph over it and everything else that came with it, the cold reality was I was not ready for it.

I didn't have a plan of how I would or should continue. For the first time, ever, I feared not being in control. Readying myself for this journey, I realized it was the one matter in life that I had ignored and put it off until "someday," in the event, it ever did occur. Now, cancer was standing at my front door, and I was facing it, totally unprepared. Not only embroiled in an emotional wrestling match in dealing with its delayed diagnosis, but some complications travel with it. Writing my will was one.

I finally did it. Denial is not a luxury people like us can afford. It is of little or no benefit for us or our loved ones. Leaving behind emotional devastation in my children's lives, as what occurred at the end of Dad's, was not a choice. I swore the same would not happen with my children.

A will relays messages to those we loved during our lifetimes, a final word, solely for them. It includes affirmations of what the relationship with them meant to us. Its importance is not to distribute wealth or material items; it is the final resolution of a lifelong relationship.

After Dad's death, I wondered if he left messages for any of us. I dreamed about what he may have written. "To my daughter, Linda, who always kept me guessing, I leave my love…" or "To my loving daughter Lindy, who is long on generosity and short-fused, to you, I leave patience…"

A year before he died, Dad called. His voice broke as he said, "Lindy, I am at my attorney's office, writing my will." He wanted to know what he could do for my siblings and me.

"She's thinking about returning to school for her master's degree," Dad said of their oldest, adopted daughter. "Would you like to go back also?" It was a sweet gesture. At forty-four years of age, I had found success in my business. I didn't see the need to return to college and complete my degree, nor did I have the time to do so. I only needed a few required classes. At over forty years old, I had other priorities.

But I loved the way Dad still thought of me as he did when I was young, during the times he was unable to see or spend time with us. He used a good part of the estate left by our grandmother that was partially earmarked for our educations to build his large homes, help in setting himself up in business, and for the properties he bought. He intended to pay it back someday.

Jim had also given his inheritance from Grandma back to the estate, so Dad and Marcella would receive an equal distribution of it. Both Dad and

Marcella advised that what Jim had earlier given, would be returned from their estates. It never occurred. The executors of Dad's estate never reimbursed it back.

During that call, I explained to Dad that Jim, Donna, and I are accomplished in our own right. We had bought our homes, ourselves. The three of us had worked our way through college, paying for it ourselves. Mom had paid for some of Donna's education, and Donna had covered the rest with student loans and grants. Jim and I covered our costs. Over forty years old, none of the three of us intended to go further, but we all had children who were doing well in school and preparing to move upward.

Jim had done well. He earned a bachelor's degree in Business and obtained a Doctor of Jurisprudence in Law. Donna was a few units shy of a bachelor's degree, as was the situation with me. We both had successful investigative businesses.

Dad and I spoke of his children and how much more dependent they were upon Dad and their mother than our children, and we ever were. He had spent the past twenty years putting his wife and her daughter through college. Their youngest daughter had just finished attending an out of state junior college, and he was trying to encourage his youngest son to continue his education.

With a family accustomed to a much higher standard of living than the way we had lived, Dad was concerned about how they would be able to adapt to a future that required them to be independent.

"What can I do for you, then, if you don't want to get an advanced degree?" Dad asked in frustration. "I want to do something."

"Dad, I don't have time for it. I'm already at the top of a demanding career. Why don't you think about setting something up for the educations of the grandkids? It would be a great gift to leave behind." Christopher was fourteen, and Judi hoped to attend college the next year. Donna's daughter was nineteen, and Jim's kids were nearing college age.

Though, according to the executor, Dad did precisely as he said he would during a telephone call that spring, not one person in our family was ever officially notified by the executors of his estate as to of his wishes. Nor did any person receive any benefits, whatsoever from what Dad had promised he would do.

Shortly after his death, we received a telephone call from an insurance claims adjustor who oversaw Dad's small $15,000 life insurance policy through Nevada Bell Telephone. We had previously asked his wife if Dad had insurance policies. She said he had not. He invested in real estate. Before he died, Dad advised us that he had listed us as beneficiaries in those policies.

Splitting the face of his insurance policy between four beneficiaries, half to his wife, and the other half to be divided between my two siblings and me at $2,500 each, upset our stepmother.

"You were not supposed to get that," she spouted angrily when we told her of the call. "It was all supposed to go to me."

I offered it back. Less than half of what I made in an average month, I cared less about the money. I thought it was sweet that Dad loved us enough to think of us.

She declined. I offered to share it with their children. They also refused, saying their mother was giving them money from "her part" of Dad's estate.

To avoid what occurred with us, in my father's family, Steve and I gave each of our children a copy of our wills, assuring transparency. We realized the devastation of losing someone we love can affect those left behind far beyond the day of the burial. The last thing we wanted was to impose hurt upon our children in the manner it occurred with us.

Dad provided us with a keen sense of integrity and character. He taught us to live humbly. Like our father, my siblings and I are self-made, as are our children. The three of us possess the ability to care for ourselves. The purpose of Dad's bequeathing college assistance to the grandchildren was a gift of love, an assurance that during his life, he did he care about them and their futures.

Stating he was proud of us, he would have also been immensely proud of his grandchildren. Of his three adult children, seven adult grandchildren, and four great-grandchildren in *our* family, collectively, they have achieved one doctorate in jurisprudence, with another now working on her doctorate, two master's degrees, and six bachelor's degrees. Six attended vocational schools in addition to some college.

Our father left us far more than a legacy of hereditary cancer, indicated by the successes in the generations of our family. Despite the adverse circumstances, the disparity we experienced, and the difficult challenges we faced while growing up, he left us with more than many fathers leave their children, integrity, and character. The positive aspects of our father's DNA flow through us, accompanied by the traditions passed through the generations of our family.

Making my final arrangements and setting guidelines for my family to follow would make it easier for them to handle my complicated desires during a difficult and emotional time of loss. I hoped it would deter from any issues of "what Mom would have wanted." So often, conflicts occur after a family member dies. I dearly wanted to avoid that for my family.

Finally, I wrote a personal letter to each of the hundreds of extraordinary people I have cared for during my lifetime, to be forwarded in the event of my death. It relayed how much I loved and appreciated them, and always will.

Left to complete was the unfinished business of the nitty-gritty details involved in researching the side effects of a subtotal colectomy and a hysterectomy. I made sure to learn all I could about the complications that occur after those surgeries so I could prepare myself to face them.

Preparation is the key to survival. Preparing for every known possibility that could occur is the most loving thing we could do for our families and ourselves. Committing to live, I needed to know what I would be facing with treatment.

I found most cancer patients experience a permanent reduction in stamina, following surgery. With the realization it would be problematic to sit through interviews or testify in court with an unpredictable colon, I contacted my clients and revealed I would no longer be available to take cases. I closed all matters and wrapped up my business affairs.

Life is one big series of negotiations, and when negotiating, there is give and take. Fighting cancer is also a negotiation. The losses I faced were more than a fair trade-off in exchange for life. I'd be off work for a long time, forever. I was willing to take the risk, no matter the cost.

The week before my diagnosis of cancer, we received the approval of our building permit that allowed us to construct our new home at the ranch. Spending over a year drawing the plans, it reminded me of Dad, as I was doing what he had done when he was building each of his three homes and the spec homes he built. It surprised me how much I remembered what he taught us, while young.

It was to be the sprawling mission-style adobe ranch home my grandfather had always dreamed of building in Santa Barbara before he contracted cancer. We were anxious to begin immediately upon receiving the approval of the construction loan, which arrived a few days before that devastating morning when we received the diagnosis of late-stage colorectal cancer.

There was no question that we needed to place our dreams on hold. With my state of health, the project would be too challenging to manage, and it would be unaffordable if I could no longer work. The uncertainty of a future suddenly hit hard. Everything we had worked on, for years, was dangling outside of our reach.

Contacting the lender, the contractor, and the building inspector, we advised them we would not be building. The building permit went back to the county, and we ate the thousands in costs. We placed the engineered plans in the attic for reconsideration, "someday."

Saving the most difficult calls for last, I dialed the number for the international investigative firm that I had performed counter-terrorism assignments since 9/11. It was difficult to report them that I was now unavailable for consideration for an assignment we had discussed only a week earlier.

My heart winced when they encouraged me to return after recovery. I did not have the heart to tell those I had worked with that it was unlikely to occur. It was doubtful I would have the stamina to work fulltime or the ability to do what I had once done for prolonged periods until recovery occurred from all the surgeries I would have to undergo. We would have to wait until we knew the side effects of the treatment. Until the years of surgeries and treatment were completed, my capabilities to continue working would be uncertain.

Postponement of life matters is painful when it involves health issues. First, we must accept and adapt to our circumstances, and then we live one day at a time until the situation becomes stationary. "Later," to treat cancer, and as we embark on the road toward the prevention of future cancers, is when we learn to adapt to the changes inside us. I found it to be the best time to create new dreams, hopes, and goals, dependent upon our recovery and abilities.

We still needed witnesses to my signature for my living will and to deliver it, along with the return of a plethora of other forms to the hospital. Drafting powers of attorney allowed Steve to act on my behalf in managing our joint assets if I was unable to represent myself. Preparing and signing quitclaim deeds that were attached to property deeds, as my father had done the week before his death, I finally tucked them into our safe. Safely setting next to the pink slips relinquishing my ownership of our vehicles to my husband, I let out a sigh of relief. Finally done, I hoped I hadn't forgotten anything. It was essential to think of everything we needed to do before my hospitalization, so I would not be a burden on anyone. I was preparing for myself to die in the manner I have always lived.

With the process of the business matters of dying out of the way, we began focusing on living. Christmas was coming, and I was excited. Steve decorated the exterior of our house with dripping lights hanging from the eaves and placed a wreath with big red bows upon the door.

That year, our Christmas tree was not the sixteen-foot pine of the past, harvested from our ranch. Steve realized I would want to take some part in decorating it. He also understood my level of stamina would not likely match my level of desire.

He went to the corner Christmas tree lot and retrieved a much smaller tree. It was a bit droopy and showed a few imperfections. My feeling was it was perfect — it reflected me. I loved it. We were both imperfect and droopy. Once decorated, that little tree sparkled. Motivating me to dress up and go downtown with Steve, just for a while, we enjoyed the town's sidewalks and the beautifully lit trees.

Christmas Eve was quiet and peaceful. I spent it with Steve and my son Chris. The next day, Steve celebrated Christmas at the home of his parents while I remained at home and read by the fire. It was the time of year when his nephew always had a cold. I could not afford to become ill, just before surgery, especially with an overworked immune system.

I was not the only person in the family who heard the clock ticking down the hours, minutes, and seconds of our lives. In their late eighties, each Christmas held more importance to them than the one prior. In my heart, I knew we would have more holidays. That year, everyone got what they wanted, however bittersweet it was.

I had never asked for anything for myself from God, making my own decisions and holding responsibility for my actions. With so much suffering of people with needs far greater than mine, I was not sure God could even hear me above the chaos rising from a needy world. But, on Christmas Day, in 2007, I found myself negotiating with him during prayer. I promised if I could live, I would do something to make my life count.

New Year's Eve arrived. Steve and I remained at home. At the stroke of midnight, we sat, beneath a clear California sky filled with twinkling stars. Readying ourselves for what was to come in the days, months, and years ahead, with the surgeries, treatments, and procedures I would need to undergo, we, again, played it safe. I could not afford to go out into the crowds and take the chance of becoming ill.

During those first days of the New Year, we cleaned, performed home maintenance, arranged for housekeeping, set-up grocery delivery, and stocked the cabinets with necessities. Appointments kept, attorneys consulted, the taxes done, and loved ones notified, we were ready to roll.

Steve redecorated our bedroom for my return. He painted it the vibrant apricot color of a desert sunrise, so every morning I would awaken to sunshine and give thanks for the day. Within it, he placed a small refrigerator, a microwave oven, a television, and a telephone; everything I needed to care for myself was right there without having to go downstairs.

Leaving for the hospital on that cold January morning, I looked back at our home and the comfort of the little Vacaville, California court where we lived. With renewed resolve, I turned and focused straight ahead as we headed down the hill toward the highway. Bring it on, I thought. I'm ready now.

Chapter Twenty-Five

SURGERY

Just because you didn't put a name to something does not mean it wasn't there. —Jodi Picoult

Ordinarily, the feeling large institutions leave patients is one that is cold and impersonal. This day, something was different about Kaiser Permanente, adding warmth to its otherwise sterility. Upon arrival, there was no standing in line to process admission papers. No stone had been left unturned. Nothing existed that would create future stress. They were ready for me.

A nurse swept me away into the sanctity of the surgical unit, where she helped me into a faded but wonderfully soft hospital gown and some bright-colored socks. Tucking into bed and cuddling under warmed blankets and fueled with the positive dispositions of everyone around me, I felt amazingly comfortable.

A compassionate and efficient team of nurses placed needles into my veins and installed tubes to machines that continuously monitored my vitals. Dr. Berndt and the anesthesiologist dropped by for a few minutes to check on me. Their positive attitudes were infectious, feeding into my determination to approach surgery confidently.

A picture of health, until age fifty, my experience with hospitalizations was minimal—twice for diagnostic testing for stress-related abdominal pain, twice for the live births of my children, and once for a late miscarriage. Living a risk-filled life, I experienced my share of accidents and dangerous situations. I always got through them without significant injury. Far from a stranger to Murphy's Law, my life was the perfect reflection of the fatalistic statement, "If anything can go wrong, it will."

Blessed with the good fortune of being a risk-taker and born with more lives than the average alley cat, I ended up walking away from most dangerous situations, unscathed. Though calamities occurred, I was different from my parents. I relied upon a hopeful optimism and a lot of laughter that got me through, while my parents relied on prayer.

As a child, I swallowed dozens of straight pins without lighting up an x-ray machine; I leaped into the icy waters of Lake Tahoe without knowing how to swim, and I shared my bed with a pet rattlesnake. At eleven, I flew past the windshield of a police car on a rope swing. Losing my grip, I fell upon the hood of their vehicle.

At sixteen, the vehicle my friends and I were riding in sailed into a lake. As water spilled inside and it began to sink, we crawled onto the roof and ended up swimming to the banks. Later, I slid through a hole in the ice. At seventeen, Sandee and I flew above the wake of her father's boat, precariously hanging onto only a rope.

Not once, but twice, I bounced off a river raft filled with burly police officers. Hurled into large boulders stretching down a quarter-mile of icy Class V rapids fed by the Sierra Nevada spring snowmelt, I was sore for a long while. A car filled with drunk men t-boned me while we were driving sixty miles per hour down a highway. Though suffering from tissue damage, I spent only a few days off work with a whiplash and back pain.

A few more events resulted from my work. A disgruntled, murderer wanted to throw me off a fifty-foot high tier; a serial killer expressed a desire to cold-cock me, and a drug dealer put a .45 caliber revolver to my head and fired. I survived the many hits issued that gang members and high-level drug dealers placed upon my life, and I received more than my share of duty-to-warn notifications from the psychiatrists treating a stable of my loyal stalkers. I had set my life up in a manner that the only thing I could have done with it, which would be challenging enough, was to work on the streets of two of the most violent cities in the nation.

Finally, only the Lord knows how many disenchanted people I left behind following my later years of investigating homicides, violent crimes, public corruption, and terrorism. After surviving all that, I did not intend to let cancer beat me.

This should be a breeze.

Humming to myself, I waited for the anesthesiologist to twist the nozzle and put me to sleep. The surgery went without a hitch. I awakened for a few seconds and listened to the conversation of the operating team as they worked on me. I felt nothing during the removal of all but seven inches of colon and quickly found myself focusing upon recovery as a lady of leisure sitting beside a morphine dispenser. During the weeks spent in bed, I sang, hummed, laughed, and wrote dozens of comedies in my mind.

Not expecting the long-ranged difficulties I experienced, my body was not in sync with my mind and spirit. Morphine could not help with that. My colon refused to awaken. To add to it, a visiting physician ordered the nasogastric (NG) tube that removed gastric fluids from the stomach, cleared, removed. I was thrilled; the NG tube was uncomfortable and annoying. Dr. Berndt was not at all pleased.

"Lindy, we're putting this back in," he said firmly.

"Please," I begged. "I don't want it."

"Okay, you have two choices," Dr. Berndt said, putting the decision upon me. "Either we put it back in, or we go back into surgery at once."

My flipping luck!

Groaning loudly, I chose a physician who did as I had once done, offering choices of doing something "the hard way, or the easy way." That reflected one of the many reasons I had faith in him. He had a stronger will than me. I resigned myself to the cold fact that no matter what, it was going back in. My only decision was how it would occur.

On or about the twentieth day of hospitalization, with my colon still on strike, he arrived early one morning and announced immediate surgery was necessary. He had waited long enough. The series of intensive tests he ordered revealed a clip on my anastomosis had slipped and needed replacement.

Surgery occurred without a hitch. I thought I was recovering well until two days later. I awakened one morning to find strangers wearing masks and grabbing at me. My lungs filled with fluid; I faced difficulty breathing.

Flooded with confusion, I did not know who those people were or what they wanted from me. My mind held a treasure trove of secrets.

About eighty percent of seriously ill patients, hospitalized for an extended period, become affected by "ICU psychosis." A disturbance of consciousness and cognition, it develops over a brief period. Comforting me was the realization Dr. Berndt was holding my hand and speaking in a soft voice, quietly repeating the questions of others. I answered him until I was no longer able to talk. Then, I spelled out my answers in his hand.

Unable to leave physically, my mind drifted to where I could not hear the noise. Within seconds, I was at our Northern California ranch, lying atop a bed of pine needles, next to a log. It was quiet and peaceful. I could hear the water of the Pit River gurgle as it rolled across stones, heading downstream. Water is life. Before my diagnosis, I spent considerable time by the river. It is where the generations of the Hammawi Pit River Tribe once hunted and fished during summer. Native women picked wildflowers while men played hand games—both stacked rocks in competitions.

A fledgling eagle laid upon the log, next to me, blinking his eyes. Sprawled side by side, two wretched forms of nature, our eyes locked. I wondered why he could not fly. Was he one of the fledglings hatched from nests of eagles that flew overhead during the past spring?

Wobbling upon unsteady legs, he repeatedly pulled himself up, sometimes collapsing, but he did not give up. Eventually, the young bird's stance became steady the more he tried. As termites and ants crawled on the log, he captured them in his beak.

Finally, fluttering his wings, he hopped up to the branch of a nearby tree. He occasionally stopped to look down upon me while hopping from one branch to another. Repeatedly, he did this throughout the morning until reaching the top. I watched as he glanced upon me one last time before taking flight and winging into the distance, leaving me alone. I wondered why I wasn't flying with him. It was then I realized I was alive.

Awakening, I saw strangers sitting at their desks, through the open windows in front of me. Their eyes focused upon computer screens. Dr. Berndt was standing in their midst, also watching the screens upon a wall. Again, a brief few seconds of ICU psychosis struck as I wondered what he was doing with those people.

Comforted by his presence, I drifted back to sleep. Dr. Berndt remained until I was stable. When Steve arrived, he found me attached to a BiPAP machine that pumped pressurized air through a mask. I awakened long enough to utter a few words before dozing off again. Intense pain roared through me as I remained in the ICU for three days.

Upon stabilization, I returned to a room in one of the recovery wards. My eyes filled with tears, as a compassionate nurse said, with a smile, "We found you a room with an eastern window."

"All good things come from the east," I heard Mom's voice whispering as the sun began to rise, its vibrant warmth pouring upon the bed. She must have been present in spirit with me that day. Quietly, as I saw her do, I whispered gratitude for the new day and the continuation of life.

I felt a surge of strength flow through me. Sliding off the bed, I stood on shaky legs for the first time in a month. Trailed by tubes, I staggered to the bathroom, pulled off my gown, and leaned against a wall, melting into it as I took my first shower in twenty-four days. After standing beneath the warm water for a good fifteen minutes, I stumbled back to bed, having scrubbed off the weariness and the uncertainty. Not only did I feel clean, but I felt my stamina returning.

Unable to concentrate on much, I spent a considerable amount of time deep in my head. Thoughts of our ancestral grandfather Lewis Green appeared. Fearless and having the stamina of a wild cat, Lewis settled in the Appalachian Mountains of Southwest Virginia in the mid-1700s, near Porter's Fort. He once experienced the same as I was enduring, but for a much longer time, and under far worse circumstances. A long-hunter of Native American, Scottish, and English ethnicity, he was tall with a brown complexion and silver-colored eyes. Colonial War documents described him as being a colonial spy who reported Indian activity. The memoirs of Daniel Boone reveal an inspiring story of his intense desire to live.

In the depths of winter, Lewis and a brother-in-law hunted some distance from where they lived near Porter's Fort, deep in the Virginia Appalachian Mountains. Erecting a cabin to protect themselves from the elements, they subsisted on bear jerky and the wild game they hung from the overhead rafters.

Outside and alone, Lewis saw a bear wander into camp. Raising his musket, he fired upon it. The bear fell over an embankment into a sinkhole. As Lewis edged carefully over the side to view it, his feet slipped on the ice. Sliding into the hole, and slamming into the bear, the angry animal mauled him, ripping out an eye. Done with Lewis, it crawled out and ambled into the forest. Returning, Lewis' brother-in-law found him. He carried Lewis into the cabin and made him comfortable in a bed of leaves and straw, under some furs.

Hanging a cooked, wild turkey overhead and leaving beef jerky and water by his side for Lewis to eat, his brother-in-law stated he was going out to hunt. Believing Lewis would die, he went home and reported to others that Lewis was dead.

The fire went out in the cabin. Alone and incapacitated, Lewis had run out and had no way of getting more firewood. To stay warm, he cut off the feathers of the turkey and tucked them around himself for warmth. Through the winter, he lived off the dried bear jerky and melted snow.

When spring rolled around, his family and others organized a party to set out and retrieve Lewis' body. En route, they stood astonished upon seeing Lewis limping out of the forest, with one bum leg, one eye, and stumbling with his arm leaning upon a stick, fashioned as a crutch to hold him up. Once home, Lewis recovered enough to resume his hunting and military activities. Terribly disfigured, he lived to be sixty years old.

Lewis' will to live contributed toward his survival in the cold, despite his mass injuries and being alone, during the depths of winter. As I laid in my warm hospital bed, I thought of my father also battling cancer alone. I hoped some of their resilience passed genetically through the family. If he and Lewis could do it under those terrible conditions, I could do it with mine. All it required was the will to live.

Chapter Twenty-Six

CHEMOTHERAPY

*Some days there won't be a song
in your heart. Sing anyway.*
— Emory Austin

Chemotherapy is tough. No amount of sugarcoating can minimize the grueling effects it wreaks upon some, while it hardly affects others. Our ability to tolerate it and whether it will annihilate our cancers is a result of the draw. Some sail through it playing on the golf course, while others like me curl up on their sofas and stare at the ceiling for months on end.

Until targeted therapies such as immunotherapy that can get right into the cancer cells become a basic standard of care, the current treatments of chemotherapy are unavoidable. 5FU and the combination treatments with other ingredients, including platinum drugs, are the medical standard for care for cancer treatment today. It is often the most used approach to the treatment of cancer until more effective drugs are approved.

Some mutations of Lynch syndrome are not receptive to 5FU and the traditional methods of chemotherapy for our cancers. An oncologist, with knowledge of Lynch syndrome, will determine what treatment they feel will be most effective and tolerated by the patient. Testing of the tumor is available to aid them in personalizing therapy for Lynch syndrome patients.

"Someday," cancer treatment will become personalized for everyone, with every tumor, studied to determine the most effective treatment approach for patients like us. It is happening now for some bladder cancers, colorectal, and other cancers. It not only saves the costs of cancer treatment, but it saves lives.

The first step in preparing for adjuvant chemotherapy (treatment administered after surgery) is to get a "port" installed. Also known as a venous access device (VAD), the port supplies a system to deliver liquid chemotherapy into the bloodstream, replacing the need for an IV.

Composed of plastic, The VAD is the size of a quarter. Containing a small chamber, topped with a raised area, interventional radiologists implant it just under the skin of the chest, and over a major artery. Its purpose is to simplify the flow of liquids into the veins and to allow for blood draws.

Relaxing in the basement hallway of the radiological procedure room, awaiting my turn to get a port installed, I overheard a conversation between a few patients.

"What type of anesthesia are you having with your port installation?"

A bell tolled inside my head. I suddenly realized I messed up. I did not know what type of anesthesia they would give me, if anything. I did not think to ask.

"Lindy," the nurse called from the doorway. Hesitating with trepidation for a few brief seconds, I reluctantly rose and followed her into the cool depths of the darkened cavern where the procedures occur. Stepping aside to allow a nurse to wheel a woman out the door on a gurney, I noticed she was stone-cold out of it, and snoring like a baby. Despite the chill in the room, it warmed my heart.

"So, it's done under anesthesia, huh?" I excitedly asked the nurse as I followed her to the table. The day was getting better.

The nurse chuckled as she shook her head. "Not for you, sweetheart."

My face dropped. I could almost hear the loud crash of my chin hit the floor.

"Uh, what do *we* use?" I asked apprehensively.

"Oh, about twenty-five milligrams of Demerol and maybe a little Valium," she answered.

I groaned. I had been there and done that before. With the birth of two kids, decades earlier, back when the medical profession believed traditional pain relief procedures would pose an adverse effect upon newborns, I had been given 25 mg of Demerol. Then, they thought it was enough to ease the pain from twelve hours of hard labor. My thought then was every male physician should go through a ritual of pushing a cantaloupe through their lips, to get an idea of what women face.

Glancing toward the procedure table at the jovial doctor, then back toward the nurse, a realization hit. It was going to be a challenging day.

"This won't hurt... much," the radiologist teased as he tugged on his gloves and prepared to start. I laughed, thinking it was funny.

Within two minutes, I was wailing. "Whoa, Doc, you're killing me here," I whined.

"Next time, make sure you get admitted as an in-patient," the assistant whispered in my ear as I tried to get my mind to go somewhere else... anywhere else but there, in that room, at that time.

Next time? No way! I'm keeping this port forever.

"Okay," I said, closing my eyes and wishing myself upon a warm sunny beach somewhere, far away from the basement of the Kaiser Permanente Vallejo facility. I made another reminder to myself to protect my port at all costs because I didn't ever want to go through this again.

Pain relief methods for medical procedures vary, dependent upon the admission scheduled for the patient. It also depends upon your health insurance coverage, your physician, and your circumstances. An inpatient registrant may get anesthesia. I was an out-patient, so it wasn't going to happen. It was Demerol and some Valium, coupled with a hefty dose of compassion from the medical staff. After receiving a topical administration of Lidocaine and a small amount of Demerol, it did not take long to understand why they administered Valium. They intended it to keep me calm enough to make sure I did not leap off the table while they tunneled under my skin. Fortunately, it was a quick procedure.

Finally, with the port installed, we were ready to roll and move on with treatment. That is after I attended a chemotherapy class and an orientation to the infusion center.

Planning to attend before the installation of the port, but in the same manner that good intentions end up tossed by the wayside, I procrastinated until the last minute. Yet another lesson learned. Attend classes early. Had I done so, I would have learned the difference and availability of anesthesia available for in-patients and that supplied to out-patients.

Steve and I attended the one said to end the mysteries of the specific chemotherapies. It offered explanations and tips on how to manage the plethora of side effects that chemotherapy presents. Still battling exhaustion from surgery and severe anemia, I slept through it, later asking Steve what they said. Steve reduced the information to two sentences. "It will be difficult," he said. "Just follow their instructions."

Groaning, I reminded myself to get into a mindset to expect that nothing comes easy when one has cancer. I had to toughen up and prepare myself for a bumpy ride.

During our travels through life, we all face challenges. Cancer is a common challenge for many. One of three people contracts cancer during their lifetimes. Some contract it once and never again. Others find themselves contracting cancer a few times. With Lynch syndrome, our predisposition to contract multiple cancers several times is not unusual.

With problems, come choices. Some sail through treatments, and others face challenges. I was still learning the lessons of Murphy's Law. What we experience during our journey in life may be circumstances, and sometimes it may be the ramifications and the consequences of how we handle those circumstances. In the end, none of that matters. What *does* matter is that we survive and find the best and the more convenient ways for it to happen, so it does not occur again, the "hard way vs. the easy way."

I managed mine by not offering myself much in the way of options. Sometimes it worked; sometimes it didn't. Again, I exercised the philosophy of choosing the hard way over the easy way. I was adamant about not repeating the choices of my father, who faced much of his journey alone. I desired to be like my aunt, who danced her way through cancer, on a tropical beach. No matter what manner we choose to get past our cancer, we must pull from that dogged determination that is in all of us to live.

The specific chemotherapy treatment prescribed was FOLFOX. It is still a standard treatment given to those who contract colorectal cancer. A concoction composed of three chemical compounds, 5FU, leucovorin, and oxaliplatin, for some people, results in a boatload of side effects, some of which may be lifelong.

How each of us tolerates chemotherapy is different, dependent upon how well we and our genetic makeup responds to it. Some experience considerable side effects while others spend their time playing on the golf course or working full-time. Some of us lose hair; some do not. I lost clumps and sprigs with it but never had a problem with nausea if I took anti-nausea medication early in the morning, an hour before breakfast, with a bite or two of toast, and then twelve hours later, before dinner.

It was my thought the side effects were mere inconveniences when considering the unacceptable alternative to not undergoing chemotherapy. My sole focus was to live. Whatever I needed to do, within my capabilities, to reach that goal, I intended to do it, including running through the gauntlet of side effects.

At first, everything was a battle. I placed considerable trust in my oncologist, Aradhana Ghosh. She was a godsend as she worked with me throughout the journey with chemotherapy.

"I think you should be evaluated for Lynch syndrome," she too had told me during our first consultation, as had Dr. Martin and Dr. Berndt. The hope I received from knowing there was progress is detecting what was causing our hereditary cancer was invaluable. Warm, knowledgeable, and energetic, she made the treatments easier, intuitively knowing when the therapy was becoming too much to tolerate.

"Patience, Linda. Time is your friend," she would say.

The most significant difficulty I faced was the thought of someone injecting chemicals into a vein leading into my heart through a plastic tube. It was immensely stressful, requiring me to place complete trust in the individual administering the treatment. Relinquishing control into the hands of others and trusting those I do not know is not natural for me.

With my feet kicked up on the footrest of the orange vinyl recliner and wrapped in an Indian blanket, I would sit in the infusion room, read for a short while, and eventually hum myself to sleep. A few hours later, the nurse removed the tubes and attached a canister to my waist to take home to continue treatment until emptied, for another forty-four hours.

Only after the chemotherapy developed a cumulative effect within my body did I realize physical problems that I did not expect. Feeling "wasted," I spent most my days curled up like a cat, looking up toward the ceiling with a blank stare. Chemotherapy offered me a new perspective on drug addiction. It reminded me of my mom when she was high… physically wasted and mentally and emotionally numbed.

It was not long before I awakened in the mornings to find small clumps of hair in my mouth, in my bed, wrapped in my fingers, and lying at the bottom of the shower. The mirror reflected little spots of bald appearing atop my head. Tossing on a baseball cap before leaving the house to hide it, I could feel myself becoming stressed with the fear that my hair would not grow back.

To reduce the increasing amount of hair loss, I slept in a soft net sleep cap, as done when young. After a while, I realized I needed to do something about it. It was well past time to act. I feared I was setting myself up to be demoralized. My mind filled with debate.

What's a little hair for a shot at a much longer life?

That little voice inside had not abandoned me. It was a fair question to ask. I appreciated the honest response sounding from somewhere deep within the depths of my heart.

The real question is, how badly do you want to live?

I got it. All the whining and the denial in the world wouldn't change the circumstances. It all came down to perspective and choice. The reality struck hard. I was the captain of my fate.

With few options available, again, considering the hard way or the easy way, I decided it was time to let the hair go. It didn't make sense to set myself up for something that was to be inevitable. Keeping a cheerful outlook is essential to the success of our treatments and our quality of life. Each day, I arose and dressed. I didn't allow myself to get too upset over the clumps of hair that fell out when I brushed it. It often happens with chemo. By cutting it short, it would be one less problem to worry about "later."

Hair grows back.

Later came a week or two after. Judi chauffeured me to her hairdresser. While lying in the chair and watching all but a few inches of my hair fall to the floor, I felt empowered. My daughter cried. It broke my heart.

The removal of my hair was symbolic of reality for each of us viewed it as exerting control over the effects of my treatment. Judi saw it as an act of devastation to her mother, and something she may later experience.

"Where would you like to go for lunch?" she asked as we left. "I'm buying."

"How about grabbing a quick hot dog?" I suggested as I stumbled into her car.

"Hot dogs? Please, Mom. I'm taking you somewhere nice," she said. I looked down at myself. I knew too many people in our small town. There was no way I could enter a restaurant looking the way I did I did. My clothing hung on me, and my pallor was gray. It took all the energy I had to get in and out of a car. Handling more than an hour away from home was exhausting. And, for days, I had been craving hot dogs, ever since I went to Target, with Steve.

That day, after entering the store, he raced off to fill his list of things he needed. Leaning heavily upon a shopping cart, and leisurely using it as a walker, I set out to get some exercise when I looked toward my right. Instantly, I stopped as I saw my reflection in an enormous mirror, gazing back at me. I hardly recognized myself.

I was wearing no makeup and my hair straight, thin, and stringy, my clothes hanging from my frame. It reminded me of one of the bag ladies I used to know in Oakland, who pushed her shopping cart up and down the city streets. The look was complete with the floppy hat, the bulky woolen sweater, and the fingerless gloves I wore, all intended to protect me from a flare-up of neuropathic pain from the store's air conditioning system.

Suddenly, my legs buckled. No place to sit and weakening, I let out another amused laugh of exhaustion as I carefully lowered myself upon the floor, wondering how the security officer would react.

Just a few minutes to gather my strength.

While sitting there, a memory struck. Years before, after a long day, a couple of women agents and police officers spent an evening emptying too many wine bottles at a local watering hole and talking "girl talk."

One of the women police officers said, "Here's to becoming a bag lady when I retire." We roared with laughter at the thought of it.

"Let's do it! We can be winos instead of widows," another suggested, raising more raucous laughter. From there, it got worse for the guys.

"Ah! Who needs men? We've got badges and retirements!"

"Don't need no stinking badges either, just the retirements," another jested.

Then, the verbal jousting was typical for women who worked in non-traditional occupations. Many had survived broken marriages and had solely raised and supported children into adulthood. There were those of us who were going through hell and others who made it through the emotional gauntlet, but who were now living with the scars.

Every one of us was continually adapting to a different lifestyle during midlife. Eventually, our buffoonery evolved into a fantasy to buy a little alley, where we would sleep in refrigerator boxes next to our shopping carts during summer and wander Caribbean beaches as homeless bums during winter.

Life would be worry-free. There would be no makeup to apply; no manicures needed; no more hairdressers to make us look "trendy." No more bills we couldn't pay or collections agents hitting us up on pagers that we no longer needed.

Ex-husbands would have to find someone else's living room where they could dump their baggage, and there would be no more yards to keep up. We'd no longer need anyone's approval, and we wouldn't have to feel the pressure of resolving everyone else's circumstances.

Dining on frothy milkshakes and convenience store hot dogs as we did when working on the streets, there would be far more joy in our lives. Expectations upon us would be nonexistent.

That morning, sitting on the cold floor of the Target store, I couldn't stop laughing, thinking of then, when we were once everything to many, and nothing to others, living under the constraints of an evolving society while being "ahead of our time."

I don't know where most are anymore. None of us were any good at sending Christmas cards. Life went on, and we continued rolling with it, keeping the memories tucked somewhere deep inside.

Sometimes escaping for just a few minutes from where we are at is enough to help us continue. An evening of drunken laughter over something so ridiculously crazy as making plans to spend our end as bag ladies can contribute to a need in later life. Here, I was, sitting on a cold floor of a discount store, unable to get up, and not caring about what anyone thinks.

Giggling, I attempted to rise. I put my hands behind me, but I didn't have the strength to catapult onto my feet. I rolled into a position to rise, but I was unable to get past a sorry crawl. Unsuccessful, I gave up and sprawled out, laughing hysterically, hoping the end of my life would not occur on that floor in Target. What an obituary that would be!

"Are you okay?" the security officer asked, his eyes wide.

"Just resting," I chuckled, as I scooted backward, to lean against a shelf until Steve arrived. The cold rising from the floor felt glorious. It soothed my inflamed body. All I needed was a hot dog and a chocolate milkshake. It sounded so good, right then.

Steve walked down the aisle, laughing as he saw me sitting on the floor with a sheepish grin on my face.

"Not as strong as I thought," I apologized.

"She's been out too long. I need to get her out of here," Steve explained apologetically to the store security officer as he helped hoist my sorry body off the floor.

"Come on, old gal," he said, leaning me up against the shopping cart. "Let's go, or we'll be late for your infusion."

"Chemo," he half-whispered to the security officer, with a wink.

Now, back in Judi's car, running my fingers through the two inches of hair on my head, I watched as she flicked on the ignition. With memories safely tucked into the back of my mind, I was still chuckling as I glanced toward my daughter, who was sitting in the driver's seat, questioning my sanity.

Not only did I laugh a lot during my surgery, but my imagination also ran wild while lying in that bed with little stimuli for distraction. I began writing screenplays in my mind, but I laughed a lot when going through chemo while hanging out in its shadows. As I learned when I worked on the streets, laughing was the only thing that kept me from crying. I had done it during an entire career when the nitty-gritty of the darker side of life had become too much to handle emotionally. We laughed when faced with adversity. What else can one do when confronted with a situation that doesn't offer the comfort of normality? That same feeling exists when one is working their way through cancer and its treatments; during a time when all we can rely upon is our faith in others and a blind sense of hope.

"Are you sure, Mom? Judi asked.

"Seriously, Judi, I *really* need a hot dog, after all this."

"Would it make you happy?"

"Thrilled," I answered. "Ever seen an unhappy person eating a hotdog?"

Judi earned her title as the queen of debate, but even she could not argue that point. I knew my body would face difficulty tolerating it. I would have fifteen minutes to make it into the driveway and another minute or two to take a mad dash to the bathroom after finishing it.

Then, I would continue to pay for it with an afternoon of solitary confinement in a room with a toilet. How bad could that be? I had worked in an institution where thousands of men lived their entire lives that way. Eating a hot dog that day was worth it to me.

So, hot dogs it was. Just thinking about them had my mouth watering. I paid for it and served my sentence dutifully. It was worth it to get my head back into a positive perspective. Rebellion can be a good thing. Just as hot dogs, on rare occasions, can be healthy, at least for the spirit.

The complications of chemotherapy continued, growing worse as the drug accumulated in my body. It terrified me when it affected my mind. That was the one part of myself that held me together. My imagination kept me entertained through the weeks of hospitalization and beyond, but now, with chemo brain setting in, I could not remember that said a moment ago. My mind filled with fog, I was unable to follow a television sitcom or recall what occurred in the prior scene without taking notes.

Losing my balance followed. At night, I walked sideways, often bumping into walls, and occasionally dropping to my knees or stumbling when descending the staircase. I turned to my computer, finding losing balance was a symptom of peripheral neuropathy. Suggesting we place night lights throughout the house, the information found in the article worked. The nighttime stumbling ended. To navigate the carpeted stairs, I sat and softly bounced to the bottom, to avoid falling.

As chemotherapy continued, the side effects worsened. While driving downtown, two miles away, which I had done for over eighteen years, one afternoon, I could not figure out how to get home. I had lost my navigational skills, just as what occurred during the shooting incident years earlier.

Pulling the car over, I did as I did then. I made myself relax and breathe deep. In and out, I inhaled and exhaled slowly. I reassured myself that everything was okay. Sitting back and closing my eyes, I rested until my memory awakened—go straight past the park, take a left past the school administration buildings, go to the shopping center, and then take a right turn. It all came back with the reduction of stress and anxiety. I managed it the way I managed PTSD. The symptoms of the two, at times, are almost identical. Nonetheless, when I got home, I hung up my car keys for a while, until the side effects disappeared.

I was once someone who remembered thousands of names and miscellaneous bits of information others. The dates of their birth of inmates, parolees, criminals, terrorists, and their commitment offenses, their addresses, their associates, and the hundreds of license plate numbers of the cars they drove. Then, my mind had been almost photographic.

Now, I could hardly remember the question my husband had asked only moments earlier that I was trying to google. While compensating for the loss of cognitive skills, it was frustrating to see the difficulty my tangled thoughts imposed upon my family, as they patiently waited for a few seconds until I could sputter out a complete thought. I was struggling with remembering familiar words and telephone numbers. Worse was my fear; it would never resolve itself.

Searching online, I found nothing to treat it. I was on my own to figure out how to manage it. I did well for a little while until it worsened and became harder to achieve. The family helped. They played a game of "Grandma Trivia," guessing what Grandma wanted to say. Everyone finished my sentences.

Systematically, we worked to decrease the adverse effects. Planning smaller sentences before speaking and carrying my tablet with me, I practiced what I intended to say. Consulting a thesaurus, I would type in a definition of the word I faced difficulty recalling.

"What is the type of loan to buy a house called?" A thousand answers popped up. I was relieved. At least, when it occurred, I could get past it, and it wouldn't be so hard on everyone else.

In a family, not just one person deals with the effects of cancer and cancer treatment. The entire family does, especially when it is hereditary. Survival is all about allowing a loved one to help you into and out of the bathtub or to comb your hair when you are not able to do it for yourself. Recovery is all about being able to adapt. Not just for us but for everyone we care for and who cares for us. While we are fighting to survive, they are also learning from us how to do the same.

I asked Dr. Ghosh, "Just how long does one need to be on chemotherapy for treatment to be effective?"

She did not know. Neither did anyone else. At that time, there had been no study conducted on the number of sessions individuals should engage in FOLFOX chemotherapy treatment for it to be effective, except those protocols used in the clinical trials when seeking approval of the drug. Because of the side effects that exist, few patients can comfortably receive all six months of oxaliplatin-based chemotherapy. Today, research findings show a reduced number of treatments for less aggressive cancers may be acceptable for some, though for severe Stage III cancers and over, the goal is to continue the standard treatment. The oncologist considers a range of factors in determining how long the patient can withstand it.

A study of 188 Korean patients showed there was a minor difference in survival rates between a four-month protocol of FOLFOX chemotherapy and a six-month protocol of FOLFOX chemotherapy. A higher incidence of peripheral neuropathy existed with a six-month length of treatments. Though a preliminary study, needing a much broader base, it is hopeful. It supplies encouragement for researchers to conduct robust research to confirm these results.

Dr. Ghosh reduced the dosage on several occasions. It eased the side effects. To increase my blood count, Steve administered injections into my stomach before he left for work each day. I slept through most of them.

The realization hit that there was little that relieved the sense of constant weariness that travels with chemotherapy. No amount of sleep helped, even after treatment ended. I called Dr. Walker, in tears, begging him, "I need sleep. It won't come."

Spending the hours of insomnia gazing through the window at an enormous California redwood towering in the backyard, I watched over the barn owl who lived there. At night and during the early morning hours, I would hoot at him, and he would respond, reassuring that he was out there, somewhere in the darkness.

The ancient ancestors of my mother associated the owl with having healing abilities. They believed it served as a warning to those who fell ill. I found his presence comforting. Desperate for any distraction to get past those afternoons of cancer treatments, I readily accepted all the help I could get from this world, and from those who existed in that beyond.

Following session after session of chemotherapy, I increasingly weakened. Mustering the motivation to continue was difficult. The waiting room was dismal, filled with sick people. Hardly a smile existed anywhere. Sitting in the lobby and waiting for my nurse to call my name was sheer agony. I feared the opening of the door to the infusion clinic to open because once I was inside, I was reliant upon others in injecting chemicals into my body. The only control I had was to accept or reject the treatments. Some choice, I thought. Neither appealed to me.

Burying myself into a magazine, but not reading, I was flipping through the pages, studying the photos. My eyes lit upon an advertisement for a television show. It depicted a federal marshal. She and her partner were standing in front of a door. With their weapons drawn, her dark eyes revealed the intensity of the depth of her uncertainty while trying to conceal her fear. A caption read, "Would you go in, knowing you might not come out?"

Catapulted into the past, I was captivated by the image. I, too, had been where that woman was, often. Having spent years doing the same during parole searches and serving search warrants, I often felt the same intense uncertainty she displayed before making entry.

For a few short moments, I was back on the streets, smelling the decaying porches and watching the litter dancing in the breeze. Memories flooded with police officers banging on the door, yelling, "Open up! Police! Search warrant, parole search!"

My body jerked as the impact of a foot kicked in a door, releasing the aroma emanating from the fresh splintering of raw wood. Acutely aware of the feel of cold, rigid steel in my hands, I cuffed up parolees and other suspects. Combined with the distinct odor of leather cleaner that wafted in the air as we unholstered our weapons, was the lump in my throat and the pumping of my heart while preparing to go through that door, not knowing what was on the other side. It was always the same, the restrained sense of fear, followed by adrenaline racing through the body. Glancing up and studying the clinic door, it didn't look any different from others I had entered. A door is simply a door. I had been through thousands.

I can do this.

Suddenly, it creaked partway open. I glanced up to see Linda, my nurse, sticking her head through the opening. She smiled and asked, "Ready, girlfriend?"

"As ready as ever," I sighed, rising, and gathering my purse. With the magazine clutched tightly in my hand, I followed her into the hallway. Having second thoughts, I turned and saw the door close behind me.

Done is done.

Walking down the hallway, we finally reached the tiny infusion room, the one with the bright orange recliner. Placing my handbag and the magazine on the table, I took a deep breath and readied myself for the afternoon. Opening the magazine to the advertisement, I placed it next to my chair, to view when the waves of uncertainty and anxiety hit. At the day's end, tearing it out of the magazine, I carefully folded it, putting it into my purse.

It was a profound experience in my life, realizing throughout it, we all enter and exit through thousands of doors, not knowing what lies beyond them. Most of the time, we make it through unscathed, suffering a little more than a few scrapes at the worst, and gaining a tremendous sense of empowerment that provides us with a sense of strength we could never have imagined. The infusions became easier to tolerate when viewing chemotherapy as just another of the thousands of doors we enter during our lifetimes.

Chapter Twenty-Seven

GENETIC TESTING

Tell me, and I forget, teach me, and I may remember,
involve me, and I learn.
—Benjamin Franklin

A few months before completing chemotherapy, my physician scheduled me for a genetic counseling session to determine if our family history met the criterion to allow me to participate in genetic testing for hereditary cancer. Lynch syndrome is a subset of hereditary nonpolyposis colorectal cancer (HNPCC). It places individuals at high risk for contracting many cancers, including colorectal cancer, endometrial cancers, ovarian cancer, and other cancers of the gastric system, breast, pancreas, biliary tract, ureter and renal pelvis, bladder, thyroid, small intestine, and brain (usually glioblastoma), including lymphoma, sebaceous adenomas, sebaceous carcinomas, and keratoacanthomas, as seen in the Muir-Torre syndrome variant.

Genetic testing is the method of determining if a defective mismatch repair gene of Lynch syndrome exists. The mismatch repair gene corrects errors in cell replication. When this gene malfunctions, it allows the creation of defective cells to form. As it tries to correct the errors, it is unable, and errors stack upon one another, creating rogue cells that eventually develop into aggressive tumors.

Eleven years ago, when I received a genetic counseling appointment, the last thing I wanted to do while undergoing chemotherapy treatments was to travel thirty-five miles, each way, to attend a traditional genetic counseling appointment. At that time, it was the nearest location offering counseling. Incredibly ill, I barely had the energy to care for my personal needs, let alone travel that distance. It occurred at a time when I could not read more than a paragraph or walk more than a block before becoming exhausted. I could not take a bath without help, watch, and understand a thirty-minute sitcom, or sit longer than an hour.

With an unpredictable colon, I needed access to a bathroom every one-half to two hours. Leaving home for an extended time was difficult, for not only was my colon unstable, but its instability created a tremendous amount of anxiety when traveling any distance. Nonetheless, it was a prerequisite to being allowed genetic testing to learn the identity of the hereditary cancer syndrome killing our family. I had to prove to my children that Lynch syndrome was no longer a ticket to the stars, as it was for the generations before ours. Today, there is little to fear if we take part in preventative cancer screenings. I live year by year, without the existence of uncertainty.

Mandated to attend a one-hour educational session with a genetic counselor to learn about a syndrome, for which they had not yet diagnosed me, didn't make sense. It was like having to learn about the parts of the heart before being given an EKG. I wondered why I could not attend the educational sessions *after* I had taken a genetic test.

Then, the standards set within the Amsterdam criteria of requiring a three-generation history of certain cancers provided an enormous barrier for genetic testing. Today, it is still almost impossible to construct a three-generation lineage of cancer, because of the secrecy developed in families, and documentation of causes of death of cancer.

From the late 1800s to 1965, many physicians documented the side effects that occurred with cancer as the primary cause of death, instead of the actual disease, to protect patients from eugenic acts. Seldom were the family histories of cancer documented. Most of the time, patients did not reveal them to them. Instead was the listing of the accompanying effects of the disease as a cause of death, such as nephritis, heart failure, bowel blockage, diabetes, tuberculosis, and other side effects of cancer during the eighty years of the existence of the eugenics movement makes it impossible.

The primary goal of a genetic counseling session is to educate the patient about genetics, supply details about the cause of the syndrome, provide necessary "informed consent," which explains the potential risks to a patient of taking a genetic test, to assess the possibility of risk of a genetic mutation, and to determine whether to allow the patient to get that test.

Fortunately, I was a member of an HMO. The average amount charged for that one mandatory counseling session, including the genetic test, in the commercial market at a clinic, hospital, or institution, exceeded four thousand dollars. It did not include the hidden costs of three to five hundred dollars for the physician's referral, the lost wages involved in missing work, the laboratory appointment, the cost of the genetic counselor, and costs of travel, and daycare provisions while attending several visits.

Today, in comparison, the costs of obtaining quality genetic hereditary cancer testing online, which includes genetic counseling, if positive, do not exceed $250 if done through the direct to consumer genetic testing company, Color Genomics. Used by physicians and organizations nationwide, it positively challenges the effectiveness and the problems of traditional methods of genetic cancer diagnostic testing.

Pulling into a parking space, I emitted a sigh of relief. It was a smaller building than expected, not the large medical centers I often visited. There wouldn't be a long walk to the building, followed by a longer trek down drafty hallways with little or no place to rest.

The outside temperatures were in the triple digits. Sweltering heat enveloped us as Steve helped me from the car and tugged my Kaiser hat down over my eyes. Gazing toward the building, I pulled on my sweater and, after taking a big breath, pulled together as much stamina as I could muster. Then, we set out to find the genetic counseling office.

The counselor was cordial. We sat upon a sofa, our hands folded upon our laps as she displayed exhibits from a book and explained the basics of genetics and Lynch syndrome (LS). I had no problem following her instructions. After my cancer diagnosis, I had reviewed hundreds of studies and articles on Lynch syndrome, written by global experts.

"What is the name of the condition you think we have is?" I frequently asked Dr. Martin. It was so long that remembering what he repeatedly told me was impossible. I felt it was what affected us. The name was so long; my father would never have been able to remember it.

"Hereditary Non-Polyposis Colorectal Cancer," he answered. "Just look for HNPCC," he patiently answered each time, finally writing it upon his business card, which I kept in my handbag. I was grateful for his patience with me. The chemo brain was tough to manage, and my mind was slow.

Once home, I tapped those five letters into the browser of my computer. About 89,500 links supplying information about Lynch syndrome, also known as hereditary nonpolyposis colorectal cancer (HNPCC), appeared.

Astonished, I leaned back in my chair and stared at the computer screen after reviewing page after page of research material. It was the same I had found a decade earlier, but with different cancers. If I could find it by entering a few search terms in Google, I wondered how all those doctors that my father, brother, aunt, and I had seen through the years, could not.

When physicians diagnosed my father with cancer, researchers had patented genetic testing for Lynch syndrome four years earlier. I received my diagnosis ten years following my father's death and fourteen years after that patenting. Today, genetic testing has existed for our specific mutation for twenty-six years. Diagnoses for LS are slow, and I meet physicians every day who have never heard of it.

It takes one full generation or thirty-four years for physicians to embrace new health practices, the same amount of time for a complete turnover of physicians, allowing a whole new breed of doctors to graduate from medical schools and take over.

Today, it has taken that long for medical professionals and the public to learn about Lynch syndrome and other hereditary cancers and disease. As a result, we have lost an entire generation to it. Many still do not know about hereditary syndromes, especially in inner cities, rural areas, small towns, and local hospitals.

"Despite knowing if you have Lynch syndrome, there are risks to genetic testing," the genetic counselor explained, reading a lengthy list of negative aspects, including not being able to obtain insurance.

My first thought was I was grateful that most HMOs do not report to insurance companies. If what she said was true, little did it matter. My employer supplied group life and health insurance through an HMO. Others in our family are not as fortunate.

Though insurance companies cannot turn down coverage for those with pre-existing conditions, patients are often charged more for the policies. Today, the average costs of health insurance equate to three weeks of minimum wages when covering a family of four. Adding co-pays and deductibles increase the patient's cost of care.

The United States and Canadian insurance companies have collaborated with the use of a database called the "MIB" that makes every investigator's mouth salivate. It collects data from life insurance applications, medical records, and claims. Insurance underwriters can search through data entries and see if anyone in a family has ever been evaluated for hereditary cancer or has contracted cancer, what type of cancer was contracted, and at what age. By tracing back family members and health histories, they can estimate the likelihood of an inherited predisposition to disease.

If no cancer information existed in the family previously, it becomes recorded when the genetic counselor bills the insurance company for the counseling appointment. That sets off a red flag for the entire family. If there is an already documented family history of cancer, the insurance companies know it, so genetic testing doesn't make much of a difference. The database alone could qualify us for a genetic test as it can establish multiple generations of disease.

Having survived cancer, I am confident a flag exists next to my name in the insurance underwriter's database, along with my siblings, my father, my aunt, and my grandfather, as well as my mother, her mother, and her mother (if they had insurance) and my grandfather and his family. That red flag would be waving wildly, at least for ten years, if I remained cancer-free. The information the database holds is a treasure chest for investigators. I continued to listen, but my investigative antennae continued to rise while I was processing every word she said.

"A possibility exists that employers and others may discriminate against you," she read.

They could say that about everyone with any chronic, life-threatening condition.

While I was pursuing genetic testing, federal legislation was pending, later signed by President George W. Bush. The Genetic Information Nondiscrimination Act of 2008 (GINA), specifically disallows insurance companies to deny insurance to those with preexisting conditions and discrimination by employers. Employment discrimination was no longer an acceptable practice.

After what I had experienced with cancer, surgery, and everything else, I was frustrated with the counseling. It seemed excessive. Coming from a family with a high rate of cancer, I knew I was already a risk to insurance companies. Frustrated, I wanted to say, "All I need is a genetic test to find out what is wrong with us."

Instead, I said, "I see," hoping the session would be over so I could get out to my car and sleep.

She continued, "If positive, it is important to undergo annual cancer screenings."

My mind was racing. Preventative care is only available to those who can afford it, costing as much as $30,000 a year, at the billing rates of health facilities to insurance companies and patients alike. The ability to obtain those lifesaving screenings depends upon many factors that are often out of control of everyday people. The hidden costs further increase the ability to obtain genetic testing and ongoing preventative testing, if positive.

Again, I said, "Okay."

Sitting in that chair, I wondered how what she said would affect my children during their lifetimes. It wasn't likely that kids turning eighteen years old would be able to afford the test and the counseling, let alone the $1000 a month (one half of a minimum wage) being charged today for health insurance for those with pre-existing conditions.

I looked at obtaining genetic testing for a hereditary cancer condition the same way as I viewed getting a test for any other life-threatening condition. What credible health care association imposes stringent criteria for diagnosis for any other life-threatening disease? The removal of mandatory counseling, as a requirement for HIV testing, occurred years before.

Overwhelmed by thoughts of the future for my family and all the processes required for genetic testing, I wished the appointment involved crisis counseling. After all that I had been through, it was something dearly needed. I found myself with another crisis.

A crisis is what many of us are experiencing as we walk into medical offices to seek help to keep ourselves and our families alive. We need an incredible amount of support, along with information, the second we enter that clinic.

At the point, before diagnosis, our biggest worry is not whether others will discriminate against us. We are what we are. What is, is. And, what was, was. It is nothing shameful.

The big question is whether we have a hereditary syndrome, and how can we test thirteen people in a family, at $5,000 each, totaling $65,000 and be able to provide all of them with regular cancer screenings at $30,000 each, per year?

It was the point where I found myself centered, trapped at the level of the cost of testing of an entire family. Initially, what I needed was to receive a single order for a phlebotomist to take my blood and send it to a lab. It would have fulfilled my desperation to know why my family was dying of cancer. Nothing more. It was the first step and the only offer of the relief I needed from the sense of anxiety I felt. It was frustrating to experience the complicated levels of the standards of care to allow individuals to test for hereditary cancer syndromes.

That one mere act would have made the journey more straightforward. It might afford my family and myself to prevent cancer and live. The rest, including that cost, I could figure out later. I knew there had to be a way we could absorb that cost, with so many needing to test. At that point, I could have cared less whether someone may attempt to discriminate against me. My concern was whether we lived through a cancer diagnosis or died from it.

Fear of not being able to obtain affordable life insurance should not be a barrier to genetic testing. The average face of a life insurance policy bought in 2018 is $160,000, an equivalent of two years of average wages in California. The facts are we will have less risk of contracting severe life-threatening cancer than the average person, with genetic testing and regular cancer screenings. Most of us will never sustain a developed, serious cancer if we submit to routine cancer screenings.

Working toward legislation to provide affordable health insurance and lobbying our legislators for programs that will offer affordable genetic testing and cancer screening tests should be our priority. Everyone should be working toward it and taking steps to protect existing legislation that requires insurance companies to continue accepting those with pre-existing conditions.

If life insurance is still a priority, but difficult to obtain at reasonable rates, there are other options available. Homeownership is the first. It is wiser to invest in two smaller homes, rather than a large one. Renting one home out can pay its mortgage payments, often with the monthly costs far less than that of the monthly payment for an insurance policy, especially at a later age. There will always be a return upon the sale of a home. The costs of insurance premiums for life insurance increase with age and then expires. By owning two houses, one would not have to sell their principal residence in a time of crisis.

Those with an employer or union offered group life insurance policies can sometimes max out those policies or convert their group policy into an individual policy. Survivorship policies, as they are referred to by those in the insurance industry, can be obtained for both the husband and the wife. They must be used following the death of one or the other. The policyholder can then add a "spouses paid-up insurance purchase option" (SPPO rider) to a permanent policy that would cover the insurable spouse. When the spouse dies, the uninsurable spouse can buy a new premium plan within ninety days.

Guaranteed issue policies and simplified policies are those that require no medical examination. They come at a higher price, sometimes as much as a mortgage payment. An affinity plan is a group plan not requiring medical examinations. Credit life insurance can be obtained on big purchases to pay off homes and large bills and used as a financial buffer.

Purchasing cancer insurance and finding group insurances are also reasonable options. Fear of not getting life insurance, disability insurance, or home health care insurance should not be a concern or a deterrent to genetic testing when so many options exist.

But more importantly, it is especially so when the opportunity to dance at my grandchildren's weddings and to experience the births of their children will exist decades from now. The best way anyone can get around the difficulties getting health and life insurance is to secure employment that offers the benefits of group health and life insurance.

Concerning ourselves with what may occur "someday," when we die, it is not productive. Getting through today and tomorrow is. Essential for our survival is affordable genetic testing, regular cancer screenings, and obtaining affordable health care coverage.

It is far more reassuring and less costly to detect and remove cancer at an early stage than it is to spend years treating it with surgeries, radiation, and chemotherapy. The odds are only a few of us will experience full-blown cancer if regularly screened. It makes little sense not to get a genetic test because of difficulties obtaining life insurance. We need to focus on working together with legislation allowing for low-cost health insurance for our families.

Disheartened with the emphasis of the negative factors in the genetic counseling appointment, I tried to conceal my impatience for the end of the session, so she would give me a referral to be tested.

Steve and I continued to listen. When asked, I provided the cancer history of the paternal side of the family. My brother contracted colon cancer before the age of fifty. Our paternal aunt contracted two colon cancers and uterine cancer, two of which occurred before the age of fifty. Our father presented with ureter cancer, renal pelvis cancer, and esophageal cancer after age fifty, and with skin cancers at age forty. My brother, my aunt, and I had contracted colorectal cancer.

The death of our paternal grandfather in 1945 was the result of stomach cancer, and Lord knows what cancers family members contracted that were said to be "heart attacks" to protect them from eugenicists. My grandmother, grandfather, and father said all my grandfather's siblings died of cancer in the second and third decades of the 1900s, during their mid-fifties, except for one in his thirties.

Tumor testing of my tumors showed they were MSI-h, which meant a high number of genetic markers, known as microsatellites or SSRs, were present in my cells. It indicated the mismatch repair gene was not functioning normally. With it being unable to repair errors in DNA replication, rogue cells develop. They quickly evolve into tumors.

"See, it meets the guidelines of the Amsterdam criteria for genetic testing," I said.

I then related to her my mother's family history. She developed breast cancer in her early forties after *her* mother died of metastasized breast cancer in her forties, and *her* mother died of a stroke after contracting breast cancer. I added that Mom's father survived a bout with gastric cancer. The family history met the criteria for testing for BRCA 1 and BRCA 2 hereditary breast cancers. Not considered, I didn't mind. I didn't possess the skills to deal with another cancer syndrome.

"Can you get me your father's medical records, please?" the genetic counselor asked. My heart immediately filled with desperation.

Oh, my God. She is not going to refer me for a test!

Anxiety flooded, I wondered why she would postpone it until I provided my father's health records. The existence of cancer is prolific in our family history. It met the criteria set in the Amsterdam II standards, issued in 1999, two years following my father's death. It set the basic rules of care for referral for testing.

Had this occurred today, in 2019, I could have ordered a test online from Color Genomics, received it within a few days, swabbed my checks, and sent the DNA I collected back. Within a few weeks, a genetic counselor would have called if the test were positive, and I would have received my results by telephone, receiving genetic counseling then. This easy, straight forward process of genetic testing not only saves thousands in costs but ends the amount of time and cost for traveling for repeated consultations and reduces anxiety for patients.

Researching the genetic counselor's decision, I found her request was following the genetics standards set within the genetics organizations, at that time. Though it was more prohibitive than that listed within the basic standards of care, it was a procedure geneticists developed to collect research information..

Emory University and many other esteemed cancer centers also had a similar policy. It read something to the effect of, "The genetic counselor will take your pedigree (family history), request medical records on any family members with cancer, explain the significance of the cancer present in your family, discuss the role of genetics and environment in the development of cancer, and the availability of genetic testing."

Not considered by them were existing HIPPA regulations that disallowed the release of medical records of deceased individuals to anyone except by the executor of the estate. Many states forbid the release of medical records of the dead to others, in the absence of court intervention. They are often challenging to obtain.

The policies of the genetics community often required patients to pay thousands of dollars to obtain the medical records of those who are deceased, by forcing court action against their families as what we would have to do. No reasonable explanation existed to deny a lifesaving test to promote research. The anxiety it created was unforgivable. It presented an appearance that health care institutions and insurance companies were rationing genetic testing to those who are not only willing to pay the thousands of dollars for each test but only to those who can provide medical records of family members. Thankfully, the 2019 guidelines, issued this year, end these barriers.

What has occurred in the past imposes a boomerang effect upon the present. It includes events such as what we experienced that created distrust toward the genetic counseling profession.

In the past few years, the Lynch Syndrome Screening Network, a nationwide organization of genetic counselors, shared an online website that expressed an intent to access and collect patients' medical records without patient knowledge or permission. They planned to bank patient records in a Michigan State Public Health Department database without patient knowledge or consent. They were under the mistaken belief they were entitled to the files of patients since they "performed research."

This irreparably created patient distrust and lack of confidence in the privacy of medical records, accompanied by a lack of trust in specific institutions and counselors. The biggest backfire was it created doubt in the minds of patients who were considering genetic testing.

My mind whirled as I tried to figure out how to obtain a referral for genetic testing. As an investigator, I knew I had to have permission from the executor of Dad's estate to receive his medical records, according to HIPPA. But our father's spouse had cut off all contact with our father's first family before Dad's estate was settled. We needed a court order to access his health records. To get one, required hiring an attorney at $400 to $600 per hour, not including the cost of filings, court costs, and expenses.

A less expensive alternative would be to pay $5,000 in cash to a doctor and get the test through a commercial testing company, despite the contract with my HMO to provide that care. The delay created by having to leap over unnecessary hurdles was frustrating. Time means everything to those of us affected by hereditary cancer. Delays create anxiety. I was incredibly stressed and anxious while undergoing medical treatment. Anxiety and stress impose adverse effects on our body and feeds into cancer. The process had taken over six months to even get to a genetic counselor. Now we had to jump through hoops to obtain testing.

Complicating issues was Dad died eleven years earlier. There were no assurances that his medical records still existed. The average retention period for keeping them is five to ten years, thus the importance of making sure to obtain a copy of the results of every single medical visit and the lab and radiological test results of a deceased family member. It was not considered by the genetics community when developing policies requiring records of deceased family members to qualify for genetic testing.

Unfortunately, not being Lynch syndrome patients, genetic counselors do not have the real-life experiences of living with a hereditary disease as patients do. They do not see or understand the family dynamics that occur in the home. They do not realize each state's laws for time constraints for records and who can get them, and under what circumstances. The counselors do not know our family members or our children. Most have never lived in a home with people facing our circumstances.

Many are young women and men who are just out of college since the profession is young. Most do not have families and do not possess life experiences in dealing with family medical crises. They don't know how we live or the challenges we face. Nor is it often discussed during their two-year master's degree training. Its focus is upon science, not psychological counseling, or dealing with social issues. The responsibilities placed upon them to counsel do not meet state-mandated qualifications to provide the service.

"I may have to go to court to get it," I said.

"Be sure and let me know when it happens," she responded.

Deflated, we drove the thirty miles back home in silence. Trapped within an emotional storm over which we had little control over the ability to detect if we were affected by a hereditary cancer syndrome, I found myself overcome with a sense of hopelessness that we would ever find why our family was dying of cancer.

Today, thanks to the NCCN Hereditary Cancer Medical Panel, who establishes the basic standard of care procedures for the diagnosis of Lynch syndrome and to Color Genomics, which provides quality, affordable tests directly to the consumer, eliminating the many barriers to traditional testing that still exist.

Today, the primary issue faced by patients is the refusal of many counselors to allow the genetic testing of children, despite their parents' wishes. Throughout the internet, their writings state the genetic counselor is to assess the psychological state of the child and the parent. This is reckless.

The underlying influences involved in families can be messy. Human behavior is unpredictable and complicated. Unless one has extensive education and background of performing psychological assessment and counseling of individuals and families experiencing crises, they should not be doing it.

Most genetic counselors are not licensed under state regulations overseeing psychological counseling and are prohibited by law to perform such assessments of individuals and their family members.

The manner of how each of us our body reacts to situations is unpredictable. Every family and every person who is a part of it are different from one another. No one person is the same. Most genetic counselors do not possess the training or credentials to evaluate and diagnose patients and their families psychologically.

We, with Lynch syndrome, need the assistance of experts. Providing specific diet information is best left to nutritionists and endocrinologists who spend years studying and practicing what is best for those affected with cancer. Trained, licensed, and state credentialed psychologists, and social workers should provide psychological and crisis counseling.

Before instituting a policy, genetics and medical associations should be consulting an attorney to determine if what they are implementing complies with the laws of the federal government and those in each of the fifty states. There has been much advancement in genetic privacy legislation and addressing genetic information on state levels. Patient advocates should be involved in the dialogue to determine guidelines and standards of care for genetic testing. They offer great insight into what is of benefit and what is not, for individuals and families affected by hereditary cancer.

Delays are fine when conducting generalized research, but they can devastate patients when applying it to the everyday lives of people whose genetic counselors deny a diagnostic test, desiring to test their tumors for Lynch syndrome. It is especially so if the patient is waiting for genetic testing results. With pending surgeries, a clock is ticking. Delays in the genetic counseling processes can result in the type of surgery needed, the extent of the surgery, and in extreme cases, the difference between life and death.

Entrapped in a Catch-22, if my family were to survive, I was willing to do what my health care system desired to get it. I did not want to deal with emotional conflict and engage in a three-year court battle to obtain it. Not only would that create more family dysfunction, but my family and I could not afford that to occur on top of all the emotional issues involved in a family with hereditary cancers.

I had no other choice. Once home, I went to work on trying to obtain my father's records. First, I called the facility where Dad received treatment. The custodian of records said it was doubtful eleven-year-old records existed. If they did, federal governmental regulations of HIPPA required I would need the executor's permission to access them.

I wrote a letter to my father's youngest son, asking if he could obtain the records for us from his mother or his sister, the executors of Dad's estate. I explained the situation and the reason behind getting them. We waited for weeks, with no response. It was heartbreaking. Two vastly different messages were sent. Ours relayed a desperate need to obtain lifesaving information for the members of our family. His lack of response that telegraphed he cared less if we lived or died. It was clear someone did not want us to have access to our father's medical records. We knew why. It had nothing to do with us.

Medical records tell a personal story about a person that they may wish to keep between their physicians and themselves. It may be for treatments they received for infections or some other sensitive medical condition.

For those who lived during the days of eugenics, it tells the stories of mandatory or voluntary sterilizations which can affect relationships with adopted children and force parents to reveal the true parentage of their children, or it can tell the story of unwanted pregnancies and other sensitive matters.

Demanding medical records creates a complicated and emotional situation for everyone involved in a family, especially for those needing medical records that can ensure survival for loved ones. This ugly situation with our stepmother, her oldest daughter, and their son was painful.

A few years later, Steve and I visited Carson City. Standing on the street, watching the Nevada Day parade, I glanced up and saw my brother walking toward us. Steve and I stood quietly, watching as he approached. Our eyes met. Upon seeing us, my brother's eyes flashed with fear. Immediately, he grabbed his new bride's hand and turned around, disappearing around the corner. There was no doubt he felt immense guilt for what he had done to our family and me.

My heart broke for him. He was the one person in Dad's second family appearing to have a spark of compassion. Dad would have been disappointed in him and his sisters, with what happened after his death.

A few years after Dad died, our mail carrier delivered a registered letter addressed to me. The return address reflected "Emerald Bay Boats," the company my father once owned. I broke into tears upon seeing it.

"It is from my father's business," I told the carrier. "He built beautiful, hand-crafted wooden boats. It closed when he died a few years ago. I don't know who sent this."

I returned it to the unknown sender. Nothing mattered to us except the importance of honoring Dad's requests, allowing his grandchildren to realize he *did* care about them. Despite Dad stating it occurred, no notification in compliance with state law was ever made to those children or their parents by the executors of his will.

The last step in the complicated process of obtaining a genetic test was to speak to an attorney and to prepare to take my Dad's second family to court to get my father's medical records if they still existed. None of them were related to him. It shouldn't have mattered.

Realizing it might be the last gasp available route in getting genetic testing, allowing us to protect *my* family and *my* children from the family cancer syndrome. The attorney said it would take months to even get into a courtroom, and years to resolve. The costs would be over ten thousand dollars. Money wasn't the issue. It was many could die by then.

From this, we learned when a family member dies of cancer, make sure to have the medical records released to you from the family or the executor of the estate, *at once*. Waiting can be devastating. Estates and money bring out the worst in people. Immediately, obtaining them can save time and the lives of loved ones.

Several weeks later, I contacted the genetic counselor, relaying to her that I would go to court to protect my family and their lives, but it would be at a prohibitive cost, to our family. I was still seeking other alternatives. If she could not do it, I stated we would deal with the HMO later.

"We can just move forward now," she offered.

A month later, we received a telephone call. "Would you like your results now?" the genetic counselor asked.

"Please," I answered, sitting down, and holding my breath.

"It came back positive for Lynch syndrome with an MSH2 mutation," she said.

My eyes filled with tears. A ton of weight lifted from my shoulders. The news was bittersweet, a blessing and a curse. Nobody wants to have a hereditary cancer condition, but if they do, they need to know how to prevent the cancers that are certain to come so they may be able to protect themselves and their families.

Today, genetic testing has evolved well past most of the barriers that we experienced. Hopefully, it will never occur with anyone else, especially with the available options for obtaining online direct-to-consumer testing, which is now available.

Recent research at Sloan Kettering Memorial Hospital in New York has evidenced half those whose tumors reflect MSI-h (high) or MSI-I (intermediate) did not meet the testing criteria for Lynch syndrome. Many others were denied testing because of strict standards, like us.

The availability of direct-to-consumer testing, and the new National Comprehensive Cancer Network standards of care issued in the spring of 2019, for the diagnostic testing for Lynch syndrome, have ended the barriers that negatively affected those with Lynch syndrome and that previously denied many of genetic testing.

The new standards of care issued by Lynch syndrome experts working with the National Comprehensive Cancer Network are shared below, exactly as published. A medical professional or genetics professional will determine if a patient should be tested if:

1) A diagnosis of a known Lynch syndrome pathogenic variant exists in the family;

2) A person whose tumor shows evidence of a mismatch repair (MMR) deficiency by microsatellite instability or loss of MMR expression should be tested.

3) Those with colorectal or endometrial cancer should be tested who meet *any one or more of* the following: A) <fifty years and diagnosed with specific Lynch syndrome cancers; B) or diagnosed with another Lynch syndrome cancer; C) or having a first-degree or second-degree relatives with a Lynch syndrome-related cancer diagnosed <50 years of age: D) or a first-degree or second-degree relative regardless of age.

4) Possessing a colorectal tumor with MSI-high histology (i.e., presence of tumor-infiltrating lymphocytes, Crohn's-like lymphocytic reaction, mucinous/signet ring differentiation, or medullary growth pattern).

The guidelines also read that genetic testing should be prescribed for individuals who meet any of the following criteria:

1. Having an initial-degree relative with colorectal or endometrial cancer diagnosed <50 years old, *or*

2. Having a first-degree relative with colorectal or endometrial cancer and another synchronous or metachronous LS related cancer; *or*

3. Having a first term or second- degree relative with an LS related cancer, including more than one diagnosed <50 years old; *or*

4. a first degree or second-degree relative with an LS related cancer, regardless of age.

These guidelines are important to know when seeking testing for one's self or their family members. Be sure and often check for updates. I cannot express enough my appreciation for the NCCN panel's decision for the need of physicians to test *tumors* of those presenting with cancers. It is not only to find if a hereditary cancer condition exists but can also determine a personalized treatment that will be most effective in annihilating that cancer. Tumor testing, in concert with testing based upon assessments of family history, is lifesaving. These policies developed by the NCCN Panel will help many with Lynch syndrome cancers to survive.

The panel at the NCCN and the quality, pioneering online, direct to consumer testing company, Color Genomics, have resolved most of the barriers to genetic testing that have existed in the past and will hopefully end much of the paternalism that previously existed in traditional genetic counseling. Those processes required two to three days off work and loss of wages to obtain a simple laboratory test. Many did not return to receive their test results.

Besides the enormous costs of over four-thousand dollars for traditional testing and the time-intensive processes required, it is more problematic, time-consuming, and expensive for the patient to get diagnosed for Lynch syndrome than it is to be diagnosed with a heart condition. Today's new standards of care have resolved most barriers except for costs.

Addressing the concerns and the needs for the dissemination of public awareness and physician information on Lynch syndrome, silos exist that are affecting positive communication. Involving the genetics community, medical professionals, and patient advocacy organizations, because of silos, they are every bit as ineffective as they were when we left Lynch syndrome International in 2014. These silos create an enormous barrier disallowing Lynch syndrome diagnoses and treatment.

This silo mentality exists when entities that rely upon one another to work successfully and to share information about resources, priorities, and processes to protect patients and families against Lynch syndrome, break down, and fail.

Failing to work together to share information disallows for the education of the medical community and the public. When the knowledge of one segment of an integral part of a system never reaches another, it is a tremendous problem; and it is detrimental to human lives. Coupled with past genetic testing procedures, and the prohibitive costs of traditional genetic counseling and testing, these factors have presented themselves to be the primary reasons it has taken so long for patients to become diagnosed with a hereditary cancer syndrome. It is why some patients have given up on the system and died.

The 2020 standards of care, determined by the NCCN for diagnosing Lynch syndrome, is promising for our families and our futures. Now, it is time for the testing companies to reduce the costs of their tests and for the genetics departments to embrace all for genetic testing by raising funding to assist those without resources.

The quality direct-to-consumer testing by Color Genomics has resolved the barriers to patient access to genetic testing by providing quality genetic testing, at a low cost, for our families.

Chapter Twenty-Eight

CREATING A MEDICAL TEAM

Everybody knows there is no such thing as normal. There is no black and white definition of normal. Normal is subjective. There's only a messy, inconsistent, silly, hopeful version of how we feel most at home in our lives. —Tori Spelling

I completed my final chemotherapy treatment in October 2008. My body could only tolerate six or seven treatments with FOLFOX. I finished the remaining sessions with Xeloda (capecitabine), an oral treatment ingested in pill form that turns into 5-FU within the body for the final sessions.

Realizing Xeloda might not work, as research efforts had not proven 5-FU to be an effective treatment against the cancers created by the mismatch repair gene errors seen in Lynch syndrome, my oncologist and I decided to take a chance. Despite its "hit or miss" reputation, it was, at that time, a generalized standard in chemotherapy treatment. We hoped that the six or seven sessions of FOLFOX that I was able to tolerate, completed with follow-up Xeloda treatments, would destroy any remaining cancer in the margins and the seven remaining inches of my colon.

With chemotherapy completed and over in October, Steve and I planned to continue our tradition of hosting Thanksgiving dinners for our family. Still not having the strength to stand for extended periods, I sat on a kitchen stool and coached as he cooked.

Teamwork had kept our family together over the past eighteen months. Having everyone back together for the holidays was an emotional experience. As I sat at our table surrounded by those we loved, I felt immense gratitude for being able to spend one more year of Thanksgiving dinners in our home.

Thanksgiving is a time of gratitude. We had much to be grateful for that first year and for all those that followed. First, we were thankful for our physicians and all the others who worked with us through a challenging time. We were also grateful that following chemotherapy, there was not any evidence of disease. The fear we experienced for After saying grace, a family tradition is for everyone at the table to make a statement of gratitude for something special in their lives. That first dinner following my diagnosis was quiet and respectful. Not so, the next year. Our children and grandchildren were more than comfortable discussing Lynch syndrome.

Taking turns, going around the table sharing expressions of gratitude became a comedic free-for-all with one grandchild wanting to give my remains to science so he could see the look upon the face of the poor medical student who opened me up to find nothing inside. Today, that comedian is a police officer and a risk-taker like the rest of us. He was the first not to be affected by Lynch syndrome. We were thrilled.

Another stated, "I am grateful Grandma has improved herself to the point that she is now correctly using a semicolon." That came from a granddaughter who is positive and who possesses faith in hope in her future. She is now pursuing her Ph.D. at one of Europe's oldest and finest universities.

The third is an aspiring lawyer, who laughed with the rest, and then made a pretty decent plea to the family to please exercise mercy with poor, old Grandma. She ended it, stating that the "Hooligans," as our grandchildren are fondly dubbed by us, to have some respect for their elders. Everyone roared at that thought.

Sitting at that table, I realized Lynch syndrome was not going to keep any member of our family down. Being able to laugh showed that most of us had adapted to experiencing the uncertainty of living within a hereditary cancer family. It showed how much can change in a year when hope exists.

We celebrated a second quiet Christmas as I still had not yet recovered from the accumulated effects of chemotherapy. It would take a while to dissipate. Winter arrived. As we tucked inside, it was a time for reflection and hope. If chemo worked and the colorectal cancer cells in my bloodstream died, all would be well. Only time could tell. We would not know for at least five years, and even then, a lifetime of uncertainty would still exist.

But I was the queen of denial wishing for full remission after five years of no evidence of disease (NED), so I could again "be normal." I was waiting for that time when I would "be cured." Yet, in my heart, I knew there was no cure. Our genetic mutation continues to produce defective genes that the mismatch repair gene tries to repair and cannot. Tumors develop from those rogue genes that form.

For a year or two, following the diagnosis of Lynch syndrome, I planned our future with that five-year goal in mind. I was waiting for the day when the threat of cancer would be "behind me." Those wishes occurred when I was undergoing chemotherapy treatments or when I wanted the risk of cancer to be "over." I knew what I wished for did not exist. We do not have the luxury of "cures" or remissions. Cancer is never "behind us." Regular screenings are lifesaving. We must exercise caution and make changes in our lifestyles that give us an edge in eliminating recurrences.

A 2011 study performed by Daniel Edelstein et al., at Johns Hopkins determined the dwell time for Lynch syndrome polyps to be 49 months and 57 months for advanced adenoma and colorectal cancer, respectively. The good news is the five-year survival rate for Lynch syndrome patients with colorectal cancer is at ninety-six percent. Countering that is a study showing a 40% risk exists of a second primary colorectal cancer within seven years of the first tumor.

There is no "getting back to normal" following cancer. Susan Morris, a Lynch syndrome cancer survivor from Australia, related that her physicians kept urging her not to be impatient. Following treatments, she *would* get back to normal. I do not doubt that it is their wish for her. Everyone who knows us wishes so much that it would be over, and we will return to the same level of health, as it was before contracting cancer. They do not realize it is impossible. Living with Lynch syndrome requires a permanent change in our lifestyles.

Susan put it this way, "One of my bybears is people suggesting that life can get back to normal. There is no going back, only an adaptation to a new normal."

Those of us with Lynch syndrome are continually adapting to change and circumstances. Each new diagnosis of cancer that we or a loved one contracts require us to adapt to accept the diagnosis, to learn about the specific disease, and the treatment involved in resolving it. Being able to adapt is critical to the goal of survival.

We can reduce those odds by taking the initiative to prevent cancer's development. Our genes are not going to change naturally. They will continue to create errors, and those errors can eventually develop into cancer. What we can do is everything possible to make certain cancer does not grow; by making lifestyle changes, reducing stress, eliminating environmental risks, drinking plenty of water, eating a proper diet, and exercising. It all contributes to fighting cancer.

By focusing on this, my brother has lived eighteen years without a second cancer, and I have lived thirteen. We have both beat the odds of contracting another cancer, so far, by being proactive.

Often, I hear from others, "How are you doing now? Are you in remission?" When I explain remission does not exist for us, it is difficult for them to accept. They do not understand we must always adhere to regular cancer screening schedules and remain alert to changes in our bodies to avoid cancer. There are always some defective cells developing in our bodies that may develop into a cancerous tumor. Regular, ongoing cancer screenings are *our* "life insurance."

"But you are okay now, aren't you?" they ask, seeking reassurance. "You *are* in remission, right?"

We are never in "remission." According to the National Cancer Institute, the definition of remission is "a decrease in or disappearance of signs and symptoms of cancer. In partial remission, some, but not all of that may have disappeared. In complete remission, it is not in existence, through cancer may still be in the body."

Since our mismatch repair genes are defective, we always have errors that occur in cell replication. Tumors may develop, but many early tumors do not survive. The occasional one that does and develops into cancer is the one we want our physicians to find, as well as the polyps, adenomas, and tumors before they become full-blown cancers. Therefore, the importance of regular screenings to detect and remove those tumors is paramount to our survival, since Lynch syndrome cancers show aggressive growth. The preventative screenings are our "superpower." Make sure to consult with your physicians and get those regular screenings, doing what our body cannot do with these rogue cells that survive. In doing so, we have less chance of contracting cancer than the average person.

Don't let anyone tell you that eating a healthy diet, getting sleep, reducing stress, eliminating environmental causes that promote cancer development, and getting regular cancer screenings to minimize odds of getting cancer won't make a difference. There is little we can do for the predisposition of the risk of cellular defects, but there is much we can do to thwart cancer development. Lifestyle changes offer us a dramatic advantage.

The difference between now and when we grew up then, is Lynch syndrome did not have a name or a treatment. Not knowing what we were fighting made it difficult to understand how to battle it. Today, we have both a name for our hereditary condition and treatment. Knowledge is power: Power to fight it or the ability to fight systems needing change so we can live.

My method of coping is to live each day as vibrantly as possible, pay attention to the warning signs in my body, stay current with my screenings, and to leave the future worries of health issues to my physicians. It makes it easier to handle.

If positive for Lynch syndrome, be sure and get treatment and regular screenings at a specialized cancer center or a large institutional health center that conducts research. It is where you will find experts in diagnosing Lynch syndrome and prescribing regular screenings personalized for the patient rather than focusing on one generalized treatment for all. Substantial numbers of qualified physicians are available to put together a comprehensive medical team, and advanced technology exists to detect cancers at an early stage. In those institutions, a strong understanding and updated knowledge of our health risks exist.

No matter where I go, I always meet someone affected by a hereditary family condition or another rare inherited disease that is life-threatening. In our New Mexico neighborhood of twenty homes, four of us have received a diagnosis of an inherited cancer syndrome. They say one in every ten persons is affected by one. Where we live during the summer, it is one in five. Therefore, I suspect it may be more, especially since seventy percent of rare diseases are hereditary. We are just one of the more fortunate in that we now have speedy and thorough diagnostic technology, sound preventative methods, and effective treatments for our cancers.

One of those treatments, Keytruda, manufactured by Merck, is an immunological method of battling cancer tumors that present as MSI-h, as our cancers do. Today, Merck is collaborating with other pharmaceutical companies on expanding this new treatment, which is especially promising for those with MSI-h tumors.

Just yesterday, I heard of another promising treatment from Susan, who has been to hell and back with a second late-stage cancer. Suffering from tumors that were not resectable, the future was appearing bleak. There seemed to be no treatment opportunities with Keytruda for her in Australia, and the state of her health made it impossible to fly to the United States to be involved in clinical trials. Her physicians tried Durvalumab.

It is an FDA-approved immunotherapy for cancer, developed by Medimmune/AstraZeneca. As Keytruda, it too blocks the programmed cell death ligand 1 (PD-L1) with PD-1

"I could immediately feel it hitting the tumors… and soon I could walk, stand, sleep, and lie down, pain-free," she advised. Today, she is showing no evidence of cancer, though she is dealing with the aftereffects of cancer and cancer treatment and is undergoing maintenance therapy.

In 2007, when I contracted cancer, the treatment options available for our cancers were resection, standard FOLFOX type chemotherapy for all, 5-FU, radiation treatments, and prayer.

Today, researchers are performing considerable research. In existence in the pharmaceutical pipelines are treatments delivered through a system using small molecules, which may, one day, allow the administration of treatments in pill form rather than infusion. The future of the treatment of hereditary cancers is hopeful.

These research studies have occurred because of the efforts of Vice-President Joe Biden and his Moonshot program. Drugs such as Keytruda have been fast-tracked through the FDA. In 2014, the White House instituted funding for the genetic testing of younger people with colorectal cancer, resulting in many with Lynch syndrome living today.

Working to prevent future cancers is a lifelong endeavor of adapting to change. My medical team is invaluable in helping me work through that process. As time elapses, I can sit at my desk for more extended periods. The chemo brain has improved, allowing reprieve. I can read and work for a few hours per day. As the months and years have passed, even eleven years after completing chemotherapy, I continue to improve.

To live with Lynch syndrome, I had to confront what I was facing, the same as I confronted dangerous situations during my career. Realizing I could not do it alone, when I worked or became ill, I needed people I could rely upon and trust to back me up. I had to assess my medical team and make sure it included compassionate and capable physicians who would do the same.

The priority was finding a general practitioner who would ensure I would have access to regular, life-saving cancer screenings. He would be the captain of the team. As a gateway physician, I would see him regularly. He would assess my symptoms if I were not feeling well to determine the root base and make referrals to specialists.

The ombudsman at my Kaiser health facility said. "I think you should consider a doctor named Chris Walker for your medical team."

Dr. Christopher Walker, an Air Force officer, had accepted a position at Kaiser Permanente as a family practitioner. At once, I called his office and asked if he had experience treating patients with Lynch syndrome. Within a minute, his assistant returned to the telephone.

"He said he hasn't treated anyone with it, but he knows how to manage it and can make certain you get the right screenings."

A surge of relief swept through me. It sounded good and offered what I needed. Few family doctors knew of Lynch syndrome. He was one.

I researched his background. Bright, respected, and well-liked, he was a father and a husband who dedicates himself to his family. Easygoing and active, he is thorough in his examinations and is compassionate. He enjoys writing for medical journals. The airmen and their families treated respected and liked him. His passion was running. He bought his running shoes downtown at a specialty store.

"If he runs, he'll want exercise from me," I groaned. It was difficult for me to garner the self- discipline necessary to participate in an intense exercise program, which is a plus to people like us. Not only does it work the heart and muscles, but it builds confidence.

Dr. Walker sounded too good to be true. A great family practitioner is invaluable to families, and the ombudsman was impressed with him. His caseload was filling up. In all fairness, exercise was something I needed. I scheduled an appointment.

While sitting on his examination table, my heart raced with the symptoms of PTSD. Since my cancer diagnosis, it was occurring more often when I attended medical appointments and chemotherapy treatments. PTSD symptoms are common among cancer patients.

The examination room came alive with vibrant energy as a tall, middle-aged, smiling man entered.

Chalk one up for him. He is positive.

"Hi, I'm Chris Walker. My specialty is caring for families. I even deliver babies. And I *am* familiar with hereditary and familial cancers,"

Chalk up another one. He is a family man. He will understand the challenges my family and I face with hereditary cancer.

"I've been working here at Kaiser Permanente for a while, and I have correctional officers and police officers as patients. I enjoy caring for them, and my family and I like living here."

Chalk yet another one up for him. He read my file, every bit of it going back, all twenty-seven years of my medical history with Kaiser.

It had been sixteen years since I moved on from Corrections. He knew where I worked and what I did, and he knew I had been in a shooting incident and had PTSD. He had far exceeded my minimum criteria. What he said next clenched the deal.

"And I understand you have had a very difficult year," he said.

Tears welled in my eyes and a lump formed in my throat. An incredible sense of relief swept within me. I at once trusted him.

He is compassionate.

"Linda, there's something that concerns me, though," he said. "Your blood glucose levels may indicate diabetes. Is there a history of it in your family?

People in my family don't live long enough to get diabetes.

"Not that I know of," I answered, surprised. Once home, I reviewed my medical records and noted the high glucose levels developed while undergoing chemotherapy. Further investigation revealed diabetes and a fatty liver might be side effects from taking the chemotherapy drug 5-FU (5 fluorouracil), with ten percent of patients contracting diabetes.

Developing both diabetes and a fatty liver increased my odds of contracting cancer and developing heart disease. People with diabetes have a 22% risk of contracting colorectal cancer. To prevent it, I reduce my intake of sugar and refined carbs, avoid foods that would boost my insulin level and take medications and a few supplements.

Developing both, I regretted not scheduling an appointment to see Dr. Walker earlier. With his level of knowledge and practice of conducting a thorough examination, we may have been able to head it off. I regretted drinking a lot of fruit juice while undergoing chemo. I have no doubt it contributed to it, I was wallowing in self-pity when that little voice piped up again from inside, intervening.

No big deal. You will adapt to this too.

With Dr. Walker scheduling preventative procedures and being "the Captain" of my medical team and Dr. Martin dealing with any gastric issues, worry dissipated. I still needed a good dermatologist for the skin cancers my brother and father have battled, as well as a great urologist to screen us for the urinary tract cancers of our father.

Dr. Suzanne Generao came highly recommended by everyone at Kaiser. She is outstanding and, like Dr. Martin, still cares for those of our family who are residing in California.

Today, at MD Anderson/Banner Health, I receive care from a world-class medical team. Dr. Boris Naraev, who is involved in clinical research, is our consultant. My endocrinologist, Iram Ahmad, has carefully teased out and balanced my cancer-related issues of heart disease and diabetes. She coordinates the team and my screening needs. Rounding out the care team is a wonderfully upbeat and energetic urologist, Chinedu Mmeje, who is passionate about Lynch syndrome. He screens me for the urothelial cancers that took the life of my father and for those frequently seen in the MSH-2 mutation. Completing the team is our passionate and positive gastroenterologist, Prathab Devaraj. When he skips into the surgical clinic in the morning, and I am ready and waiting for my screenings, I can't help but feel upbeat and positive with his great attitude and level of competence. Our blessing has been to have two incredible teams of physicians who have kept me healthy and vital for the past thirteen years.

Chapter Twenty-Nine

WOMEN'S CANCERS AND PREVENTION

The Italians having a proverb, he that deceives me once, it's his fault, but twice is my fault. —Anthony Weldon

During the spring of 2009, I sat upon more than my share of medical examination tables. With chemotherapy completed, the next step was to prepare for a cancer-free life. Waiting for the cumulative side effects of chemotherapy to dissipate, I was anxious to schedule a prescribed hysterectomy and removal of my ovaries and fallopian tubes.

Women with Lynch syndrome face up to a sixty-five percent risk of contracting uterine cancer and a thirteen percent risk of contracting ovarian cancer. The recommended guidelines for women dictate they should submit to a total abdominal hysterectomy and a bilateral oophorectomy (removal of bilateral ovaries) following childbearing years. The risk of contracting women's cancers was high. Past that age and living on borrowed time, I was not looking forward to another surgery or even discussing it with my gynecologist.

Despite being one of the three physicians with whom I shared my family history, and who provided the order to allow me to get my blood drawn and sent into a hereditary-cancer research project in Ohio, my gynecologist did not refer me for genetic testing. Had he done so, I would have been receiving regular cancer screenings and never would have contracted a later staged cancer. I was upset with him.

Grumbling, I fumbled with the buttons of my clothing as I sat upon the bed. Getting dressed was a challenge. My fingers were numb, my feet ached, and my balance was unstable due to the neuropathy contracted during chemotherapy.

"Why does everything have to take effort?" I mumbled as I struggled to zip up and button my jeans.

When going somewhere, I had to start my day an hour earlier to allow more time to prepare to leave the house. Knowing it would continue until I recovered, all I wanted to be my "old self again, though, with us, it is impossible. There's no going back, just forward.

While recovering, it was essential to keep my head in the right place to get through it all. I made myself consider treatment of cancer as a "minor inconvenience," reminding myself it could be worse.

The stamina I once had no longer existed. I could not lift my arms to brush my hair without having to rest halfway in-between, and I could still smell the odor of chemotherapy releasing through my skin, necessitating bathing several times a day.

Sitting in my gynecologist's sterile examination room, with my legs dangling over the edge of the examination table, I noted that he appeared as uncomfortable having to see me as I felt having to see him.

Perched on his stool, he alternated between running his fingers through his goatee and focusing upon his lap as he spoke, watching his thumbnail rubbing beneath his other nails, instead of looking up at me while speaking. It was clear he did not want to be there, either.

He was one of the two physicians who, for years, knew about my fear of cancer yet did not stay on top of women's issues with hereditary cancer syndromes and was not interested in prescribing genetic testing for anyone. The reasons did not matter. The fact is he did not protect me.

However, little choice existed for me. I had to see *him*. He was the chief in charge of the gynecological department, and everything would go through him, anyway. There was no avoiding it.

"You say here your mother had cancer?" he asked.

"She had a breast tumor removed," I again told him, as I had done every time that I had seen him during the past two decades. "They described it as emerging cancer."

"Emerging cancer?"

"Yes."

"Not full cancer?"

"I don't know," I answered. I didn't know what a full cancer was, but I was familiar with emerging cancers. They were cancerous cells that were developing into a tumor in my mother's body.

"Well, what did she die of?"

"I don't know."

"You do not know how your mother died?" he asked, shaking his head in amazement.

"No, I don't," I answered, shaking my head back at him.

His questioning felt like a confrontation. An uncomfortable silence prevailed as he sighed and typed something into his computer. In the past twenty years, I had told him about Mom's breast cancer, and what we knew of her death. I declined to take hormonal therapy due to it. We had discussed her life and death during earlier appointments. Her sensitivity and allergies to medications were worrisome. Her family's history of breast cancer concerned us.

I knew nothing about my mother and her life except for what I could glean from her in two brief conversations by phone, one in the summer of 1982 and one in 1984, twenty-five years earlier when she needed information for a court matter. When she called in 1982, I did not expect her voice.

"Mom, where are you?" I asked, my voice breaking.

"We are here in Spain," she answered, her voice restrained.

"We didn't know where you were."

"Lindy, we're in the book," she said, as though she was living across town and not four thousand miles away, on an island in the Mediterranean Sea. "Some bad men tried to do some terrible things to us," she added, justifying her immediate departure.

It was clear that Mom was facing severe mental health issues. It broke my heart, hearing her speak like a child. My doctor would never understand that. He could never even fathom the circumstances of what my family or I lived with due to our mother's addiction.

However, none of that mattered anymore. My mother was dead. Chuck and our adopted sister were in the wind. Hospital records on the Mediterranean island where she lived showed one medical visit in the late 1970s. She received care elsewhere, on another island, or in Barcelona. Medical records were confidential and unavailable, but I was able to obtain access to them, anyway. They were easier to get than her death certificate has been to locate. Upon request, we received no response. And, here I was, sitting in his office, again faced with all the irrelevant questions and comments he had repeatedly asked over the past twenty years.

Diagnosed with Lynch syndrome, I needed preventative surgery to stay alive. As I sat in that examination room, my gut sank deeper as uncomfortable tension filled the room. I figured the base of his hostility was due to litigation I filed due to the delayed diagnosis. It addressed the fact I had told him and others of our family history of cancer.

He *was* one of the three who did not know about Lynch syndrome. I wrote my family history on the form we had to fill out every time I saw him. He should have known. The chief of gynecology and obstetrics, I had believed him when he promised to monitor me for cancer.

It took a minute for him to soften up. At least he looked at me when he asked, "Linda, can you do me a favor? Can you tell me more about this Lynch syndrome?"

I felt guilty for coming down so hard on him. The guy thought about how calloused his comment was. He could have felt bad because he did not know much about LS. Every reason to rationalize his actions and comments flew through my mind. I had to remind myself it was not *my* responsibility to second guess what he knew or did not know. *He* was the doctor.

"It's the result of a gene defect…"

"Like BRCA1 and 2?" he interrupted.

"Not really," I said. "There is a lot more risk for different cancers with Lynch syndrome. For example, the risk of colon cancer is…"

"But there are also real risks of cancers with BRCA 1 and 2," he again interrupted.

"BRCA 1 or 2 is irrelevant," I uttered, frustrated with his interruptions. "I know all about it. Please listen about Lynch syndrome and what I need from you to live," I begged.

He glared at me. My stomach again dropped. As I sat silent, my eyes remained intent upon his.

Take a step back.

"I need a total abdominal hysterectomy with a bilateral Salpingo-oophorectomy," I said, keeping eye contact.

"Why?" he asked.

Oh, my God! You do not know by now? How could you not know?

I had just spent eight months going through hell, fighting for my life because of a later stage cancer that occurred after he claimed to be "monitoring" it. I spent a month in the hospital, followed by taking part in hellacious chemotherapy treatments, and he *still* did not know the specifics of my risk of future cancers?

"It's a basic standard of care," I said, mustering every bit of restraint I had. "I have more than a sixty percent lifetime risk of contracting uterine and endometrial cancer, and a thirteen percent risk of ovarian cancer."

"I could monitor you," he again offered as he had promised me years before I contracted cancer.

What?

I could feel the roots of my hair standing on end. I cocked my head at him as our eyes locked.

"Are we going to go through this again?

"All right," he relented, breaking the silence. "There are people ahead of you. There's a long waiting list."

"I can do that. It will give me a chance to rest."

"There are people out there who are far more ill than you," he said.

Whoa! First, was a comment intended to make me feel like a bad daughter for not knowing how my mother died, and then this?

"I realize that. But, do you realize you did not say one word about the last year and a half? Not one question, and from what I gather, you have not even read my file. You know nothing about me or about the medical problems I am facing," I said, rising and collecting my purse.

"You'll get a call when there's an opening," he called out as I left.

A few months later, I underwent gynecological surgery. Not only was my uterus, fallopian tubes, and ovaries removed but also the cervix. It was the gynecologist's recommendation. I appreciated it. Despite his marginal patient skills, he was an expert surgeon.

I remained in the hospital for about twenty-six hours. It was far too long. Hospitals are not good places for healthy people who are seeking interventions to stay healthy. They are where sick people go. I was not ill, nor did I wish to be. It was a procedure to enhance life. The sooner I could get home, the better. My odds of a successful recovery would improve with an early release.

When my daughter saw him, after his experiences with me, she asked if she should submit to genetic testing, telling him her mother had Lynch syndrome. She stated he recommended she not test.

When physicians face difficulty listening to patients, often it is because they are busy, tired, distracted, contemplating a severe case, or thinking about someone they are about to see.

Today, they face intense pressure to keep their visits under fifteen minutes. If they do not meet your needs, speak with them. There is nothing wrong with discussing concerns with your doctor. It is only fair. We have too much at stake to close doors on those who do good. On the other hand, it is not only necessary but potentially lifesaving to leave the care of a marginal physician who is not providing the care we need.

Chapter Thirty

DEALING WITH CHANGE

As to diseases, make a habit of two things —
to help, or at least, to do no harm.
—Hippocrates

S ometimes it takes something serious to shake up our lives and bring about change. No longer was I dependent, nor was I reliant upon just any doctor to care for members of our family or me. Nor would I ever again settle for "any doctor."

Kaiser Permanente has spent the past decade doing an incredible job with physician recruitment. Following my diagnosis, great specialists appeared out of the woodwork—each one upbeat, confident, competent, and compassionate. It is only because of them and of the outstanding medical team at Banner Health-MD Anderson in the past few years that I am living well today. I am grateful for the great physicians and nurses who have cared for our family. I no longer felt a sense of uncertainty with an outstanding medical team.

There is nothing like navigating through decades of fear and finally feeling the release of its grip, later spending each day with immense gratitude for the gift of life. Words cannot express the joy of creating memories that last longer than the one afternoon of sitting in a meadow of wildflowers or soaking one's feet in a bubbling creek with a loved one. Nothing can compare to the newfound appreciation for the overwhelming love felt while holding new life in your arms, dancing at your children's weddings, or listening to the laughter of loved ones as they gather at the table, and no longer having to wonder about their futures. There is nothing more empowering than having a fighting chance at life.

A few weeks after undergoing my hysterectomy and the third major surgery, which followed six months of chemotherapy over a total period of eighteen months, Steve and I took a break from everything and traveled to Kauai to relax, decompress, and spend time with Aunt Marcella. I wanted to remove the memories of two years spent in surgery after surgery, recovery after recovery, and enduring the painful treatments. It was time to replace it all with positivity.

Our eighty-two-year-old aunt and I were both recovering and learning to live with the long-termed effects of colorectal cancer treatments together. She survived two earlier cancers. Her age and experience offered a wealth of information on how to live with uncertainty.

The few days of peace were heavenly. Spending time in a stress-free environment and eating healthy made a difference. I felt great. I loved watching Steve duck in and out of waves while I sifted my toes through warm sand and read. The water was too cold for one with neuropathy but relaxing on a beach or the bank of a river felt soothing.

"Lindy, want to try this?" Steve asked, handing me a brochure on zip lining he picked up at Princeville Ranch. I read it, set it down, discounting it, and then, upon second thought, picked it up again. It tugged at my heart.

"Come on; you know you do," he teased.

"Wanting to do it and being able to do it are two different things," I said as my fingers toyed with the brochure. I needed something extreme, challenging, and that might revitalize empowerment.

"Okay, let's check it out," I answered.

The afternoon involved four and one-half hours of hiking up and down slopes, to and from nine zip lines. The final zip line was provocative. Dubbed "King Kong," it boasted twenty-six-foot-high tower to climb, leap off and fly across 1,200 feet of double zip lines extending over an enormous canyon.

"I don't know if I have the stamina to hike miles of hills," I said to Steve. "And what about my port?"

A group of army officers, physicians assigned to the base outside Honolulu, were sharing our table. They overheard our conversation. "It's upper-weight bearing. You should be fine," one military surgeon interjected, looking up at Steve, in support. "Girl, you can do this!"

A few bathrooms existed along the trail. In between, there was always prayer. My colon was not as cooperative as my heart wished it to be. A commercial airline pilot and my husband both offered to drag me back up the hill if my stamina gave out. Steve's eyes caught mine.

"All right," I relented.

Caving in, I hoped it would not be something I would regret. It was one challenging afternoon, full of fun and laughter, though it was far from easy. I asked for a difficult challenge I could master, and I got it.

The highlight was beating Steve while racing him across the canyon on the final leg of the line. The only casualty was a shredded sole on one of my shoes as we landed.

After trudging back up the hill later that afternoon, I sank into the front seat of the car and instantly fell asleep. Staggering to our room and flopping on the bed, I did not awaken until the next morning. It was well worth it.

That day was a pivotal point for the future. It brought about the realization that there was much I could not do that I had done before, but I recognized a renewed sense of empowerment that there was much I could do. I am a vital human being who is more fortunate than many. I am alive.

It delivered an understanding of why Dad moved to Carson City, needing to escape everything around him and why I spent most of my life doing what I did until I burned out and slowed down in the early 1990s. We were compensating and masking the fear of "someday." Incessant workaholics, we were entrenched in our work while racing against time.

My mind was whirling, thinking about the families I knew who had seen generations of lives passing without hope and existing in dignified silence, with many who lived in the shadows with extreme uncertainty while waiting for when cancer would hit them and their loved ones.

Reading thousands of studies and interviewing experts about Lynch syndrome opened a door that released an immense amount of fear held inside. I wondered what would happen if there was a mass public-awareness campaign, programs to educate physicians at their conferences, an open support system available to families, and fundraising for research and recruitment of patients for clinical trials of Lynch syndrome.

"What would happen if it were to occur throughout the world?" my husband asked.

He worked at major international biotech companies specializing in the maintenance and repair of ultralow-temperature laboratory systems and advanced medical research equipment. His dream of Lynch Syndrome International was grander than mine. He saw the global potential of an organization that could save hundreds of thousands of lives from hereditary cancers.

"It is a terrific way to honor your father," Steve said.

Working with Kate Murphy, a Lynch syndrome advocate, we determined our mission would include educating medical professionals, creating public awareness of Lynch syndrome, offering support to families, and supporting research endeavors.

Contacting Dr. Henry Lynch, the pioneer founder of Lynch syndrome, who had collaborated with me on a legal matter, I asked if he wished to be involved. The idea thrilled him.

"Of course, it is wonderful!" he exclaimed. We could save thousands of lives. This is huge!"

Dr. Lynch and his son, Dr. Patrick Lynch, set up the Scientific Advisory Board. Both donated a substantial amount of time presenting at our educational programs.

Developing an active board of directors with a fiduciary duty to oversee compliance with the bylaws was essential to preserve the intent and the livelihood of the organization. The directors of any nonprofit organization bring funding into it. They cannot allow it to become stagnant. We developed specific board member terms to allow for constant change and a fresh perspective to deter stagnation. A good board lends credibility to a nonprofit and compels others to become involved, to donate, and to invest in the Lynch syndrome cause. Ours consisted of patients, medical professionals, and genetic counselors, each holding an equal vote. Every effective nonprofit rotates its board members regularly to allow for fresh perspectives and individuals with fundraising and community service expertise to advance the mission of the organization.

In July 2009, the birth of Lynch Syndrome International occurred when Steve and I recorded the organization as a nonprofit organization with the State of California and with the Internal Revenue Service. Within weeks, we were speaking with hundreds of benevolent administrators of health care systems and battling with those who were unreceptive. Many in the medical profession and others embraced the organization. However, there was resistance. Most came from genetic counselors. Some were not receptive to patient advocacy and an international organization. They did not feel there was a need to organize. They told us, "You do not know what you are doing." and "You have no right to do our job."

We had shaken things up, raising issues over the standards of care that questioned the qualifications to prescribe genetic testing. We insisted on the reduction of wait times of patients needing appointments for genetic counseling to allow physicians and patients the ability to decide the extent of organ removal patients need to prevent future cancers. It is a critical issue that deters the occurrence of second surgeries to allow for prevention, following the surgical removal of tumors. Major communication issues and debate continued with some genetic counselors over parental rights in the testing of minors.

We challenged the policies of insurance companies that were removing diagnostic roles from physicians. Our feeling was that mandating their contracted provider perform genetic counseling was a severe conflict of interest.

Hereditary cancers are life-threatening for patients and their families. For others, it is their "bread and butter." Always keep that in mind when testing, getting genetic counseling, receiving treatment, and especially when receiving pharmaceutical drugs. For many, it is a living, a business.

At first, the paternalistic attitudes of some genetic counselors were difficult to accept. A few complained to our scientific board members about our organizational stance of supporting parents who wished to have their children test. Genetic counselors felt they, themselves, should make the decision and were denying testing. They told us we, as patients, were too inadequately equipped to understand our condition and to make those decisions for ourselves and our families.

Counter-balanced by the many outstanding genetic counselors who did not feel the same, we realized any medical system would have some marginal and paternalistic providers. Most approach their work with passion and see their profession as a mission for their patients and not as a self-interest to advance their own beliefs. These are the genetic counselors you will want to work when seeking diagnosis and counseling for Lynch syndrome.

We addressed the difficulties in patients diagnosed with cancer but who could not get prompt appointments for genetic testing. Some had to wait six months and longer to see a genetic counselor. Many gave up, eliminating their surgical options. Some even had to decide to have their colon resected without being provided the knowledge of whether they were at risk for Lynch syndrome. Others had to undergo two surgeries, rather than one, and to spend twice the amount of time in surgeries and recovering. Not only is this difficult for the patient, but it also creates stress for the surgeon. On several occasions, I played interference for patients facing this situation.

Passionate genetic counselors and those at cancer institutions listened to our concerns and worked to resolve them by defining the issues affecting patients. They set up appointments closer to homes, changed hours to accommodate working patients, and offered online and telephone counseling to avoid the patient necessity of taking extended time off work and away from home. Eliminating the second appointment, they began providing test results over the telephone.

To ease the anxiety and uncertainty of patients, physicians and clinics responded to our recommendation to supply programs for ongoing cancer screenings that extended over a two to three-day period each year, rather than schedule them weeks and months apart. Those affected by Lynch syndrome spent their time off work, engaging in screening procedures.

Institutions, offices of physicians, and research hospitals developed programs for those with Lynch syndrome. Communication expanded. Education efforts took place on the internet through podcasts, Skype, or other systems to educate physicians and patients. Many called requesting brochures for their offices and engaged in public awareness and educational programs for medical professionals and the public.

Trying to run an all-volunteer organization, on a shoestring, was difficult. Steve and I supplied the significant funding for it for five years, using funding from Kaiser Permanente that compensated us for the delay in care. When that money ran out, we emptied two retirement accounts to pay the bills, writing it off as a donation. Between that, the funding received from Myriad Genetics and Lynch syndrome families, and what we saved by having Steve and I volunteer fulltime services instead of paying wages to employees, we were able to meet our mission during the early years. We had enough to achieve our goals. We had planned well and were ready for the difficult, slim years. If it did not grow in five years, then it was time to disband.

Building a solid foundation, our board involved genetic professionals, medical professionals, and patients. By creating a public awareness campaign and a series of consistent back-to-back positive campaigns, the international organization went viral. We had accomplished our goals.

Our commitment to performing full-time volunteer services ended on July 1, 2014. During the five years of involvement with managing LSI, over thirty thousand physicians learned of Lynch syndrome from volunteers providing medical professional awareness at their specialized conferences. Tens of millions learned about it through direct advertising and the efforts of Lynch syndrome families in their communities. We worked with cancer centers, institutions, clinics, hospitals, and genetic counselors to introduce the resources they made available to those in their communities.

Attending a minimum of four major medical conferences per year and many other smaller meetings, we focused on educating gateway physicians, dermatologists, urologists, family physicians, gynecologists, and general practitioners. Gastroenterologists hopped onboard. Diagnoses skyrocketed wherever we concentrated our efforts.

Lynch syndrome advocacy movements developed in the Netherlands, Canada, Belgium, Norway, France, Germany, Spain, Australia, and in the UK. After we left, it expanded to Finland, Ireland, and Scotland. The passion involved was overwhelming.

Chapter Thirty-One

BREAST CANCER HITS HOME

Once I knew that this was my reality, I decided to be proactive and to minimize the risk as much as I could. I made a decision to have a preventive double mastectomy. —Angelina Jolie

Not only concerned about the substantial risk my family and I may face in contracting Lynch syndrome cancers "someday," but I felt concerned about the elevated risk of breast cancer contracted by the generations of the women in my mother's family. By 2012, every woman on the maternal side of our family, through three generations, had contracted breast cancer, except me.

Having battled Lynch syndrome colorectal cancers, I was not ready to focus on yet another life-threatening genetic condition. Contracting breast cancer had not been so much as a thought as I struggled with learning to live with Lynch syndrome.

Since 1993, when the government granted patent protections for genetic testing for Lynch syndrome, controversy has existed among researchers and genetic professionals about whether breast cancer is part of LS. I met many women with Lynch syndrome who stood adamant that it was part of the syndrome. Studies have shown Lynch syndrome breast cancer results in a threat much higher than the already elevated risk of contracting a sporadic (not hereditary related) breast cancer.

Recent studies have found women with Lynch syndrome *do* have an elevated risk; it occurs with all mutations. Those with MSH-6 and PMS2 mutations face the highest elevation of risk, while a two to three-fold risk exists in those with MLH1 and MSH2 mutations.

My brother and I hoped our sister, Donna, may be the one person in the family to be free of Lynch syndrome cancers. I hoped she would be healthy and unaffected. All of us, through our generation, had contracted cancer, except for her. All that ended one evening when the telephone rang.

"Lindy, I have cancer," Donna said. I could hear the fear in her voice. "Colon cancer, endometrial cancer, and breast cancer. I am so sick. I don't know what to do. I don't think anybody is listening," she cried. "Can you talk to them and make sure they give me what I need?"

Besides battling cancer, she faced immense challenges with her genetic counselor. Getting the breast tumor assessed to determine if it had the characteristics of Lynch syndrome was a priority.

"Could you please test the tumor to determine if it is MSI-h?" I asked.

"What? That can't be done," the genetic counselor stated.

Huh?

The genetic counselor adamantly insisted there was no such thing as Lynch syndrome breast cancer, and there was no method to test the tumor. I sighed, knowing better.

I had read dozens of studies from Australia, Ireland, Finland, Lebanon, Iran, and the United States, citing the statistics known to date by testing the tumors. Her knowledge was years behind. She had not been keeping up with the research findings that were occurring daily, whereas I had worked with many women affected with Lynch syndrome breast cancers.

When you cannot get that which you need to live from a health care provider, and that person will not listen to reason, I am a strong advocate in moving up the chain of command to protect yourself and your family. I face no difficulty in doing it. No person should feel uncomfortable doing advocating for themselves and their family when dealing with hereditary cancer in one's family. It can be lifesaving. A key to survival is to be one's own advocate.

"We can do it. We just have to find a lab that has the capabilities," the supervising geneticist said. Expecting this, I had made the call to Dr. Noralene Lindor of the Mayo Clinic, one of the world experts in Lynch syndrome, who has extensively studied the relationship between breast cancer and Lynch syndrome.

Dr. Lindor, a clinical researcher, has partnered with Stanford University and with Australian Lynch syndrome researchers. Passionate about protecting patients from Lynch syndrome cancers, they are churning out valuable information and results. They are doing it with less money and resources required by most U.S. institutions.

Following pathological testing, the tumor reflected MSI-H (microsatellite instability-high) status. It identified it as a Lynch syndrome tumor, as I suspected. A second test to rule out BRCA1 and BRCA2 hereditary breast mutations proved negative.

Donna and her geneticist determined that she should undergo a lumpectomy. Having spent a few years counseling families with Lynch syndrome breast cancers, I knew dozens of women whose breast cancers kept returning, despite treatment. The tumors of Lynch syndrome ordinarily developed in the ducts of both breasts.

Meeting the same reaction from many of their physicians and genetic counselors as Donna did, they, too, were told their breast cancer was *not* a part of Lynch syndrome and refused to test it. It still occurs today.

We assisted with getting their tumors evaluated. If the tumor presented as MSI-h, it enabled them to receive a more effective and personalized treatment approach for their cancer. Every single breast tumor that underwent a microscopic examination of women with Lynch syndrome showed it to be MSI-h.

Donna changed her mind and decided on a bilateral mastectomy. During surgery, they detected breast cancer developing in the duct of the unaffected breast. Having more extensive surgery with the removal of both breasts may have saved her life.

At that moment, it became necessary for the women in our family to assess the risks of breast cancer. With the unknown occurrences of breast cancer affecting three generations from my mother's side and the risk of having Lynch syndrome from Dad's side, experts expressed concern that the two may interplay with one another since the prevalence of contracting cancer was so extensive.

My daughter was the first to undergo a prophylactic bilateral mastectomy, the total removal of both breasts. In 2013, after discussing it with my oncologist, I too determined to undergo a bilateral mastectomy to end my risk of breast cancer. Choosing to do so was an emotional journey. The decision was not only difficult for me but also for my surgeon. Being unable to receive access to breast cancer screening tests had been a challenge for me. Having to debate the need with a few physicians, each time, had become challenging and emotional.

I could not allow myself to take the risk and cave in and negotiate for less than I needed. Finding myself forced to go into a battle once again with another physician who insisted I was not at risk for breast cancer, I found myself burned out. After refusing to allow me an MRI to detect early developing breast cancers, he attempted to turn my objections into a personal issue.

"You are just mad because I won't let you get one," the radiologist said instead of focusing on my argument that it was a basic standard of care that I was requesting. Again, like others, he did not take a family history, nor was he receptive when I attempted to explain our history of cancer.

Hanging up, I called his boss, the Chief of the Imaging Department, and explained to her that I was the *only* woman in three generations of our family not to contract breast cancer. Revealing the circumstances of my sister's breast cancer, that it had tested as MSI-h, and evidenced a deficiency existed in our defective genes, I confided I felt concerned. I shared with her how difficult it was to deal with the numbers of physicians who had little knowledge of hereditary cancers, and who were quick to minimize patients and deny preventative measures against cancer.

Being able to advocate for one's self is the most critical survival tools we have at our disposal. Most patients do not have my level of desire to debate or to negotiate standards of care guidelines with physicians, especially when ill. It is difficult and still is hard for me to do, though it does become more comfortable with experiences and after learning to protect one's self. Granted, we should not have to do it. We should be able to trust our physicians to do what is best for us. But, to live, we must first learn to fight. I learned from Angelina Jolie. It can be lifesaving. Her journey to protect herself from BRCA hereditary cancers inspired me. Of all of us, she is one who had the most to lose and the most to gain from undergoing preventative prophylactic surgery. Her courage in going public with her decision helped me to make mine.

Not all of us are the same. We do not meet a "one fits all" standardized model of care. Some need less, and some need more, like women with a family history of breast cancer, a history of the lesser cancers of LS, those with variants, and those whose tumors are unusual and aggressive. I did not feel I was asking for anything unreasonable. Neither did the Chief. She ordered an MRI. From this, the first thing I learned was I did not want to experience this situation again. Steve and I discussed ways to avoid it. We decided it would be best for me would undergo a radical bilateral mastectomy and have both breasts permanently removed.

The woman who decided to undergo a double mastectomy without breast reconstruction and the younger woman who faced a later staged diagnosis with colorectal cancer eight years prior were two different people. Both are far different from the woman I am today.

With age and experience, we evolve. My biggest regret was not paying as much attention as I should when Dr. Carlos Perez, my surgeon, as I should have when he explained breast reconstruction. Today, I would pay more attention to listening to the opinion of experts.

Experiencing reconstruction, several years later, entailed a much longer process. It took a year to complete. I wished I had consulted the many I knew who underwent the procedure. However, when I was intent on risk reduction, I did not care. I wanted my breasts gone, so I would not face the Lynch syndrome hereditary breast cancer like that of my sister.

Chapter Thirty-Two

TODAY

The beginning is always today.
— Mary Shelley

Amazed, I am alive; I am thankful for these past twelve years of being cancer-free. I never believed I would live this long. There were many times of hopelessness. Like others, I questioned my level of stamina and ability to endure. The support of my medical team and the love of my family kept me going. As a result, those moments never lasted. The sparks of hope igniting inside provided a strong motivation to do whatever I could to protect my loved ones and myself.

Today, following diagnosis, most of us are living longer than ever before with Lynch syndrome, even after facing cancer. Recent studies indicate most patients survived ten or more years after sustaining their first bout. The only exceptions are for those with the pancreatic, bile duct, and brain cancers that need more research.

Affected by hereditary cancers, we have a responsibility to carry forward what we have experienced and learned, to protect and guide future generations through this journey. It is crucial to reach out to others to pass on what we have learned and to provide reassurances that they will have far more than a fighting chance if they act as advocates of themselves and their families and engage in regular screenings.

Inspiration comes from many places. We receive it from our care teams and our family members. Our parents, grandparents, and the stories of our ancestors provided me with it throughout this journey. Reflecting upon the insurmountable challenges faced by them, and what I learned from the strengths and the weaknesses they demonstrated, was invaluable during my time of adversity. The thousands with Lynch syndrome that we collaborated with during our years involved in the founding and growth of Lynch Syndrome International inspired me. Across the globe, many worked hard to protect Lynch syndrome families and save lives. I cherish every one of them. I hold in my heart the memories of the survivors and those who did not make it but who used their strength, courage, and dedication and their time left in life to make it better for others.

After my diagnosis with Lynch syndrome, the next concern I had was encouraging our children and grandchildren to test. Many with Lynch syndrome face difficulties in getting their loved ones to take part in genetic testing. For the younger generations, traditional testing, with having to take time off work for three visits, is difficult for them.

Like us, the future generations live their lives with urgency. Today's lifestyles feed into it. We exist in a world that operates upon instant gratification. Anything we desire is available on a computer. We need not leave our homes to get tested. We can research products, communicate with others, and order what we want. Whatever we desire is generally delivered to us within days.

It is no different for obtaining a genetic test today. Quality genetic testing and counseling services *are* available online. When considering an online consumer testing company, it is essential to research the companies and their leadership.

The one reputable commercial testing company we chose for testing our next generation is Color Genomics (Getcolor.com) to examine the mismatch repair genes of nine of the next generation. The tests were completed in a record amount of time, reducing anxiety, and they were accurate. Everyone was pleased with the convenience of the testing, and the genetic counseling they received following being diagnosed. A dedicated "direct to consumer" genetic cancer testing company, their CEO comes from a hereditary cancer family. Living in a hereditary cancer family, he understands what families experience and personally knows the issues and barriers patients face in getting genetic testing.

Developed as a philanthropic corporation, they not only offer panelized testing for thirty different hereditary cancer genes but supply complimentary genetic counseling if one tests positive for a hereditary cancer syndrome. The low cost of $250 per test often allows for the remaining family members to test for the same mutated gene for fifty dollars each. An entire family can engage in genetic testing for less than ten percent of the cost of the testing of one person at a commercial laboratory.

We are indebted to them. In our family, all but two of nine of the next generation that needed genetic testing were receptive to testing online through Color Genomics. Jumping through the complicated hoops required with the traditional methods of genetic testing that require multiple personal visits to institutional genetic counselors was not attractive to them. They are young. They did not have the time, and they could not afford to take off work.

Two tested negative, and five tested positive. As we learned, and as our children now realize, with genetic testing, the opportunity exists that they can now choose careers and life partners while understanding their cancer risk. Online direct to consumer testing allows individuals to test without fear of a breach of confidentiality, and at a fraction of the cost of traditional testing. No invoices are sent to insurance companies. It alleviates the concern of bearing a child affected by BMMRD by testing future, long-term partners. It reduces the options for future complications to occur and protects families and saves lives

Lynch syndrome is a huge topic to bring up in conversation for everyone, including kids. It needs to be discussed. Growing up as a child in a hereditary cancer family, we realize kids are every bit as savvy about health risks as most adults. They, too, understand what may occur in the future, much the same as we did, and as the children did, during my father's time, while living during the age of eugenics a hundred years ago.

I am now sixty-seven years old. My husband and I embrace life. As seniors, we are beginning to experience health challenges, like diabetes and heart disease that travel with hereditary cancers and their treatments. Even considering a diagnosis of both, after contracting colorectal cancer and undergoing surgical resection of my colon, gall bladder, ovaries, uterus, fallopian tubes, cervix, and my breasts, I am still incredibly healthy. I hold immense gratitude for that. The thousands who lived before us did not have a ghost of a chance offered to us today. We live better and longer than ever before.

My brother and I are now aging naturally, thanks to the excellent care we receive from our health care providers. It is not so for my sister, who suffered a cancer-induced stroke, and faces related cognitive issues. Those regular screenings make a world of difference in cancer prevention and in easing those nagging feelings of uncertainty.

Having faced many challenges during my lifetime, I learned that not all crises we experience are life-threatening. It does not matter whether our problems involve serious illness, living as part of a dysfunctional family, navigating through grief or loss, venturing into unsafe havens, or if we are facing significant changes in life's circumstances. Survival, in all situations, requires adapting to those situations. The ability to adapt is the key to getting through those challenging times.

Our genes do not manage us; we manage them. By removing negative environmental factors and making positive changes in our lifestyles, we can increase our odds of living a cancer-free life.

Living with Lynch syndrome means adjusting our lifestyle choices and living and eating in moderation. After watching our Aunt Marcella battle three cancers, I learned environmental and lifestyle changes *can* enhance survival. It includes eating a proper diet, getting plenty of sleep, reducing stressful situations, drinking a lot of clean water, being active, engaging in exercise, breathing fresh air, keeping a cheerful outlook, and absorbing Vitamin D from sunlight. Fulfilling these needs may play a significant role in switching genes on or off.

Getting a regular good night's sleep is one of my most significant challenges. For years, I have faced difficulty with it. I have found when I sleep well; it is following those days when I have been active. Walking, hiking, or doing something that keeps me moving, ordinarily resolves it. Racing through a few stores can create enough distraction for me to get those 2000 steps a day that I need to remain healthy.

Reducing stress is key to survival. We moved from a busy, crowded, San Francisco East Bay suburb to the Mojave Desert where traffic, noise, crowds, lines, convenience foods, and dirty air do not exist. There are only three stoplights on the residential side of our little village. It is quiet. Life is slow and easy-going. As a result, living there is comfortable.

We spend our summers high in the Sangre de Cristo Mountain range in the Southern Rockies of New Mexico. In our tiny, resort town named Angel Fire, I feel energized amid nature, breathing clean air, and living a stress-free lifestyle.

Modifying my diet was a significant lifestyle change. I am a junkie when it comes to fried foods, country cooking, and sweets. My mouth drools at the thought of fry bread, Indian tacos, fast food cheeseburgers, and french fries. While my taste buds are in heaven, my body does not respond well to them. As a result, if I eat those foods often, I become sludgy and less active, except for the twelve times each day, when I race to the bathroom. My seven inches of existing colon is not cooperative in processing them.

Therefore, I dine on them one or two times a month. Like many others who have undergone colon resections, I end up paying for it by having to stay at home and close to the bathroom for the day. Urgency means "now," every bit as much as it did in the first few years following surgery.

What we choose to do to adapt is different for each of us. After a while, it becomes easier to accept the changes in us. With time, we learn what our body will tolerate and what it will not. Scheduling being away from home and traveling becomes an art for those who are newly diagnosed.

It was following chemotherapy that Dr. Martin discovered I had developed a fatty liver that had developed fibrosis. Ten percent of those who undergo a 5-FU based chemotherapy for colorectal cancer develop diabetes or a fatty liver. My liver appeared to be advancing toward cirrhosis. Today, it is scarred.

A fatty liver can cause abdominal swelling of the abdomen and ascites, enlarged blood vessels just beneath the skin's surface, an enlarged spleen, reddened palms of the hands, and jaundice that creates a yellowing of the eyes and the skin.

Dr. Walker found I had contracted diabetes. For a while, I allowed myself to feel sorry for myself until I began beating myself back into a positive attitude. Nonetheless, I still had reason to be grateful. I was alive. That was all that mattered. I would learn to live with it.

Supplementing a diabetic diet with milk thistle and turmeric, and drinking iced water to reduce inflammation and swelling, seemed to help reduce it. I cut back the amount of Metformin I had been taking for over a decade to see what would occur. A slew of side-effects disappeared, creating a higher quality of life, and offering more energy. From that, I learned to assess my medications regularly and discuss them with my endocrinologist.

In January 2018, Dr. Naraev, the captain of my medical team at Banner Health/MD Anderson, ordered a CT scan to develop a baseline for future cancer screenings. From this, he could easily recognize any changes in my body that may hint at early cancer development, and head them off.

The fibrosis of the liver, noted by Dr. Martin, was still present. Also noted were mesenteric (inflamed) lymph nodes upon the anastomosis (where the rest of the large colon attaches to the small bowel, following resection.) They detected more of those inflamed lymph nodes upon the "inlet patch" in my esophagus.

An inlet patch is a congenital anomaly formed of the gastric mucosa that appears as a velvety area near or next to the upper esophageal sphincter. Most do not present with symptoms; however, our physicians should monitor them since the research is new in determining the level of risk and the effects they can cause, including esophagitis, ulcers, reflux, or other anomalies. Seldom do they present with cancer.

Our efforts in making lifestyle changes paid off. Recent tests indicate the liver is within reasonable guidelines with some scarring, and the inlet patch is not at issue. Dr. Naraev and Dr. Deveraraj are continuing to monitor both. As with my colon, bladder, kidneys, and other cancer risks, my physicians will monitor both the liver and the inlet patch.

Ten years following the diagnosis of diabetes, my body is responding better to introduced medications. As the body changes, so do the effectiveness of our medicines. Trial and error are an essential part of managing the disease, along with making lifestyle changes in diet and exercise. It took a little while for me to get it right if I have.

That seven to ten inches of the remaining colon is touchy, so to help it along, I eat a banana each morning before breakfast. It solidifies my stools, along with half a piece of whole-grained or sourdough toast, and a poached egg that I often add for protein. Occasionally, for a rare treat, I do add a bit of bacon to it. How we eat is a big part of our level of quality of life. "Once in a while" is okay and good for the spirit. I love sipping on a small glass of a crisp Sauvignon Blanc or a good Fume Blanc. I have found nothing is as comforting as taking a few sips of Bellini after dinner. I occasionally allow myself that luxury.

While in the UK, I fell in love with their European bacon. It is less fatty and more like ham, only not as salty. It not only tasted delicious, but my body tolerated it well. I include it in my list of rare treats and buy it online at the Irish and Scottish food stores.

Because of the sub-total resection, my body rapidly digests food. Within forty-five minutes to two hours after eating, I am in the bathroom, and within an hour or two later, I am again ravenous. Eating five smaller meals a day works better for me, especially while taking medications.

During midmorning, I scavenge and eat what I want, if it is not a "bad carb" or containing sugar. Being active, it does not matter what I eat if it is healthy. Sometimes my body will tolerate my eating smaller amounts, more often. By noon, my colon has usually stabilized. Then, I feel more comfortable leaving the house for extended periods. Before doing so, I scout the locations I intend to visit and determine whether they have user-friendly bathroom accommodations. In doing so, I make a rough estimate of the amount of time to get from Point A to Point B, making sure "I don't get myself into something I can't get myself out of." Planning my days has become an art in understanding how my colon works. It takes time to get it right. Only after doing it a few times was I able to get the hang of it and to feel comfortable leaving my home. I wasn't going to let an unpredictable colon limit my lifestyle. Eventually, we adapt, and we learn to work within its limits.

"Balance, Lindy," Dr. Ahmad, my endocrinologist, reminds me when we discuss my anti-cancer and diabetic diet. She is a Godsend. Her advice has enhanced my quality of life, as well as my diet.

At night, my plate is half-filled with fresh, leafy greens and colorful vegetables. One-quarter of it (equaling about three ounces, the size of the palm of my hand) holds protein, meat, fish, chicken, or beans, while the final quarter holds a "good carb." Good carbs include quinoa, buckwheat, oats, sweet potatoes, beets, oranges, apples, whole grained wheat, brown rice, and vegetables.

A study of 47,000 adults revealed those eating a diet high in refined carbs (sugars, grains stripped of nutrients and fibers, such as white bread, cookies, pancakes, syrups, waffles, pizza dough, white rice, sweets, concentrated fruit juices, jellies, white flour, pretzels, pasta, granola bars, and a good number of breakfast cereals and more) are more apt to die from colon cancer than those who consumed a lesser amount. Having been there and battled that, I don't want to contract cancer again. I have no problem passing on refined carbs. A particularly useful reference on what to eat for an anti-cancer diet is the website of the American Institute for Cancer Research has a decent section on anti-cancer foods, and a sizeable list of what qualifies as refined carbs is located at diagnosisdiet.com.

Researchers have explored the risks of consuming substantial amounts of processed meats (smoked, salted, aged, marinated, cured, dried, or canned meats). It was found they pose an increased risk of twenty to fifty percent of colorectal cancer for *regular* meat-eaters, with a raised level of eighteen percent for those eating bacon and hot dogs.

A 2002 Holland study of 267 people, of which 69 persons had Lynch syndrome showed eating red meat in moderation, is not that much of a risk factor, though others are adamant it is. (They define "moderation" as consuming less than eighteen ounces a week.)

A lesser risk of cancer exists when eating red meat that is *not* processed. Compromising, I'm hedging bets by consuming three to four ounces of non-processed red meat once a week as the main entrée. I try to use it as an ingredient in spaghetti sauce or casseroles. During the rest of the week, I prepare fish, chicken, and eggs in place of red meat.

Hot dogs, hamburgers, milkshakes, coffee, French fries, fried eggs, and other foods, including fried potatoes (or anything fried) sweets, and bacon are not my friends. They are a staunch enemy of the seven inches of the remaining colon. During the rare occasions when I eat fast food, I get it "to go," and I consume it at home. I know from experience that I will pay for it by spending a good part of my day studying the bathroom fixtures.

To my disappointment, I have recently discovered that researchers believe that those engaging in a diet that includes increased glucose levels face a higher risk of stomach, breast, and colorectal cancers. As a result, I seldom eat sweets. To sweeten coffee, I use Stevia instead of processed sugars and chemical-filled sweeteners. Stevia, like sugar, is plant-based. It has no calories and may contain other benefits. A study published in the journal Nutrients in 2017 shows that cookies prepared with Stevia inhibited a diabetes-related digestive enzyme and promoted a sense of fullness after eating, while sugar offsets blood sugar levels. Containing antioxidants, Stevia may help the immune function and lower inflammation. Removing sweets from an everyday diet is difficult, but what I have found is it becomes more comfortable in time, and my choice of all the evils of sweeteners is a natural one.

We need to understand food preparation and its risks and benefits. Studies indicate we need to exercise caution when cooking meats. They show preparing them at elevated temperatures using methods of barbecuing, frying, and broiling can produce compounds that may contribute to inflammation that may lead to the development of cancer.

These compounds, known as lipid oxidation products (LOPS) and heterocyclic amines (HCAs), often develop in foods high in fat and processed meats (the sausages, the bacon, and those other meats high in fat.) It occurs when preparing red meats, some cheeses, fried eggs, butter, some oils, and dairy foods at high temperatures. Marinating meats may reduce the amount of LOPS and HCAs and the charring of foods that presents us with a higher risk of cancer.

To avoid this, in preparing our meals, we often use a slow cooker several times a week. The all-in-one pressure cookers, incorporating a crock pot, a pressure cooker, a rice cooker, and the other processes of food preparation are invaluable. After tossing ingredients into them in the morning, a healthy home-cooked dinner is ready when one gets home from work.

These "cookers" prepare foods at lower temperatures. Make sure whatever cooking instrument you use is lead-free. The manufacturers' tags should read "lead-free," or have an FDA rating attached to them to determine if the level of leaking lead is low enough not to pose a danger. While at it, you may want to check your other cookware to make sure it, too, is lead-free. Cooking with Pyrex type glass, stainless steel, cast iron, and enameled cast iron can reduce this risk.

Dairy foods may carry a risk of prostate cancer in men. Researchers speculate the hormones from pregnant cows may cause a predisposition to prostate cancer. More research is needed; however, in the meantime, it may be prudent to discuss this concern with your physicians.

So, what *can* we eat?

We can eat whatever we want. We live in a free country. But, if we are going to live healthy and well, we should eat in moderation and exercise the use of appropriate portions. Below are examples of foods that are anti-cancer foods. I eat as much of them as I can, and most of them, if prepared correctly, is surprisingly good. If our meals are healthy and not derived from processed foods, and if we avoid eating an excessive amount of red meat and other fatty foods, we should be fine. If we listen to our bodies, they will tell us what we can and cannot tolerate. That said, if we focus on portioning our foods, and how we place it upon plates, then practicing an anti-cancer diet becomes more comfortable. Then, all needed is to learn what consists of an anti-cancer diet.

Vegetables and fruits are high cancer-fighting foods. Many contain antioxidants. Researchers have found leafy greens contain sulforaphane reduces the size of tumors in research animals by over fifty percent. While some believe tomatoes and carrots may reduce the risk of prostate, stomach, and lung cancers, others insist eating oranges or other citrus fruit may decrease the risk of contracting stomach cancer by twenty-eight percent, if we consume three servings weekly.

Studies have found that spicing up what we eat may reduce the risk of cancer. Cinnamon may have anti-cancer qualities. I put cinnamon on sourdough toast in the mornings and occasionally eat it as a snack in the evenings. In yet another study, researchers found when taking 4 grams of curcumin (turmeric) daily; it reduced cancer lesions by forty percent. This study was small, involving only 44 persons who were not receiving cancer treatment. More research is necessary.

I take 500 mg of turmeric twice a day, morning, and night, with a bit of pepper to enhance its efficiency. What I have found is its anti-inflammatory qualities hopefully not only work as a cancer deterrent, it *does* work as an excellent pain reliever after it accumulates in my body. It provides relief with my sciatica and back pain when sleeping at night. And, it has helped assist the immune system in fighting infections.

There is no compelling evidence that sugar increases the risk of cancer. But it may be an indirect link to it. The cells in our bodies need sugar as fuel. Distributed through our bloodstream, the sugar I need comes from foods that hold carbohydrates, vegetables, fruits, and whole-grain bread and dairy products. Amazingly, some of it comes from protein. Eating excessive amounts of foods that contain sugar can create weight gain. That is what puts us at a much higher risk of contracting cancer; the body fat we have and that which comes with the development of diabetes and heart disease. It puts us at a higher risk of cancer. There is some evidence that consuming large amounts of sugar can lead to a higher risk of developing esophageal and other diseases.

Allicin, a key ingredient in garlic, holds qualities that researchers feel may stymy cancer. Thus, it may be a significant part of the thought of eating a Mediterranean diet may prevent cancer. Between that and an aspirin a day, I can attest to it, and stretching exercises also help to keep my sciatic nerve damage, the peripheral nerve damage, and developing arthritis and muscle pains in check.

A few things worth mentioning are "anti-cancer" foods that solidify stools. Those of us with colon resections live with the touchy remnants of a once functioning colon. It can still work. It is something that takes a while to resolve. To solidify stools, I eat a banana each morning. It allows me to relax over a cup of coffee without fear. At night, I eat mashed potatoes, yams, sweet potatoes, brown rice, bananas, sourdough bread, beef, and beans that help solidify the next morning's stools. High in fiber, studies suggest these foods may also protect against colorectal cancer.

Using olive oil in food preparation rather than vegetable oils may result in a 42% lower risk of cancer. I found it difficult to digest at first, with my resection. It resulted in the colon becoming more unpredictable. Balancing it with other foods is tricky. Adapting to it takes a little while, and I no longer have any problem with it.

Being overweight creates another risk factor for contracting cancer. It can cause over thirteen distinct types of cancer, five of which fall within the spectrum of Lynch syndrome. It may also contribute to a higher rate of inflammation, causing cells to divide. Fat cells can increase estrogen levels that may put one at risk of women's cancers.

Therefore, moderation with eating and exercise is the key to weight loss and helps what remains of the colon to adapt to change following cancer surgeries and treatment. It also promotes a night of better sleep. After an active day, and a lighter evening meal, my body ignores the 3:45 A.M. wake-up call that plagues me when I am not busy.

I have worked hard to do my part to prevent cancer. It is my belief it helped in deterring cancer development for the last twelve years, along with getting exercise, Vitamin D from sunshine, reducing stress, and taking part in regular cancer screenings. My brother has done the same, and he has lived nineteen years without contracting a second cancer. His recovery is remarkable, as it is well above the average rate of recurrence.

Everything else is up to the capabilities of our medical teams, modern technology, and to whatever higher power to which we subscribe. Our genetics decides what we are and what we will be. What works for me may not work for you, or it may work better for you than it does for me! Who knows? We differ in how we structure our lives; each of us does what works for us. Figuring that out, however, is the tough part.

It is difficult for us to adapt to changes. Creatures of habit, we need to be kind to ourselves and be patient. In the beginning, I missed eating sweets. Dr. Walker and I decided to allow me to indulge in consuming them once a week, again, in moderation. It worked.

Nonetheless, weaknesses still present themselves and challenge my sense of self-discipline, like that beautiful time of summer, when the peaches ripen, and for a brief period, are in abundance. I must remind myself, "everything in moderation" (except for summer.) It is my mantra.

For anyone with Lynch syndrome, I cannot recommend enough the services of an experienced endocrinologist and a nutritionist who can help with diet and with other prominent cancer risk reduction methods. Cancer is not our only problem. Unfortunately, for some of us, diabetes travels with cancer, and heart disease travels with diabetes—everything interplays with one another. Be sure and get those glucose levels checked regularly and have your doctor monitor your blood pressure and cholesterol.

Ask if your insurance to cover the services of an endocrinologist who will help with determining your cancer risk and help with information on which diet, supplements, and medications to take. Elevated levels of insulin and blood glucose can contribute to an increase in inflammation, in addition to Lynch syndrome's already highly inflammatory tumors.

I take a few supplements daily to reduce inflammation and encourage insulin production. Included in my regiment are a multi-complex vitamin, a Vitamin B12 complex, 500 mg of turmeric in the morning, and another 500 mg at night, with a low dosed Bayer 81 milligram aspirin.

The turmeric reduces the inflammation and pain in my joints, back, and hip. It has resulted in not having to take prescription pain relievers. Aspirin is being studied in the United Kingdom by families with Lynch syndrome to determine the dose needed to keep cancer development at bay. Initial findings revealed that an aspirin a day does stymy the development of cancer. Researchers are now investigating the most effective dose.

Taking a statin to avoid heart issues, I also inject myself with Victoza to get the pancreas pumping insulin and to manage diabetes. Taking medications at night prevents feeling the annoying side effects of the drugs during the day.

As one becomes older or faces health issues, it becomes a challenge to balance an anti-cancer diet. Add in other health problems, and it requires a complicated balancing act. Whatever situation you may have, remember to do the best you can. It is easy to become frustrated. Keep at it. Convince yourself it *will* make a difference.

In my impatience, I often forget no one intended living to be easy. I often need to remind myself to slow down and work my way through trial and error to "get it right." After a while, I figure out what I can and cannot eat, what I can live with, and what I cannot live without. With time, it becomes easier. I consider Lynch syndrome to be a minor inconvenience. It could be worse.

Again, it is worth repeating; I do not smoke. There was a time I did. For years, I smoked. I would stop for a few years and, in a moment of weakness, allow myself to become caught up into starting again.

The day of my colon resection was the day I quit smoking for good. There is something about spending twenty-nine days in the hospital, with four days in ICU, and seven months undergoing chemotherapy that offers a great incentive to quit. When I feel the temptation to smoke, all I do is recall my four years of back-to-back surgeries and subsequent recoveries, cancer treatment, and other interventions. And I relive my experiences with my father, who smoked when he was dying of cancer. Living through the hell of cancer surgeries and procedures is a great deterrent that I wish I did not have to experience. Another great deterrent was the heartbreak of watching loved ones die. The second to the last time I saw my father, he lit up a cigarette while speaking with me. My face fell. He noticed it.

"What's it going to do, kill me?" he asked, noting my disappointment.

"No, I guess not," I said. In my heart, I had thought Dad had done everything to stay alive, even quitting smoking. But he had not. Like Mom's dependence on drugs, his addiction was with cigarettes, and he was unable to stop when those around him smoked.

Reading the hundreds of studies that evidence smoking cigarettes is the most common cause of cancer, or taking a good look at all the famous rock stars and others who died at an early age, who are and were dependent upon drugs, nicotine, and alcohol, the evidence of the danger of smoking is indisputable.

Smoke, whether it be cigarette smoke, marijuana smoke, or smoke from a fire, reduces the amount of oxygen in the body. It changes the makeup of cells and negatively affects most of our organs. It creates inflammation, which promotes the growth of cancer cells.

One-third of cancer deaths are due to smoking. *Cancer has no one cure.* Don't buy into the marijuana hype that it cures cancer. Smoking marijuana is *not* a cure for cancer. There is no one cure for cancer. Everyone's cancer is genetic; therefore, each person's disease differs from everyone else's. The "cure for all" hype that smoking marijuana cures cancer is nothing more than falsehood.

In 2016, researchers at Johns Hopkins found patients with aggressive tumors, where treatments that starved cancer cells of oxygen died off, may face worse outcomes. Low oxygen (like that caused by smoking) encourages cancer stem cells to multiply, like that of embryonic stem cells. It creates a difficult cancer to treat.

Cancer faces difficulty thriving in an oxygenated environment. A 2016 study published in the Journal of Addiction Research and Therapy, Pharmacology of Marijuana, showed smoking marijuana created a link to contracting certain cancers, including gliomas, prostate, and cervical cancer. In pregnant women, it may increase the risk for leukemia, rubbed-myosarcoma, and astrocytomas.

Lynch syndrome tumors are often inflammatory, as mentioned throughout this book. Inflammation is our immune systems' response to the growth of cancer or from other injuries. It means it is battling against something harmful to us. Smoking anything also creates inflammation, increasing the risk of cancer.

The new medication, Keytruda, an immunological treatment, is promising. It has been shown effective in treating many Lynch syndrome tumors. A simplified explanation of the way it works is our MSI tumors are genetically unstable. They carry various mutations that set off neo-antigens that are newly formed antigens not previously recognized by the immune system. They can develop from altered tumor proteins created from tumor mutations, and they can attract lymphocytes (white blood cells that are also one of the body's primary immune cells.) These inflamed tumors have responded to Keytruda.

Keytruda blocks the PD-1 pathway that releases a protein that binds itself to T-Cells and controls the body's immune responses. The binding of the PD-1 protein to one called PD-L1 keeps the T-cells from killing cancer cells. When Keytruda blocks the PD-1 pathway, it leaves tumors vulnerable, allowing the immune system to do its job, annihilating cancer. These immunological treatments are our greatest hope for cancer survival.

It is comforting to know we now have an effective treatment and to know Keytruda is standing in the wings if another cancer occurs, but I am not waiting for it to happen. I don't want to play Russian Roulette with another bout of cancer. I am doing everything I can to prevent its development. I practice deep breathing exercises, drink fifty-plus ounces of water daily, exercise several times a week, stretch out, and get a significant amount of quality sleep. I try to remain positive, and I eat well.

There are times we can't do this alone, as our father attempted. We need help and support from others. Speaking with friends, attending psychological counseling, chatting on bulletin boards with survivors, getting resources from advocacy organizations, building our faith in a higher power, or consulting with our medical teams are all effective support systems that are available to us.

The challenges Lynch syndrome families face are not solely cancer-related. Many of us are independent out of necessity due to the way we grew up due to difficulties faced by the previous generations. A lot of us came from broken families. There are times I still must remind myself not to conceal fear; that expressing fear is not showing weakness. Recognizing fear enhances survival. And, many of us seek approval, like my brother and me. Often, we compensated for Lynch syndrome by counterbalancing it with being independent, engaging in risk, and acting as codependents who cared for others to fulfill our need for self-validation. Today, I am the second oldest woman in my father's family to have lived to my age; in the last four generations, I no longer subscribe to fear.

Our Aunt Marcella lived to eighty-six years old. She would have been around longer if she had recalled the removal of her ovaries fifty years earlier. Her death from ovarian cancer reminds us to keep copies of our medical records and those of our loved ones *forever*.

During the past twelve years, and all it has wrought, I have come full circle with Lynch syndrome. From the time of my genetic diagnosis, and contracting a later stage cancer to submitting to prophylactic surgeries to prevent colorectal, urothelial, breast, uterine, and ovarian cancers, I found the surgeries, treatments, and preventative measures I underwent were not the most challenging part of living with Lynch syndrome.

The most challenging part of learning to live with it was my difficulty adapting to the side effects of treatments and to accept the uncertainty of the high risk of another cancer.

Living with Lynch syndrome is a lifelong process. Complicated at first, after a while, it becomes less so when we realize our lives do not differ much from others, many of whom also must adapt to other serious life challenges and life-threatening survival situations. When we expand our viewpoint to peek into the circumstances of others, as Dad drilled into us, we don't have to look far to find someone worse off than us.

Living, as we knew it to be before diagnosis, is different once diagnosed. It becomes even more so when we contract cancer. It always will be. People change—times change. Families change. Circumstances change. As we age, we better learn how to adapt to those changes. If we believe in ourselves and work closely with our medical teams, we most often get by. The now thirteen more years of life I have received so far, may not seem like much to an ordinary man, but it is significant in that it is fifteen percent of an average lifespan.

Cancer has affected a child of our next generation. His physician did not pay attention when he told him his family had a history of Lynch syndrome; that he was at an elevated risk for colorectal cancer. Everyone has stood behind him as he has battled stage four cancer. Today, with Keytruda treatments, his cancer is gone, and there is no noted evidence of disease. The relief brought tears.

My siblings and I were at the far spectrum of middle age when we tested for Lynch syndrome. Our kids are younger. They take more time to decide if genetic testing is right for them. Of the seventeen of us, two have tested negative, the first we have known in four generations that are *not* affected by Lynch syndrome. Thirteen of us are positive. One is awaiting testing, and one has chosen not to test because of her religious preferences.

When the elders in our family contracted cancer, it was unavoidable. A whirlwind of advancements in cancer research has since occurred. Then, diagnostic testing and preventative screenings were not as effective and streamlined as today. Our children will be the first in our family *not* to contract life-threatening cancers if they engage in preventative measures.

And our children's children? With preventative screenings, not only will they not contract cancer, they can stop the cycle of Lynch syndrome in their family, if they choose, through in-vitro fertilization (IVF). It involves the selection and implantation of pretested fertilized embryos that do not possess Lynch syndrome genetic mutations.

If we keep up to date with our screenings, most of us will have a lesser chance of developing a "full-blown" cancer than those in the general population. Our children realize little need to worry about "someday" as we once did. They can navigate through life, not having to confront the difficult challenges we faced, and still face today, whether it be cancer because of Lynch syndrome or anything else threatening our survival. From us, they will learn to protect themselves, as we learned from others.

Developing survival techniques is as essential for everyone living in this fast-paced world of ours, as it was during the day of our ancestors. Most of us gain the skills in survival through finely tuned lessons we learned as children. What Jim and I gained from our parents, was later found to be invaluable as we have confronted our circumstances.

Often, we do not realize what we have learned may be an essential building block that could contribute to our ongoing survival. All that we need to endure is to build a metaphorical house made of bricks, with a robust base, a solid foundation, and an excellent support structure. Neither we nor a home can stand on its own without it.

We must develop the ability to put negative and stressful thoughts out of our minds. Much good comes from focusing on the immediate and the positive. It does no good to lament over what we cannot do; it does a world of good to take joy in doing that which we can. Our subconscious controls ninety-five percent of our lives. It is what provides us with a strong instinct to survive. Our genes do not control our health. *We* manage it.

Mustering the courage to face the challenges in life, we should not succumb to the fear of asking for help from those who can give it. We need to take on the responsibility of standing up for ourselves and our family members in situations that create uncertainty. Finally, the creation of interventions to reduce stress can be lifesaving. To complete any of these steps, we need no one's approval.

We can do amazing things when we get involved in activities that are greater than ourselves. Survival requires resilience, the ability to adapt to changes, and the realization that we can do anything we want if we believe in ourselves. It relies upon us having the strength to seek the big picture and to accept the losses, understanding that life is a negotiation and that each day we experience it is a gift.

In life, we take risks every day. We walk through doors into rooms filled with uncertainty all the time. Fighting cancer is one of those risks. We throw everything into the air and catch as much of it as we can when it comes back down. When taking risks, it is essential to hedge one's bets by never giving up hope and learning when to let go.

In the autumn of 2017, our hearts broke when we left the care of Kaiser Permanente. Members living outside their established boundaries could not remain enrolled. We were six-hundred and fifty miles from our care facility and our doctors. Losing our medical team was akin to losing members of our family. It is difficult to say "goodbye" to people who have held you up and saved your life. My eyes teared when Dr. Martin reassured, "I will take care of your family, I promise. Please don't worry."

The time had come to find a new team. It was a challenging mission to search for physicians as outstanding as our Kaiser team. Finding the right caregivers and the right institution where we would feel comfortable, and that possessed the resources to supply us with the top, and the newest technology was tough. Deciding to travel to a dedicated cancer center, we selected the Banner Health/MD Anderson Cancer Center in Gilbert, Arizona, where many come to receive world-class cancer care.

In January 2018, Steve and I arrived for orientation and my annual screenings. Stepping through the glass doors that opened onto a large lobby, our eyes at once caught upon the Tree of Hope set in the entrance, covered with thousands of colored ribbons. As I tied mine to the tree, I thought of those I worked with through the years with Lynch Syndrome International. I could have spent days tying thousands of ribbons upon that tree... in honor of those I know who live the same as us and of those who are gone. Beyond, sets a peaceful atrium where patients quietly converse. Everything reflects comfort.

When we are ill, we count the little things as our blessings. They organize the chairs in the waiting rooms in a manner to encourage patients to converse with others. Coffee tables, topped with jigsaw puzzles, kept patients and their families distracted from uncertainty. The exterior of planters, filled with lush vegetation, held big-screen televisions on their surface, allowing people to watch it without having to hold their heads back to view it up high upon a wall. Intermittently placed were electrical charging stations. It was impressive seeing the lobby taking into consideration the physical and psychological needs of patients.

While waiting for my appointment, Dr. Naraev's assistant offered a warm blanket to cuddle under while a volunteer wandered the halls, providing patients and their families water, juices, books, and a compassionate smile. The volunteers are familiar with cancer. All are survivors or have cared for family members.

A tight schedule of two days of annual screening tests was designed for me, considering the cancers occurring in our family and my specific mutation. Each appointment runs like clockwork, escalating with the more challenging procedures, allowing each of the medical team to review recent lab and imaging results as they occur. It saves time, costs, and provides our caregivers with the opportunity to work together to determine our risk over two days, rather than spread over a year, when, with us, anything can change. We instantly knew these physicians, and their staff would be as dear to us as those at Kaiser always will be.

Traveling five hours to receive our annual screenings and Lynch syndrome care from experts who receive daily up-to-date information on hereditary cancer care, have access to research occurring within their health system, and who possess high-quality imaging equipment is well worth taking the extra effort to be seen at their institutions. The more people they see, the more they learn about our disease.

Fueled with hope, I have always held confidence and faith that "someday" will be different for my loved ones than it was for our parents and us. That was once a dream. Today, it is a reality.

Hope is a powerful emotion that fills the voids of fear and uncertainty, offering us the strength to move forward and continue. Hope is a dynamic tool that inspires us to survive. I remind my children and grandchildren to keep it close and never lose it. It is lifesaving.

The gratitude I hold for those who care for us; is immense. Working through the challenges posed by hereditary cancer and those occurring every day, faced by ourselves and our loved ones, we have learned that we can battle hereditary cancer and will prevail if it is detected early. Thankful for research efforts, we now have streamlined procedures for diagnostic testing, regular cancer screenings, effective treatments, and a chance at life; everything that did not exist during my father's lifetime.

My heart beats with gratitude whenever I reflect upon the result of the opportunities given to me during this one life. Every challenge we face makes us stronger and more appreciative of what we, in our family, have and what we are... alive. I feel nothing but gratitude for all we have encountered during this journey, from the advocates to the researchers, to our passionate medical teams who work to make sure we remain cancer-free, and to our families and friends, I am genuinely thankful.

Their dedication, passion, and courage have instilled hope in us, offering far more certainty than that Dad and the generations living before him could have ever imagined. Life, today, is good...

Today, we live.